Evidence-Based Decisions and Economics

Health care, social welfare, education and criminal justice

Edited by

Ian Shemilt

Senior Research Associate
School of Medicine, Health Policy and Practice
University of East Anglia
Norwich, UK

Miranda Mugford

Professor of Health Economics
School of Medicine, Health Policy and Practice
University of East Anglia
Norwich, UK

Luke Vale

Professor of Health Technology Assessment
Health Economics Research Unit and
Health Services Research Unit
University of Aberdeen
Aberdeen, UK

Kevin Marsh

Head of Economic Evaluation
Matrix Knowledge Group
London, UK

Cam Donaldson

Yunus Chair in Social Business and Health
NIHR Senior Investigator
Glasgow Caledonian University
Glasgow, UK

SECOND EDITION

WILEY-BLACKWELL

A John Wiley & Sons, Ltd., Publication

BMJ|Books

This edition first published 2010, © 2002, 2010 by Blackwell Publishing Ltd

BMJ Books is an imprint of BMJ Publishing Group Limited, used under licence by Blackwell Publishing which was acquired by John Wiley & Sons in February 2007. Blackwell's publishing programme has been merged with Wiley's global Scientific, Technical and Medical business to form Wiley-Blackwell.

Registered office: John Wiley & Sons Ltd, The Atrium, Southern Gate, Chichester, West Sussex, PO19 8SQ, UK

Editorial offices: 9600 Garsington Road, Oxford, OX4 2DQ, UK
                     111 River Street, Hoboken, NJ 07030-5774, USA
                     The Atrium, Southern Gate, Chichester, West Sussex, PO19 8SQ, UK

For details of our global editorial offices, for customer services and for information about
how to apply for permission to reuse the copyright material in this book, please see our website at
www.wiley.com/wiley-blackwell.

The right of the author to be identified as the author of this work has been asserted in accordance with the
Copyright, Designs and Patents Act 1988.

ISBN: 978-1-4051-9153-1

A catalogue record for this book is available from the British Library.

Library of Congress Cataloging-in-Publication Data

Evidence-based decisions and economics : health care, social welfare, education,
and criminal justice. — 2nd ed. / edited by Ian Shemilt . . . [et al.].
       p.;   cm. — (Evidence-based medicine)
   Rev. ed. of: Evidence-based health economics / edited by Cam Donaldson, Miranda Mugford, Luke Vale.
c2002.
   Includes bibliographical references and index.
   ISBN 978-1-4051-9153-1
   1. Medical economics.   2. Evidence-based medicine.   I. Shemilt, Ian.   II. Evidence-based health
economics.   III. Series: Evidence-based medicine.
   [DNLM: 1.   Economics, Medical.   2.   Evidence-Based Medicine. W 74.1 E93 2010]
RA410.5.E956 2010
338.4′33621—dc22
                                                                                              2009046383

Set in 9.5/12pt Minion by MPS Limited, A Macmillan Company

Printed in Singapore

1 2010

Contents

Evidence-Based Medicine Series

Updates and additional resources for the books in this series are available from:
www.evidencebasedseries.com

List of contributors

* Denotes attendance at the LSE workshop

Morten Aaserud
Senior Adviser
Norwegian Medicines Agency
Norway

Asmaa Abdelhamid
Research Associate
University of East Anglia
UK

Keith Abrams*
Professor of Medical Statistics
University of Leicester
UK

Rob Anderson*
Senior Lecturer in Health Economics
University of Exeter, Exeter
UK

Barbara Barrett
Lecturer
King's College London
UK

Francesca Borgonovi
Analyst, Organisation for Economic Cooperation
and Development
France

Stephen Birch
Professor of Health Economics
McMaster University
Canada

John Brazier
Professor of Health Economics
University of Sheffield
UK

Massimo Brunetti*
Health Economist
Local Health Unit Modena
Italy

Sarah Byford*
Senior Lecturer
King's College London
UK

Anna Cantrell
Information Specialist
University of Sheffield
UK

Gordon Cleveland*
Senior Lecturer in Economics
University of Toronto at Scarborough
Canada

Nicola J. Cooper*
Senior Research Fellow
University of Leicester
UK

Doug Coyle
Professor of Health Economics
University of Ottawa
Canada

Cam Donaldson*
Yunus Chair in Social Business and
Health
and NIHR Senior Investigator
Glasgow Caledonian University
UK

Michael Drummond*
Professor of Health Economics
University of York
UK

Richard Dubourg*
Economic Adviser
Home Office
UK

Jennifer Francis*
Research Analyst
Social Care Institute for Excellence
UK

Mike Fisher*
Director of Research and Reviews
Social Care Institute for Excellence
UK

Julie Glanville
Project Director - Information Services
York Health Economics Consortium
UK

Karen Gerard
Reader in Health Economics
University of Southampton
UK

Karianne Thune Hammerstrøm
Trials Search Coordinator
The Campbell Collaboration Social
Welfare Group
Norway

Kirsten Herrmann
Study Coordinator
ICF Research Branch of the
World Health Organisation CC FIC
Germany

Karen M. Lee
Health Economist
Canadian Agency for
Drugs and Technology in Health
Canada

Chantale Lessard*
Canadian Institutes of Health Research Fellow
University of Montreal
Canada

Joanne Lord*
Reader in Health Economics
Brunel University
UK

Jacqueline Mallender*
Chief Executive
The Matrix Knowledge Group
UK

Kevin Marsh*
Head of Economic Evaluation
The Matrix Knowledge Group
UK

David McDaid*
Senior Research Fellow in Health Policy
and Health Economics
London School of Economics
and Political Science
UK

Miranda Mugford*
Professor of Health Economics
University of East Anglia
UK

Andrew D. Oxman
Senior Researcher
Norwegian Knowledge Centre
for the Health Services
Norway

Suzy Paisley
Senior Research Fellow
University of Sheffield
UK

Diana Papaioannou
Research Associate
University of Sheffield
UK

Anita Patel*
Senior Lecturer
King's College London
UK

Juntana Pattanaphesuj
Researcher of Health Intervention
and Technology Assessment Program
Ministry of Public Health
Thailand

Mark Petticrew
Professor of Public Health Evaluation
London School of Hygiene and Tropical Medicine
UK

Silvia Pregno
Public Health Physician
Italy

Craig Ramsay
Senior Statistician
University of Aberdeen
UK

Gerry Richardson*
Senior Research Fellow
University of York
UK

Francis J. Ruiz*
Technical Adviser on Health Economics
National Institute for Health and Clinical Excellence
UK

Franco Sassi
Senior Health Economist
Organisation for Economic Cooperation
and Development
France

Ian Shemilt*
Senior Research Associate
University of East Anglia
UK

Jane Sisk*
Director for Health Care Statistics
Centers for Disease Control and Prevention
USA

T.D. Stanley
Bill and Connie Bowen Odyssey Professor of
Economics
Hendrix College
USA

Yot Teerawattananon*
Program Leader of Health Intervention
and Technology Assessment Program (HITAP)
Thai Ministry of Public Health
Thailand

Luke Vale*
Professor of Health Technology Assessment
University of Aberdeen
UK

Damian G. Walker*
Associate Professor
Johns Hopkins Bloomberg School of Public Health
USA

Ed Wilson*
Lecturer in Health Economics
University of East Anglia
UK

Kath Wright
Information Service Manager
Centre for Reviews and Dissemination
UK

Preface

This book is about how the activities and outputs of evidence synthesis, systematic review, economic analysis and decision making interact within and across different spheres of health and social policy and practice. It is intended to be of interest and use to policy makers and practitioners who use evidence to inform policy and practice decisions, analysts who produce or synthesise the evidence used to support such decisions, and students studying in these areas.

The book is an entirely new edition of the earlier *Evidence-Based Health Economics: from effectiveness to efficiency in systematic review*, published by BMJ Books in 2002. A central objective for this new edition has been to expand the scope to encompass methods developments, proposals and controversies in the applied fields of social welfare, education and criminal justice, alongside those in health care. As far as possible, we have attempted to build on common experiences across these fields in the application of approaches to evidence synthesis that combine economics and systematic review methods. Equally, we have sought to recognise and explore their distinctive features that are likely to require divergent methodological solutions.

We invite readers to decide for themselves the extent to which this central objective is fulfilled in this volume. In our judgement, our success is limited by both the extent to which research practices in non-health care fields currently reflect an integration of economic and systematic review methodologies, and also by limitations in the current reach of our research and professional networks. This is felt most acutely with respect to the education field. We therefore offer this volume as a first but important step in a journey towards a fully networked, multidisciplinary approach to develop evidence bases with strong economic dimensions to inform optimal policy and practice decisions. We also invite criticism and dialogue with readers and potential collaborators.

This book has been developed from material first presented at an international workshop held at the London School of Economics and Political Science, UK, in November 2008. We would like to thank David McDaid, Anji Mehta and colleagues at the LSE for hosting this workshop and also to acknowledge the funds provided by the School of Medicine, Health Policy and Practice, University of East Anglia, UK. Finally, we would like to acknowledge the invaluable support provided by Mary Banks, Simone Heaton and Lewis O'Sullivan at Wiley-Blackwell.

Ian Shemilt (i.shemilt@uea.ac.uk)

On behalf of the editors:
Ian Shemilt, Miranda Mugford, Luke Vale, Kevin Marsh and Cam Donaldson.

Disclaimer

The views expressed in this book are those of the chapter authors, which do not necessarily reflect the views of the editors.

CHAPTER 1

From effectiveness to efficiency? An introduction to evidence-based decisions and economics

Miranda Mugford[1], Ian Shemilt[2], Luke Vale[3], Kevin Marsh[4], Cam Donaldson[5], Jacqueline Mallender[4]

[1]Health Policy and Practice, University of East Anglia, Norwich, UK
[2]School of Social Work and Psychosocial Studies, University of East Anglia, Norwich, UK
[3]Health Economics Research Unit, University of Aberdeen, Aberdeen, UK
[4]The Matrix Knowledge Group, London, UK
[5]Glasgow Caledonian University, Glasgow, UK

'The question we ask today is not whether our government is too big or too small, but whether it works - whether it helps families find jobs at a decent wage, care they can afford, a retirement that is dignified. Where the answer is yes, we intend to move forward. Where the answer is no, programs will end. And those of us who manage the public's dollars will be held to account - to spend wisely, reform bad habits, and do our business in the light of day - because only then can we restore the vital trust between a people and their government.'

(President Barack Obama, Inaugural Address, 20th January 2009)[1]

Introduction

'Evidence-based policy and practice' is a phrase commonly used to refer to public policy and professional practice informed by the application of rigorous methods to the search and review of evidence – a process often described as a 'systematic review of evidence'.

Although previous methodologists had already advocated the use of experimental evidence and synthesis of this evidence for practice decisions in many

fields, the term 'evidence-based decision making' achieved widespread use in the field of medical policy and practice.[2,3] The epidemiologist Archie Cochrane, who challenged the medical profession to base their practice on evidence from randomised controlled trials (RCTs), stimulated this.[4]

Inspired by Archie Cochrane, the Cochrane Collaboration was established to prepare, publish and regularly update systematic reviews of the effects of health care interventions.[5] Cochrane reviews have been available since the early 1990s.[6] More recently, similar reviews of interventions in social welfare, education and criminal justice are appearing as a result of the work of the Campbell Collaboration, which is named in honour of DT Campbell, an evaluation methodologist with a particular interest in the value of experimental approaches to understanding the effects of interventions.[2,7] Like the Cochrane Collaboration, the Campbell Collaboration publishes its systematic reviews electronically.[8] However, advocacy for providing a summary of comprehensively sourced, replicable and quality-filtered information for trustworthy policy decisions, and development of methodologies for doing this, has a longer history, and this work underpinned the foundation of the Cochrane Collaboration and the Campbell Collaboration.[3,9–11]

Methods for systematic reviews of evidence have concentrated mainly on the question of 'What works?'

Evidence-Based Decisions and Economics, 2nd edition. Edited by I. Shemilt, M. Mugford, L. Vale, K. Marsh and C. Donaldson. © 2010 Blackwell Publishing.

or 'Is this intervention effective in achieving a specific outcome?'. The questions 'Is it worth it?', 'At what cost is the outcome achieved?' and 'What will be the economic impact of this intervention?' have not been emphasised as much in the meta-analysis and systematic review literature to date. However, the concept and methods of economic and other forms of evaluation of the health and social impacts of interventions are well established and such approaches are being applied in evaluation of public sector projects across a range of policy areas.[12–14] In an attempt to standardise approaches to the evaluation of public projects, governments have published methodological guidelines on the use of economic evaluation.[15–24]

As the opening quotation to this chapter suggests, the need for evidence-based decisions that take account of both efficiency and fairness in society has received new emphasis as we prepared for this book. The challenge to researchers is not only to offer the tools for these decisions, but that the methods we advocate also meet President Obama's acid test: that they are efficient, effective, transparent and fair.

Evidence-based policy 'helps people make well-informed decisions about policies, programmes and projects by putting the best available evidence from research at the heart of policy development and implementation'.[25–27] However, the ultimate purpose of evidence-based policy and practice could be rephrased as being to 'optimise the configuration and delivery of services in order to maximise individual and public welfare'. Economics has been defined as the study of the optimal allocation of limited resources for the production of benefit to society.[28] Decisions based only on highly focused evidence-based methodologies that consider only one dimension of the economic decision (i.e. whether the intervention works) may contribute to inefficient policy and practice and greater inequalities through lack of consideration of these potential trade-offs.[29,30]

At the same time, a decision based on an economic study that does not utilise the most reliable evidence of effectiveness will also be flawed. In the field of health care in the UK, Archie Cochrane and Alan Williams were two influential leaders of their disciplines who acted as advisors to the Department of Health at the same time. Their own accounts of events illustrate how they agreed on the need to incorporate economic viewpoints, and how their work paved the way for the

National Health Service (NHS) to embed both health economics and evidence-based decision making into research and policy making in the UK.[4,30,31]

In spite of the recent increase in recognition of the important role of economics in decisions across broader areas of policy and professional practice, as well as in the health care field, aspects of both systematic review and economic analysis make it difficult to neatly combine these approaches. This book is intended for those involved in decision making, whether your role is to provide evidence to support decisions or to use evidence to make decisions. Therefore, we do not assume depth of knowledge of either economics or systematic review. To set the scene for the book, the remainder of this chapter introduces some key concepts of systematic review and of economics. The final section introduces the structure and the contents of the book.

A brief introduction to systematic review

Systematic reviews attempt to collate all empirical evidence that fits prespecified eligibility criteria in order to answer specific research questions. They involve the use of explicit, systematic and replicable methods to assemble, select, critique and synthesise reliable and up-to-date evidence, from published and unpublished sources, on the effects of interventions.

The main purpose of systematic reviews of interventions has been to provide reliable, up-to-date evidence about the beneficial and harmful effects (outcomes) of interventions when compared to an alternative practice or form of care.[3,32,33] The need for such an approach was advocated both by Archie Cochrane for the health field in 1972 and by DT Campbell for the field of educational psychology in 1963.[2,4,34] The purpose was to overcome disagreements among experts on best practice that arise from reliance on unsubstantiated expert opinion, single studies, and incomplete or unsystematic reviews.

These views were further supported by methodologists such as Light & Pillemer, who elegantly illustrated the biases that can be introduced in attempts to sum up evidence for policy decisions, including examples on the educational debate on the effect of class size on students' performance, where misleading conclusions can be gained by simply counting the number of studies with significant findings for or against smaller classes, for example.[10] Light & Pillemer also emphasised the importance of drawing on a range of sources of evidence, including both qualitative and quantitative research.[10]

Application of systematic review methods on a large scale was pioneered in the health field by the Cochrane Collaboration, which has been publishing and maintaining reviews of the effects of health care interventions since 1992, followed by the establishment of the Campbell Collaboration, in 1999, to do the same in the fields of social welfare, education and criminal justice. Both organisations explicitly recognise the importance of best evidence in economic decisions. Neither organisation currently requires that its reviews necessarily include economic questions or methods; however, the fact that authors of reviews wish to do so is recognised by the inclusion of economics methods guidance in methods handbooks for reviews published by each Collaboration.[35,36] The need to further develop guidance to assist authors and editors to make their reviews more useful for policy decision makers, and for economists to understand and engage in this process, is one of the principal motivations for development of this book.

In this book, a central focus is on systematic review as defined by the Cochrane Collaboration and the Campbell Collaboration, in which a protocol is developed and published that describes questions and methods to be used. Then, as laid out in the protocol, a comprehensive search for evidence is conducted, also seeking relevant unpublished findings. In this process a 'map' of research evidence that is known to have been published to address a specific question, and what is missing, is formed. When there is enough research evidence that meets preset criteria for inclusion, the evidence is synthesised from a subset of sources that minimise the risk of bias in the comparison of options. This can include meta-analysis of critically assessed RCTs and other types of robust comparative study.

A brief introduction to economics for the non-economist

Resources, such as people's time and skills, raw materials, land and energy, are needed as the inputs for providing goods and services. Economics is about how resources are used to meet needs and wants at different levels, including the individual, the household or the state. The efficient economy has been defined as one where no change in resource use can make anyone better off without making someone else worse off. This principle was first proposed by the economist Vilfredo Pareto (1848–1923). It works up to a point where there is spare capacity in the system, but in a busy, already 'Pareto-efficient' economy, trade-offs need to be made when new policies are introduced. That is, if all resources are fully used, some existing production must be changed, and output lost, with an associated loss of benefits from that use. This loss is known to economists as 'opportunity cost'. Judgements about costs and benefits are then needed between stakeholders who 'win' (benefits) and those who 'lose' (costs).

Where resources are bought and sold, there is a price for each unit of resource (such as staff salaries, rent for buildings, the price of computers, books, medicines, etc.). Money, which is used as an indication of value and a medium of exchange, is an important part of most economies, oiling the wheels of exchange of goods and services. Economic theory, based on a strict set of assumptions, suggests that unregulated economic markets can provide an optimal allocation of resources. In practice, these assumptions are not met, and most markets for goods and services fail to clear themselves efficiently or equitably for all those involved.

Markets are rarely (many would say never) 'perfect' for many reasons. There is lack of information to both producers and consumers about the nature and quality of goods and services and about consumer needs and wishes, both now and in the future. Some buyers and sellers in the market can individually determine price levels through monopoly power. Other factors cause barriers to market entry by producers, such as trade association or professional agreements, or the viable size of production units needing prohibitively large investment or a lack of mobility of resources. Consumers of services are also constrained in how they participate in the market by their personal resources (e.g. income, support networks and ability) and by whether there are any alternatives to the good or service they are seeking. In addition, there are some goods and services, known as 'public goods', that are seldom regarded by entrepreneurs as worth producing and selling in the free market because, once they exist, they benefit everyone whether they have paid or not. Examples of public goods include public sanitation and crime prevention initiatives.

Because markets fail in areas of social and political importance to individual and public welfare, such as health, social welfare, education and criminal justice, governments intervene in different ways and degrees around the world. Services and funding are provided through publicly regulated organisations in various ways. Although it is unusual in most economies for state provision to be managed at all levels with no element of market activity or private sector involvement, it is also recognised at government level that other 'non-market' approaches for optimising economic welfare are needed to aid decision makers choosing policy and guiding practice in public services. For this reason, among others, both economic analysis and evidence-based approaches are used.

Guidance on methods to inform policy and practice decisions

How should we go about compiling the best evidence on the economics of interventions in addition to their effectiveness? Can the systematic review approach aid reviews of broader types and bodies of evidence, including economic evidence? Can economic evaluation and other forms of economic analysis be conducted systematically and transparently? What guidance do we have and what are the strengths and limitations of different approaches?

Decisions on policy and practice take place at many levels, from individual practitioners and service users to governments. Although groups informing consumers and professional and regulatory bodies do not all take the same approach to decision making, they are all interested in the best, least biased evidence and in optimal use of resources. Around the world, governments have published guidance to evaluators so that the evidence used to inform decisions is based on comparable methods. For example, in the United States, the Office of Technology Appraisal published guidance between 1975 and 1995 that has been used as the basis for many international variants on guidance on technology appraisal in different countries, especially in the health care field.[15–18] This guidance includes emphasis on the need for systematic reviews of effects and economic evaluation. In the UK (as in several other countries), the Treasury publishes a handbook for evaluators of public

projects, which includes reference to both quality of evidence and the approach to be taken for economic evaluation.[19]

Further review of the guidance on evaluation across policy areas highlights many areas of difference, all of which pose important questions for those who, like the authors and editors of this book, are engaged in efforts to guide the systematic review community in providing economic evidence relevant to decisions about interventions implemented in more than one policy domain and in (or, in some cases, across) different economic systems, which takes account of the distribution of costs and benefits within (or across) populations.[21–23]

Overview of the book

This book is about how the activities and outputs of evidence synthesis, systematic review, economic analysis and decision making interact within and across spheres of health and social policy and practice. It is also about the challenges that arise from these interacting processes.

In 2001, a group of economists and reviewers took part in a workshop in Banff, Alberta, funded by the Alberta Heritage Foundation, which led to the publication of the book *Evidence-based Health Economics* by BMJ Books in 2002.[37] This new volume, an entirely new edition, was prepared following a similar workshop at the London School of Economics and Political Science in November 2008. It follows the progress of the issues raised in the previous book and also takes a broader perspective, reflecting the importance of evaluation methods and decisionmaking beyond the health sector.

This book aims to:
- describe the current state of the art in approaches to evidence synthesis that combine economics and systematic review methods within and across the health care, social welfare, education and criminal justice fields
- examine the case for evidence-based principles in economic analysis, and the need for such principles to include an economic dimension.

The next three chapters build on this introduction to provide further insights into core methodological concepts and principles (Chapters 2 and 3) and the use of economic evidence in decision making (Chapter 4).

Chapters 2 and 3 take alternative perspectives. In Chapter 2, the focus is on how evidence is assembled and synthesised in decision models for economic evaluation, whilst Chapter 3 considers how economic perspectives and evidence drawn from previous studies can be assembled and synthesised in evidence reviews for policy decisions. Both chapters highlight questions of where economic thinking fits into evidence gathering and synthesis processes, and how systematic review methods relate to economic analysis methods. Chapter 4 builds on the preceding two chapters by providing an overview of how outputs from decision models and economic evidence reviews are currently used in the formulation of public policy and practice in different jurisdictions. The way in which policy makers and practitioners use information for decision making determines whether the work of evaluators and reviewers is likely to influence policy, practice and the delivery of services.

The next chapters cover a range of specific methodological issues facing evidence reviewers and economists. Two overarching concerns often expressed about systematic reviews and economic analyses are that their results may not be generalisable or transferable to other settings, and that they fail to consider the fair distribution of benefits and costs. Chapter 5 considers how an internationally used review, such as a Cochrane or Campbell review, might be relevant in different specific contexts, taking account of the complexity arising from the range of variables that can influence the final best answer. Chapter 6 illustrates and discusses how reviews and evaluations could, and should, go beyond the simple question of effectiveness and efficiency to consider equity.

Chapters 7–10 present developments covering several issues highlighted in the first edition of this book. Chapter 7 examines the evolution of literature search methods to identify evidence for systematic reviews and decision models that aim to support cost-effectiveness decisions. Chapter 8 addresses parallel issues in the identification and synthesis of health state utility values, which are commonly used to inform measures of the value of outcomes of health care interventions. Chapter 9 examines the use of evidence in decision models and how the use of different sources of evidence can influence model results. The authors propose hierarchies of sources of evidence to help limit the potential for bias in results.

The question of bias and quality is further addressed in Chapter 10, which presents frameworks for grading evidence on resource use, costs and cost-effectiveness and presenting these types of evidence flexibly and usefully for users of reviews.

Although it is common that health care and other systematic reviews place emphasis on the results of controlled trials of interventions, because this method is applied widely and provides least-biased evidence of treatment effects, it is also often the case that in the health field, as in other areas of social policy, the only and best evidence available is from observational datasets, such as those collected for administrative purposes or government surveys. Whilst the statistical and econometric methods used to analyse these data to detect the effects and costs of practices are unfamiliar to many analysts, meta-regression and other techniques are increasingly applied to help sum up findings in evidence reviews. Chapter 11 illustrates how meta-regression analysis can be used to explore the findings of studies, whatever methodology they employ.

A systematic review may find little or no relevant evidence, but this does not mean there is no policy decision to be made and, as such, analysis of evidence in reviews and economic evaluations can be used to estimate the value of new research. Chapter 12 profiles the use of evidence in value of information analysis to estimate the economic value of new research to answer policy questions.

Further criticism of the overall assumptions behind evidence-based approaches includes their failure to consider political priorities, and especially the impacts on inequalities in the distribution of benefits and access to services. Chapter 13 challenges the orthodoxy of assumptions underlying current approaches to evidence synthesis and presents the conceptual framework for a new approach.

Chapters 14 and 15 draw key implications of all the preceding material for current practice and future research. Chapter 14 summarises and discusses current recommendations for analysts utilising approaches to evidence synthesis that combine economics and systematic review methods. Chapter 15 presents a summary and discussion of priorities for further empirical research needed to develop the evidence base that underpins current and future research practice. Finally, to assist the reader, Chapter 16 provides a glossary of selected key terms used throughout the book.

Summary and invitation

The theoretical case for wanting to integrate economic analysis and systematic reviews is strong. In some cases, such integrated analysis can prove relatively straightforward and provide important results. However, the conduct of economic evaluation and other forms of economic analysis is not always straightforward. It will be seen in this book that different approaches to the same underlying issue can lead to different results, that there are significant negative consequences to not utilising the best evidence available at the time an economic analysis is conducted, and that there is not always a consensus on the best way forward.

In preparing this book, the editors and authors were aware that the first edition was firmly based in the health care field but that many of the policy issues faced in other related fields, including social welfare, education and criminal justice, are similar. Some of the authors and editors of this book are already working in these applied fields, and we have sought examples of applications from these fields. Our success or failure in this is reflected in the content of this book, and we are aware that there are areas that have less coverage than we hoped. Two specific areas we have identified are: methods for and examples of economic analysis in the field of education, and discussion of the role of econometric studies in policy formulation. Our success or failure has probably reflected the limits of our own networks, however systematically we have searched, and we look forward to finding like-minded colleagues willing to participate in our future work as a result of this book.

It is important that systematic reviewers and economists alike are aware of such issues, and that there is no single best way of integrating economic analysis and systematic review methods. In addition, it is necessary to think about the limitations of both economic analysis and systematic review more generally and, also, of the limits of integrating the two methodologies. If you are interested in some or all of the above, we invite you to join us on a journey 'from effectiveness to efficiency' and enjoy reading this book.

How this chapter should be cited

Mugford M, Shemilt I, Vale L, Marsh K, Donaldson C, Mallender J. Chapter 1: From effectiveness to efficiency? An introduction to evidence-based decisions and economics. In: Shemilt I, Mugford M, Vale L, Marsh K, Donaldson C (editors). *Evidence-based decisions and economics: health care, social welfare, education and criminal justice.* Oxford: Wiley-Blackwell, 2010.

References

1 BBC News. *Transcript of Barack Obama's inaugural address, 20 June 2009.* London: British Broadcasting Corporation, 2009. Available from: http://news.bbc.co.uk/1/hi/world/americas/ obama_inauguration/7840646.stm.

2 Campbell DT, Stanley J. *Experimental and Quasi-Experimental Designs for Research.* Boston: Houghton Mifflin, 1963.

3 Cooper H, Hedges LV (eds). *The Handbook of Research Synthesis.* New York: Russell Sage Foundation, 1994.

4 Cochrane AL. *Effectiveness and Efficiency: random reflections on health services.* London: Nuffield Provincial Hospitals Trust, 1972.

5 Cochrane Collaboration. *The Cochrane Policy Manual.* Cochrane Collaboration, 2010. Available from: www.cochrane.org/admin/manual.htm.

6 Cochrane Collaboration. *Cochrane Database of Systematic Reviews.* Cochrane Collaboration, 2010. Available from: www.thecochranelibrary.com.

7 Campbell Collaboration. *A Strategic Plan for The Campbell Collaboration.* Campbell Collaboration, 2008. Available from: http://camp.ostfold.net/resources/ policy_documents/ strategic_plan.php.

8 Campbell Collaboration. *The Campbell Collaboration Library of Systematic Reviews.* Campbell Collaboration, 2010. Available from: www.campbellcollaboration.org/library.php.

9 Stokey E, Zeckhauser R. *A Primer for Policy Analysis.* New York: Norton, 1978.

10 Light RJ, Pillemer DB. *Summing Up: the science of reviewing research.* London: Harvard University Press, 1984.

11 Wolf FM. *Meta-Analysis: quantitative methods for research synthesis. Quantitative Applications in the Social Sciences No. 57.* Newbury Park: Sage, 1986.

12 Levin HM. Cost-effectiveness analysis in evaluation research. In: Guttentag M, Struening E (eds) *Handbook of Evaluation Research.* New York: Sage Publications, 1975.

13 Mishan EJ. *Cost-Benefit Analysis.* London: Unwin Hyman, 1988.

14 Sugden R, Williams A. *The Principles of Practical Cost-Benefit Analysis.* Oxford: Oxford University Press, 1978.

15 United States Congress Office of Technology Assessment. *The Implications of Cost-Effectiveness Analysis of Medical Technology.* Washington DC: United States Congress Office of Technology Assessment, 1980.

16 United States Congress Office of Technology Assessment. *The Implications of Cost-Effectiveness Analysis of Medical Technology: methodology issues and literature review (Background Paper No.1).* Washington DC: United States Congress Office of Technology Assessment, 1980.

17 United States Congress Office of Technology Assessment. *Benefit Design in Health Care Reform: Report 1 - clinical preventive services (OTA-H-580)*. Washington DC: US Government Printing Office, 1993.

18 United States Congress Office of Technology Assessment. *Identifying health Technologies That Work: Searching for Evidence (OTA-H-608)*. Washington DC: US Government Printing Office, 1994.

19 HM Treasury. *The Green Book: appraisal and evaluation in central government*. London: The Stationery Office, 2003.

20 National Institute for Health and Clinical Excellence. *Guide to the Methods of Technology Appraisal*. London: National Institute for Health and Clinical Excellence, 2008.

21 UK Civil Service Policy Hub, National School of Government. *The Magenta Book: guidance notes on policy evaluation*. Ascot: UK Civil Service Policy Hub, National School of Government, 2010. Available from: www.nationalschool.gov.uk/policyhub/ evaluating_policy/magenta_book/index.asp.

22 World Bank, Operations Evaluation Department-Evaluation Capacity Development. *Monitoring and Evaluation: some tools, methods and approaches (Independent Evaluation Group Working Paper)*. Washington DC: World Bank Group, 2004. Available from: http://lnweb90. worldbank.org/oed/ oeddoclib.nsf/InterLandingPagesByUNID/A5EFBB5D776B 67D285256B1E0079C9A3.

23 US Department of Commerce, National Oceanic and Atmospheric Administration (NOAA), National Marine Fisheries Service. *Guidelines and Principles for Social Impact Assessment*. Washington DC: US Department of Commerce,1994. Available from: www.nmfs.noaa.gov/ sfa/ social_impact_guide.htm.

24 Gold MR, Siegel JE, Russell LB, Weinstein MC (eds) *Cost-Effectiveness in Health and Medicine*. New York: Oxford University Press, 1996.

25 Davies PT. What is evidence-based education? *British Journal of Educational Studies* 1999; 47(2): 108–121.

26 Davies PT. *Is evidence-based government possible?* Jerry Lee Lecture, presented at the 4th Annual Campbell Collaboration Colloquium, Washington DC, 19 February 2004. Available from: www.nationalschool.gov.uk/policy-hub/downloads/JerryLeeLecture1202041.pdfGray 1997.

27 Gray JAM. *Evidence-Based Health care: how to make health policy and management decisions*. London: Churchill Livingstone, 1997.

28 Samuelson PA, Nordhaus WD. *Economics*. London: McGraw-Hill, 2005.

29 Maynard A. Cost effectiveness and equity are ignored. *British Medical Journal* 1996; 313(7050): 170.

30 Williams A. The cost-benefit approach. *British Medical Bulletin* 1974; 30(3): 252–256.

31 Williams A. How Archie Cochrane changed my life. *Journal of Epidemiology and Community Health* 1997; 51(2): 116–120.

32 Egger M, Altman D, Davey-Smith G (eds) *Systematic Reviews in Health Care: meta-analysis in context*. London: BMJ Books, 2000.

33 Higgins JPT, Green S (eds) *Cochrane Handbook for Systematic Reviews of Interventions*. Version 5.0.1(updated September 2008). Oxford: Cochrane Collaboration, 2008.

34 Shadish W, Cook TD, Campbell DT. *Experimental and Quasi-Experimental Designs for Generalised Causal Inference*. Boston: Houghton Mifflin, 2001.

35 Shemilt I, Mugford M, Byford S, *et al*. Incorporating economics evidence. In: Higgins JPT, Green S (eds) *Cochrane Handbook for Systematic Reviews of Interventions*. Version 5.0.1 (updated September 2008). Oxford: Cochrane Collaboration, 2008.

36 Shemilt I, Mugford M, Byford S, *et al*. *Campbell Collaboration Methods Policy Brief: economics methods*. Oslo: Campbell Collaboration, 2008.

37 Donaldson C, Mugford M, Vale L (eds) *Evidence-Based Health Economics: from effectiveness to efficiency in systematic review*. London: BMJ Books, 2002.

CHAPTER 2

The role of review and synthesis methods in decision models

Kevin Marsh
The Matrix Knowledge Group, London, UK

Introduction

The decision model has been defined as an analytic tool used to support systematic approaches to evaluating the impact of alternative interventions on costs and other outcomes under conditions of uncertainty.[1,2] Given the paucity of economic evaluations in a number of policy areas, if the goal is to support decision making with economic evidence, decision models will need to lead the forward line. In health economics, leading proponents of economic evaluation have argued for several years that modelling – the art of synthesising the best available evidence on the costs and consequences of representations of 'real-world' choices between alternatives – is an 'unavoidable fact of life'.[3]

In the first edition of this book, Donaldson and colleagues provided an introduction to economic evaluation and gave an overview of how systematic review and evidence synthesis methods can be employed to inform economic evaluations, including decision models.[4] This chapter provides an update to that paper. Specifically, it attempts to answer two questions. First, has any progress been made in answering the methods questions raised by Donaldson and colleagues? Second, can the insights provided by Donaldson and colleagues with respect to the evaluation of health care interventions be applied to other fields, in particular social welfare, education and criminal justice?

The first section of this chapter introduces economic evaluation and provides a summary of Donaldson and colleagues' recommendations about how systematic review methods can be employed to inform economic evaluation, including decision models. The next two sections address the questions posed above. Finally, the chapter concludes with recommendations for how systematic review methods can be applied to economic evaluations conducted using decision models. Signposts to other chapters in this volume, which present further, detailed discussions of many of the issues introduced in this chapter, are provided throughout.

Using systematic reviews in economic evaluation

Systematic reviews of evidence on the beneficial and adverse effects of interventions have become an important source of information for decision makers.[5–8] However, in many cases decision makers need to consider not only whether an intervention works or harms, but also whether its adoption will lead to a more efficient use of resources.[9,10] For this reason, comparative analysis of both the costs and effects of interventions (i.e. economic evaluation) provides important information for decision makers.[11,12]

Resources are scarce and policy makers need to choose the most efficient intervention in order to maximise some objective, such as health or societal welfare. However, the effectiveness of an intervention is insufficient evidence on which to base decisions,

Evidence-Based Decisions and Economics, 2nd edition. Edited by I. Shemilt, M. Mugford, L. Vale, K. Marsh and C. Donaldson.
© 2010 Blackwell Publishing.

because the cost of the intervention may outweigh its benefits or an alternative intervention may achieve the same outcome for a lower cost. There is also empirical evidence of the importance of economic evaluation to decision making. For example, Marsh and colleagues have demonstrated that considerations of both the costs and benefits of criminal justice interventions produce different policy recommendations compared to analysis of their effectiveness alone.[13]

Economic evaluation is concerned with the 'opportunity cost' of a policy or intervention (see also, *inter alia*, Chapters 1, 3 and 4). Opportunity costs express the effects of an action in terms of the foregone benefits of the next best alternative use of the resources needed to implement that action.[14] That is, resources are used efficiently if there is no way to increase benefits (financial, quality of life, etc.) by shifting resources from one intervention to another.

In some cases, it is relatively clear that an intervention represents an efficient use of resources. This is the case if an intervention is able to achieve the same outcome as the next best alternative but at a lower cost or if an intervention costs the same as the next best alternative but produces greater benefits. In these circumstances, the intervention can be judged, unequivocally, to be a better use of resources than the alternative (in economic terms, the intervention is dominant and 'more technically efficient').

In other cases, the relative efficiency of interventions is less clear; for example, when an intervention both costs more and produces greater benefits or, conversely, when an intervention produces fewer benefits but is also less costly. In these circumstances, a further judgement is required about whether the extra benefits are worth the extra cost (or, conversely, whether the benefits foregone are justified, given the reduction in costs); this is an 'allocative efficiency' question. To inform this judgement, a comparative analysis of the incremental costs of an intervention with the value of its incremental benefits (i.e. an economic evaluation) is needed.

Economists have developed a number of techniques to value benefits (outcomes) for this purpose. For example, the use of cost-utility analysis (CUA) is common in the economic evaluation of health care interventions, such as those undertaken on behalf of the National Institute for Health and Clinical Excellence (NICE) in the UK.[15] In a CUA, measures of the health benefits of compared interventions are valued in terms of quality-adjusted life-years (QALYs), a composite measure of length of life and health-related quality of life, and interventions are compared in terms of their incremental cost per QALY. Alternatively, HM Treasury suggests that a cost-benefit analysis (CBA) is undertaken for evaluations of public sector initiatives within and across several sectors.[16] In a CBA, measures of the outcomes of compared interventions are valued monetarily based on estimates of people's willingness to pay for these outcomes, which is calculated using stated preference methods (contingent valuation), revealed preference methods or the human capital approach.[17,18] Examples of the use of monetary valuation techniques to undertake a CBA can be found in the evaluation of criminal justice interventions.[19,20]

Donaldson and colleagues identified a number of approaches to the use of systematic reviews to inform economic evaluations of health care interventions.

• Systematic review of all (economic) evaluations containing relevant data.
• Systematic review of effectiveness studies, with cost data obtained from any available economic evaluation.
• Systematic review of effectiveness studies, with cost data obtained only from economic evaluations performed alongside robust study designs.
• Systematic review of effectiveness studies where key 'cost drivers' (areas of resources use) are identified as review outcomes, which may or may not subsequently be costed by combining with relevant (local) prices.
• Performance of a secondary economic evaluation where the systematic review of clinical effectiveness is the main source of data but secondary searches and primary data collection may be performed to identify resource use, cost and utilities.[4]

They argued that, whichever approach is adopted, each requires the collection of data on the types, quantities and values of resources and outcomes (i.e. description, measurement and valuation). Specifically, three types of data are required

1. The *main event pathways* that have distinct resource implications or outcome values associated with them. For a health care intervention, this might include estimates of the probability, length and intensity of inpatient admissions, surgical or medical interventions, medication and outpatient consultation, as well as health outcomes.

2. The *probabilities* associated with the main event pathways.

3. The *resource consequences* and *utilities or values* associated with the event pathways.[4]

Donaldson and colleagues also acknowledged, however, that there are challenges to identifying the above data through the use of systematic reviews.[4] For instance, while randomised controlled trials (RCTs) often include data that can be used to calculate the probabilities of outcomes, similar data are not necessarily available in RCTs for resource use or costs (see also, *inter alia*, Chapters 3, 7 and 9).[4] Further, data on utilities associated with outcomes are seldom reported in RCTs (see also Chapter 8).[4]

Drummond and colleagues arrived at a similar conclusion in their review of NICE health technology appraisals to assess the extent to which these systematic reviews of clinical literature inform economic evaluations.[21] The authors concluded that economic evaluations can benefit from systematic reviews of clinical literature – as expected with appraisals undertaken for NICE, all the 41 technology appraisals reviewed contained a systematic review. However, they also concluded that there are challenges to employing systematic reviews of clinical literature in undertaking economic evaluations. For instance, given the lack of reporting of utilities in RCTs noted by Donaldson and colleagues, much of the data required to estimate composite measures of health gain (in this case, QALYs) is not contained in systematic reviews of such studies (see also Chapter 8). Systematic reviews may also present summary statistics in a form that is not appropriate for use in economic evaluations (e.g. median survival time rather than mean survival time).

Given the limited data on resource use, costs and utilities reported alongside trials of health care interventions, Donaldson and colleagues concluded that overcoming these gaps in the evidence requires use of decision models, which combine effects data obtained from trials (or systematic reviews of trials) with data on baseline risks, resource use, costs, and (in health care) utilities collected from a range of other sources, such as administrative datasets, observational studies and other primary research (see also, *inter alia*, Chapters 7, 8 and 9).[4] However, they also concluded that it was not immediately clear how this should be done:

'What is not clear, however, is which is the most appropriate source for the different types of data required (resource use, prices, patient outcomes) to conduct the evaluation.'

(Donaldson et al., 2002:22)[4]

The remainder of this chapter builds on this discussion of the use of systematic reviews to inform economic evaluations in two ways. First, it considers whether methodological developments since 2002 offer insights that can help researchers to overcome the lack of guidance on decision modelling identified by Donaldson and colleagues. Second, it asks whether the approach outlined by Donaldson and colleagues for health care interventions is also applicable in other fields or whether different policy areas require alternative approaches.

Decision models: methodological developments

Decision models are frequently used to conduct economic evaluations alongside systematic reviews, as only rarely is all the evidence required for an economic evaluation available from one source (see also, *inter alia*, Chapters 7, 8 and 9).[22,23] Decision models provide an explicit, quantitative and systematic approach to decision making, and synthesise data from different sources to allow the cost-effectiveness of alternative interventions to be assessed using cost-effectiveness analysis (CEA), CUA or CBA. This approach to conducting economic evaluations is recommended by a number of prominent organisations worldwide, including the NICE in the UK and the Canadian Agency for Drugs and Technology in Health (CADTH). NICE methods guidelines state that:

'... it will be necessary to construct an analytical framework within which to synthesise the available evidence so that estimates of clinical and cost effectiveness can be made that are relevant to the clinical decision-making context. This framework will usually require the development of a model using aggregated or individual patient data to estimate parameters.'

(NICE, 2008:28)[15]

Decision analysis splits the measurement of cost-effectiveness into a number of components, which can be evidenced from different data sources. Under this methodology, the possible chains of events (from initial choice of intervention, through intermediate events, to final outcomes) are identified using an explicit structure that clearly specifies their sequence. Data are analysed by giving each possible event a valuation (either in terms of resource use, health outcome or both), and by weighting valuations of interventions, events and outcomes by the probability of their occurrence. Examples of decision models that use a decision tree structure from education and criminal justice are presented in Figures 2.1 and 2.2.

Cooper and colleagues have identified a number of specific reasons why decision models are employed in health economic evaluation.[23]

- To extrapolate primary data beyond the endpoint of a trial.
- To make indirect comparisons between treatments for which no 'head-to-head' trials exist.

- To investigate how the cost-effectiveness of clinical strategies/interventions changes as the values of key parameters are altered (often not observable in primary data analysis).
- To link intermediate endpoints to ultimate measures of health gain (e.g. QALYs).
- To incorporate country-specific data relating to disease history and management.

Decision models are parameterised using diverse sources of evidence including, *inter alia*, RCTs, observational studies, administrative data and expert opinion (see also Chapters 7, 8 and 9).[24] Systematic reviews are often employed to identify and synthesise evidence on the effects of the interventions compared in a model. However, strategies for identifying evidence for other parameters (i.e. baseline risks, resource use, unit costs, and, if applicable, utilities) are not always made explicit in practice (see also Chapters 7, 8 and 9).[23]

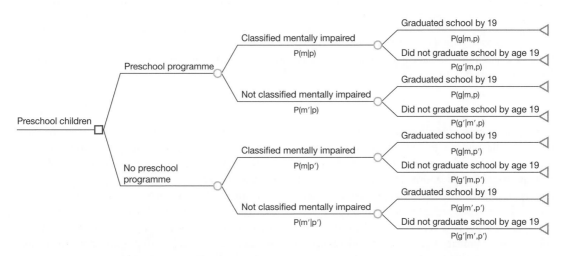

P(m|p) = Probability that the child will be mentally impaired given that they attended the preschool programme

P(m'|p) = Probability that the child will not be mentally impaired given that they attended the preschool programme

P(m|p') = Probability that the child will be mentally impaired given that they did not attend the preschool programme

P(m'|p') = Probability that the child will not be mentally impaired given that they did not attend the preschool programme

P(g|m,p) = Probability that the child will graduate school by age 19 given that they were classified as mentally impaired and attended the preschool programme

P(g'|m,p) = Probability that the child will not graduate school by age 19 given that they were classified as mentally impaired and attended the preschool programme

P(g|m',p) = Probability that the child will graduate school by age 19 given that they were not classified as mentally impaired and attended the preschool programme

P(g'|m',p) = Probability that the child will not graduate school by age 19 given that they were not classified as mentally impaired and attended the preschool programme

Figure 2.1 Illustrative decision model for a preschool programme designed to improve subsequent school attainment (decision tree structure).

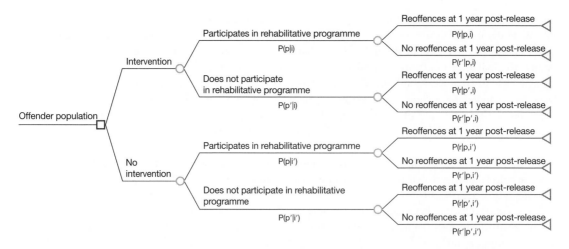

P(p|i)	=	Probability that the offender will participate in the rehabilitative programme given that they received the intervention
P(p'|i)	=	Probability that the offender will not participate in the rehabilitative programme given that they received the intervention
P(p|i')	=	Probability that the child will participate in the rehabilitative programme given that they did not receive the intervention
P(p'|i')	=	Probability that the offender will not participate in the rehabilitative programme given that they did not receive the intervention
P(r|p,i)	=	Probability that the offender will have reoffended at 1 year post release given that they participated in the rehabilitative programme having received the intervention
P(r'|p,i)	=	Probability that the offender will not have reoffended at 1 year post release given that they participated in the rehabilitative programme having received the intervention

Figure 2.2 Illustrative decision model for an intervention designed to increase uptake of a rehabilitative programme (decision tree structure).

A number of recent studies have identified the use of systematic reviews to measure treatment effect parameters in decision models for health economic evaluation. As noted above, Drummond and colleagues reviewed 41 technology assessments published between 2003 and 2006 and concluded that all contained a systematic review to measure treatment effects.[21] In a similar study, Cooper and colleagues reviewed economic decision models developed as part of the UK Health Technology Assessment (HTA) programme between 1997 and 2003.[25] The authors of this study concluded that systematic reviews are often used for the estimation of relative treatment effects and are the most common approach.

Use of systematic reviews to measure treatment effects in decision models is, however, far from universal. In a review of drug therapies, Hanratty and colleagues found that only a small proportion of published economic studies used systematic reviews that would have been available at the time the studies were conducted.[26] They concluded that there is a consequent risk that estimates of cost-effectiveness could be biased, due to the failure to utilise the most precise estimates of treatment effects available from meta-analyses.[26,27]

A similar observation was made by Demicheli and colleagues, who concluded that their analysis demonstrated that 'a significant proportion of evaluations rely on estimates of effect derived from single, small, non-randomised studies or, possibly even worse, expert opinion'.[28] Drummond and colleagues have identified a number of possible reasons for systematic reviews not being employed to inform decision models, including authors being unaware of the availability of existing reviews, there being no review available, and the time and cost associated with undertaking a new review.[21]

The remainder of this section considers two specific challenges facing the construction of decision models that are of particular relevance to the use of systematic review methods: how should evidence on model parameters be identified and analysed and how should the quality of such evidence be assessed?'

It is important to note that methodological guidance published to date offers limited and somewhat inconsistent answers to these specific questions. Whilst a number of published papers offer general guidance on good practice and model quality in decision modelling for health economic evaluation, a review of 15 such papers conducted by Phillip and colleagues concluded that they offer conflicting guidance on key issues.[1,3,24,29–41] Furthermore, most published methods guidelines do not address methods for the identification of parameter estimates or assessment of the quality of data inputs. This situation is, however, starting to be addressed (e.g. Chapters 7, 8, 9 and 10 of this volume offer methods proposals, based on recent and ongoing research, that aim to address each of these two specific questions).

Identifying and analysing evidence

In their 2005 study, Cooper and colleagues identified a lack of guidance on methodologies for identifying evidence to inform model parameters (other than clinical effects parameters, for which there are well-established search methods – see Chapter 7) and a lack of clear reporting of the sources of evidence used to inform model parameters.[25] Any guidance for identifying decision model parameters should answer a number of questions, including: What sources of evidence are available to estimate model parameters? What search strategies should be adopted? How should search strategies be reported? How should the evidence collected be analysed?

Sources of evidence

As stated above, decision models need to be populated with estimates of their specified parameters (main types of parameters are beneficial and adverse effects, baseline risks, resource use, unit costs, and, if applicable, utilities). For example, to estimate costs, locally applicable estimates of both amounts of resource use associated with compared interventions and their unit costs are needed. For decision models, prospective data collection or analysis of reliable administrative data for the specific study or, alternatively, recently published results of prospective data collection or a recent analysis of reliable administrative data, collected from the same jurisdiction, have been proposed as the best sources of evidence to inform estimates of resource use parameters (see Chapter 9). Similarly, unit cost calculations based on reliable databases or data sources conducted for the specific study or, alternatively, recently published cost calculations based on reliable databases or data sources, collected from the same jurisdiction, have been proposed as optimal sources of evidence to inform estimates of unit cost parameters (see Chapter 9).

As such, prospective data collection, administrative datasets and published (or unpublished) economic analyses may all be considered as potentially useful sources to inform resource use and unit cost parameters in a decision model (see Chapter 7). Research into the unit costs of health and social care, combining data collected from each of these types of sources, has resulted in compilations of unit costs data being made available in some jurisdictions (e.g. in the UK the Personal Social Services Research Unit provides an annually updated volume of unit costs of health and social care and the Pharmaceutical Benefits Advisory Committee provides similar sources in Australia).[42,43] Other compilations of health care unit costs data in the UK include National Schedule of NHS Reference Costs volumes and British National Formulary volumes.[44,45] Comparable compilations are available for other jurisdictions, for example, within Diagnostic Related Groups (DRG) systems in Germany.[46]

Similar compendia are currently being developed for other policy areas and jurisdictions. For instance, the Personal Social Services Research Unit (PSSRU) is developing a 'UK unit costs of crime and justice' volume.[47] Also, the Centre for Child and Family Research (CCFR) at Loughborough University is working on UK education unit costs as part of a project to develop a 'children's services' cost calculator for UK local authorities.[48]

A number of sources of published economic analyses of health care interventions are suggested in the literature, including the NHS Economic Evaluation Database (NHS EED), the Health Economic Evaluation Database and Econlit, the American Economic Association's electronic bibliography.[9,49–51] We are, however, not aware of equivalent databases covering the fields of education, criminal justice or social welfare (see also Chapter 7).

Search strategies

As noted above, systematic review methods are often employed to identify evidence on treatment effects for use in decision models for health economic evaluation, but are rarely fully implemented to identify data used to estimate other model parameters (see also Chapters 7, 8 and 9). This is in part because of the cost and time that would be needed to undertake a full systematic review for all model parameters, but primarily because specific features of decision model development processes mean that systematic review methods are not directly applicable in this context (see Chapter 7 for a comprehensive discussion of this issue).

Consequently, Cooper and colleagues suggest a number of search strategies that may improve the efficiency of searches for data to estimate decision model parameters (see also Chapters 7, 8 and 9).[23] First, focused, systematic searches should be conducted around those parameters that have the largest influence on model results, using expert opinion, previous studies or initial models to inform judgements about which parameters these searches should focus on. Second, an iterative approach to searching should be adopted (see also Chapter 7). Examples of iterative approaches to searching include citation searches, 'pearl growing'(i.e. using relevant articles to identify other relevant articles) and 'berry picking' (i.e. using each newly identified piece of information to redefine the initial query, resulting in an ever-modifying search strategy) (see also Chapter 7).[52,53]

When adopting iterative approaches to searching rather than full systematic reviews, it is important to know when 'sufficient' evidence has been collected (see also, *inter alia*, Chapters 7, 8 and 12). Cooper and colleagues suggest that 'sufficiency' can be defined in terms of parameter uncertainty (i.e. incorporating additional evidence does not affect parameter uncertainty) or in terms of a precision/bias trade-off (i.e. while incorporating additional information reduces uncertainty, it does so at the expense of increasing bias, as the additional data are less relevant or of poor quality) (see also Chapter 7).[23] The framework of value of information (VoI) analysis also provides the possibility of quantifying how further information will reduce decision uncertainty (see Chapter 12).[54]

Analysis

A well-conducted meta-analysis of RCTs with direct comparison between alternative interventions has been proposed as the least biased source of data to inform estimates of beneficial and adverse effects parameters in decision models for health economic evaluation (see Chapter 9).[25,55] However, there are limitations to the application of such methods to the synthesis of data to populate cost, resource use and (if applicable) utilities parameters.[9,10]

Meta-analysis requires that a common metric is available across two or more studies. Attention therefore needs to be paid to the equivalence of the meaning of estimates of costs, resource use and utilities (or other outcome values) across studies prior to any decision to pool these estimates (see also Chapter 9). Estimates of resource use, costs, and outcome values are sensitive to features of local contexts, such as prices, preferences and the configuration of service delivery (see also, *inter alia*, Chapters 3, 4, 8 and 13).[17,56,57] This may limit the generalisability and transferability of such estimates across settings. Therefore, selection of the best available sources of locally applicable data for a specific context is (subject to availability), arguably, likely to be preferable to (adjusted) estimates based on data collected in other settings and to pooled estimates derived using a synthesis of (adjusted) data collected from several studies conducted in different settings (see also, *inter alia*, Chapters 3, 4 and 9).

Reporting

Assessment of the appropriateness of a search strategy undertaken to populate a decision model requires that the strategy employed is clearly reported (see Chapter 7 for a detailed discussion of this issue). This also enables the search to be reproduced and updated. Cooper and colleagues observed that search strategies employed in the development of existing decision models are in general poorly reported.[25] It is important that the method for identifying evidence on all model parameters is reported, including a clear description of inclusion and exclusion criteria, as well as an assessment of the quality of the evidence used (see Chapter 7 for a detailed discussion of this issue).[58]

Assessing quality of evidence

As decision models use data from diverse sources, which may themselves be subject to varying degrees of different forms and sources of bias, it is important that the quality of the evidence included in models is assessed. Chapter 9 of this volume proposes a hierarchy of data sources for evidence to inform estimates of different parameters in decision models for health economic evaluation (and may also provide a useful starting point for development of hierarchies applicable to decision models of social welfare, education and criminal justice interventions). Use of such hierarchies may in itself limit the potential for bias in decision models. However, where evidence for decision models is derived from previously published or unpublished studies, there is a further need to undertake detailed assessments of risk of bias in, and methodological quality of, each source study.

Given the range of types of parameters in a decision model and the range of study designs that may be drawn upon to collect evidence to estimate each parameter, a battery of different tools may be needed for this purpose. Several tools have been suggested in the literature for use to inform assessments of different study designs. For example, Cooper and colleagues identified instruments such as the Jadad Scale for assessing the quality of RCTs, and the Newcastle-Ottawa Scale for assessing the quality of non-randomised/observational studies.[23,59,60] Other potential tools include the Cochrane Collaboration's tool for assessing risk of bias and the EPOC Risk of Bias Guideline (to inform assessments of both RCTs and various forms of non-randomised/observational studies).[61,62]

Jefferson and colleagues identified a number of tools to inform assessments of the quality of economic evaluations, including guidelines for authors and peer reviewers of economic submissions to the *British Medical Journal* (BMJ checklist) and the Quality of Health Economics Studies (QHES) checklist.[63–66] The Campbell & Cochrane Economics Methods Group recommends a two-stage approach to assessment of health economic evaluations, utilising the Cochrane Collaboration's tool for assessing risk of bias (stage one) and, depending on the approach to economic evaluation, the BMJ checklist and/or the criteria list for assessment of methodological

quality of economic evaluations (CHEC criteria list) or the quality assessment in decision-analytic models (Philips checklist) to inform each stage.[9,24,64,67] However, there are many other quality checklists that could be applied to those economic evaluations that provide data used in decision models. Chapter 10 of this volume refers to an unpublished review that identified more than 20 published checklists designed to inform assessments of the methodological quality of economic evaluations conducted alongside single, empirical studies, as well as several more designed to inform similar assessments of previously published and unpublished decision models (including some based on methods guidelines cited earlier in this chapter).

Given that decision models may draw on data from several previously published studies that utilise different study designs, a challenge facing quality assessment of studies in the decision-modelling context is the need to assess quality *across* study designs.[68] For example, when is a good-quality quasi-experimental study better than a poor-quality RCT? Most of the checklists and guidance currently available do not facilitate such comparisons. However, the GRADE system, described in Chapter 10 of this volume, *does* provide a comprehensive framework for rating the quality of evidence on both health and other effects, collected from RCTs and observational studies, as well as evidence on resource use and costs, drawn from previously published economic evaluations (excluding published decision models). Moreover, in the UK, NICE has developed checklists to inform assessments of the applicability and quality of decision models, including the sources of evidence they use, which draws on the GRADE approach (see Chapter 10 for a full description).

How should potential biases in the data used in a model be dealt with? First, sensitivity analysis should be conducted to assess the impact of the quality of the evidence included in the model on its results. Should this analysis reveal that the results of the model are sensitive to different qualities of evidence, a number of solutions have been proposed to attempt to adjust for biases.[23] First, evidence obtained from studies that fall below a prespecified quality threshold can be excluded. Second, weights can be given to the studies according to their quality. Third, random effects modelling of bias can be employed. Fourth, full bias modelling can be employed in an attempt to identify all sources of potential bias in the available evidence, obtain external information on the likely form of each bias and construct a model to correct the data analysis accordingly. Each of these methods requires a judgement about how study design affects reliability. Cooper and colleagues suggest that adjustments for study-specific biases may be obtained by employing clinical and/or epidemiological experts to judge the validity of each data source.[24]

Beyond health care

Debate on the use of review methods to inform economic evaluations, including decision models, has almost exclusively taken place in relation to health care interventions, which have consequently been the main focus of this chapter. This section explores the extent to which non-health care policy areas, such as social welfare, education and criminal justice, pose distinctive methodological challenges for such methods or whether the methods are broadly applicable to other areas.

An important opening observation is that health care interventions have been the subject of much larger numbers of economic evaluations compared to social welfare, education and criminal justice interventions. For example, a systematic review conducted Sefton and colleagues found that, between 1996 and 2000, an average of approximately 30 economic evaluations was published each year in the social welfare field, compared to 15–20 times that number in the health care field.[69] A comparable total number of economic evaluations of criminal justice interventions were identified in a study by Marsh.[70]

Consequently, social welfare, education and criminal justice policy makers and practitioners wishing to include considerations of economic evidence for a given decision are likely to be able to draw on evidence from previously published economic evaluations much less often than their health care counterparts. This suggests that Donaldson and colleagues' recommendation that decision models are required for economic evaluation of health care interventions applies equally to non-health care interventions.[4] After all, recognising that decisions still need to be made, decision models offer a systematic approach to

evaluating the impact of alternative interventions on costs and other outcomes under conditions of *uncertainty* and in the *absence* of ideal evidence.[1]

It also seems reasonable to suggest that the data requirements for economic evaluations of health care interventions outlined by Donaldson and colleagues apply equally to non-health care interventions.[4] There is nothing subject specific about the need to understand the event pathways associated with compared interventions, the probabilities associated with these pathways, and their associated costs and values. However, a further implication of the relative lack of previously published (and unpublished) economic evaluations in the social welfare, education and criminal justice fields is that reviews conducted for the purpose of populating decision models are, at present, less likely to be able to draw on data collected from previous economic evaluations. This suggests that decision models of non-health care interventions are currently more likely to rely on evidence on resource use, costs and monetary (or other) valuations of outcomes that has been obtained from analyses of administrative datasets, published compendia and expert opinion (assuming primary data collection is not a feasible option).

There are also important differences between the health care and non-health care fields that will need to be taken into account when designing reviews to inform decision models (and empirical economic evaluations). Within the UK, many such differences are evident in current debates regarding application of the NICE reference case to economic evaluations of public health interventions.[15,71,72]

Some differences are of degree rather than form. For example, a key challenge identified in the previous section, that relates equally to decision models developed in health care and non-health care fields, is the need to develop quality assessment methods that incorporate non-experimental study designs. This challenge is particularly pertinent to policy areas such as criminal justice, where the use of experimental methods may be limited in practice by ethical or logistical concerns.[73]

Other differences present a more serious challenge to the conduct of reviews to inform decision models in social welfare, education and criminal justice. First, given the general lack of formal analyses of the costs of interventions described above, it is likely that alternative approaches are required to identify these data, including primary data collection and use of new, review-based methods to identify resource use data within comparative effectiveness research studies, to inform cost analyses.[74] Second, there is a lack of agreement on appropriate measures of outcomes. This poses a challenge to the synthesis of outcome data, as studies often do not measure the same outcomes or adopt different metrics to capture the same outcomes.

Two further differences between health care and non-health care policy and practice contexts, which have serious implications for the conduct of economic evaluations and reviews to inform decision models that warrant further discussion, are analytic perspective and valuation methods.

Analytic perspective: which costs and effects should be included?

Delivery of social welfare services involves a range of funders and decision makers. For example, in the UK, social care funding comes from a combination of central government grants, tax revenues and user charges. Social care policy involves a range of stakeholders, including local authorities, health care practitioners and users, who all play a key role in determining which services are provided in practice. The multisector nature of social care provision and the increasing importance of users as decision makers mean that it is not only important that the costs and benefits accruing to all stakeholder groups are included in an economic analysis, but also that the costs and benefits accruing to *each* stakeholder group are presented separately (as well as trade-offs between costs and benefits accruing to different stakeholder groups). This is essential to allow each stakeholder group to assess the impacts of an intervention on costs and other outcomes from their own perspective.

Given that stakeholders normally operate within fixed budgets to achieve a specific objective, such as maximising health outcomes or reducing crime, Claxton and colleagues have argued that, in such circumstances, adoption of a multisector analytic perspective is appropriate.[75] The decision rule thus becomes that an intervention should only be recommended if either benefits are greater than costs from the perspective of *each stakeholder group* necessary to deliver the intervention or if those stakeholder groups

that gain from the intervention can compensate those that lose (in the latter case, a mechanism is needed to allow stakeholders who gain to compensate those who lose).

Adoption of a multisector analytic perspective in policy areas such as social welfare has implications for data collection for decision models. In particular, it is likely to increase the number of parameters that need to be estimated in a given model, which in principle might increase the research resources needed to identify data for this purpose. This places greater emphasis on the need to develop efficient approaches to identification of the data needed to estimate model parameters (see also Chapters 7 and 8), as well as methods for identifying when sufficient data have been collected.

How should outcomes be valued?

One of the key challenges in the use of systematic reviews of RCTs to inform decision models of health care interventions is that evidence on the impact of interventions on health state utilities is not restricted to RCTs (see Chapter 8). This challenge is exacerbated in non-health policy areas, as health state utilities do not necessarily capture the value of outcomes associated with social welfare, education or criminal justice interventions, and no equivalent measures have yet been fully developed in these fields. Furthermore, the philosophical basis for measures of utility employed in health care is often rejected by those working in non-health policy areas.

The valuation of public sector outcomes, such as improved health or well-being, raises difficult questions about what is 'good'. In particular, two such questions stand out.

1. Whose judgement about the value of outcomes has legitimacy – the general public, service users or decision makers?
2. Should values be derived from people's preferences or from their experiences?

Health economics research often employs the QALY, a composite measure of length of life and health-related quality of life, as a standard measure to value health benefits. When deciding whether to recommend a new health care technology, in England, NICE has chosen to assess the incremental QALYs associated with the new technology (compared to alternative interventions) to determine whether this

QALY gain justifies the cost of the technology. This entails adoption of what is sometimes referred to as an 'extra-welfarist' approach, which places an implicit legitimacy for valuing outcomes on past decisions. Implicit in this approach are answers to the above two questions. Specifically, decision makers' preferences determine what is good. Critics of this approach argue that values derived from past decisions are influenced by political and affordability issues rather than the preference of the population.[76]

Two alternative approaches to deciding what is 'good' are available. The 'welfarist approach' states that value judgements should be based on individuals' welfare and that individuals are the best judges of their own welfare. From this perspective, individuals' willingness to pay is the appropriate way to value outcomes. This is the position adopted by HM Treasury's guidance on how to undertake economic evaluations and is a position that has been adopted by a number of economists working on criminal justice interventions.[16,77–79] However, a number of commentators have criticised the validity of techniques employed to elicit people's willingness to pay, arguing that they are based on unrealistic underlying assumptions about the functioning of markets or are subject to a range of biases.[80]

Both the 'welfarist' and 'extra-welfarist' approaches emphasise the importance of people's preferences in deriving valuations of outcomes. New techniques that use measures of subjective well-being (i.e. people's responses to questions such as 'how satisfied are you with your life?') to value policy outcomes accept the welfarist principle that value judgements should be based on individuals' welfare, but reject the welfarist principle that individuals' *preferences* are the best way to assess welfare. Instead, the focus is on people's *experiences* and how these relate to their evaluations of their lives.[81] A key argument in favour of such an approach is that people are poor predictors of what mechanisms will improve their well-being. Thus, rather than ask people about their preferences for certain outcomes, a direct measure of their experiences of the outcomes on well-being is argued to provide a more accurate picture of the likely value of interventions.

The resolution of this debate is beyond the scope of this paper. However, it is sufficient for present purposes to acknowledge that policy makers and researchers in non-health care fields may adopt a different approach to valuing policy outcomes to their health care counterparts. For example, as noted above, economic evaluations in the criminal justice field often employ monetary values of crime outcomes that correspond with a welfarist view of the world. Economic evaluation in education often employs the human capital method for valuing outcomes. Furthermore, policy makers have recently begun to look with increased interest at the possibility of using measures of subjective well-being to evaluate public policy. For instance, the OECD recently convened a conference of academics and policy makers to discuss the use of such measures in policy making.[82]

The likelihood that non-health care fields adopt different notions of value to those currently adopted in health care has potential implications for the employment of reviews to inform decision models. For instance, quality grading scales may need to be developed for studies of the subjective well-being impact of outcomes, or studies of the monetary value of such outcomes, or alternatively these study designs need to be integrated into existing evidence grading frameworks that accommodate a range of study designs (see, for example, Chapter 10).

Discussion

The limited data on resources use, costs and utilities reported alongside studies of the beneficial and adverse effects of interventions (e.g. RCTs) mean that supplementary reviews need to be conducted to populate decision models for the economic evaluation of interventions. However, published decision models raise a number of concerns. First, use of systematic reviews as the framework for analysis of evidence on beneficial and adverse effects is far from universal in decision modelling. Second, strategies for identifying evidence for other key model parameters are rarely made explicit. Third, development of decision models rarely includes rigorous quality assessment of the sources of evidence they utilise.

Solutions to these challenges have been limited to date by a lack of consistent guidance on decision modelling methods. However, this situation is starting to be addressed as proposals begin to emerge from recent and ongoing research (see, *inter alia*, Chapters 7, 8, 9 and 10). First, the costs associated with undertaking reviews of evidence to inform model parameters mean that more efficient search strategies are being developed. There is an emerging consensus that searches should focus on those parameters that have the largest influence on model results and also use more iterative approaches. Second, the literature identifies a number of tools that can be used to identify the quality of the data employed in models. Third, the importance of clear reporting of the methods employed is emphasised.

However, a number of important questions remain to be answered before guidance on the use of review methods to inform decision models comes of age. In particular, further work is needed to define and measure when 'sufficient' data have been collected to build a decision model (see also Chapter 7). Also, further research is required on how the quality of data inputs affects the reliability of the results of decision models (see also Chapter 9). Finally, further guidance is needed on methods for addressing potential biases within the data employed in a decision model.

Much of the debate to date has focused on methods for use in decision models for economic evaluations of health care interventions. Many components of the methodologies proposed in the health care literature are relevant for the economic evaluation of non-health care interventions. If anything, the limited evidence base in other policy fields places more emphasis on the need for decision models and the use of diverse sources of data to inform their development and population.

However, distinctive features of non-health care fields mean that some challenges facing health care are exacerbated in other applied fields. These challenges currently restrict the synthesis and use of evidence on the efficiency of interventions and further methodological research and development are needed before they can be overcome. First, the limited evidence base and relative dearth of high-quality research on the costs and effects of interventions are a major barrier to the development of decision models to evaluate the efficiency of non-health interventions; thus more economic analyses are needed. Second, both real and imagined obstacles to conducting experimental studies on social and behavioural interventions place greater emphasis on the need to develop quality assessment methods and analytic approaches that incorporate non-experimental study designs.

Third, the multisector analytic perspective indicated in policy areas such as social welfare is likely to increase the complexity of decision models, which will demand a corresponding increase in the urgency to develop efficient search strategies and clear guidelines to inform judgements of when sufficient data have been identified. Fourth, different notions of value employed in non-health care policy domains mean that greater attention needs to be focused on the development of quality grading scales to accommodate assessments of studies of the subjective well-being impact and monetary valuation. Finally, the resources available to assist those developing decision models in non-health care fields are limited. Therefore, investment is required to develop specialist database(s) of previously published economic analysis and compendia of the unit costs of resources used in social welfare, education and criminal justice sectors.

Acknowledgements

Other contributors to this chapter: Nicola J Cooper, Senior Research Fellow, University of Leicester, UK; Gordon Cleveland, Senior Lecturer in Economics, University of Toronto at Scarborough, Canada; Ian Shemilt, Senior Research Associate, University of East Anglia, UK; Luke Vale, Professor of Health Technology Assessment, University of Aberdeen, UK.

How this chapter should be cited

Marsh K. Chapter 2: The role of review and synthesis methods in decision models. In: Shemilt I, Mugford M, Vale L, Marsh K, Donaldson C (editors). *Evidence-based decisions and economics: health care, social welfare, education and criminal justice*. Oxford: Wiley-Blackwell, 2010.

References

1 Soto J. Health economic evaluations using decision analytic modelling. Principles and practices – utilization of a checklist to their development and appraisal. *International Journal of Technology Assessment in Health Care* 2002; 18(1): 94–111.

2 Briggs A, Claxton K, Sculpher M. *Decision Modelling for Health Economic Evaluation*. Oxford: Oxford University Press, 2006.

3 Buxton MJ, Drummond MF, van Hout BA, *et al*. Modelling in economic evaluation: an unavoidable fact of life. *Health Economics* 1997; 6(3): 217–227.

4 Donaldson C, Mugford M, Vale L. Using systematic reviews in economic evaluation: the basic principles. In: Donaldson C,

Mugford M, Vale L (eds) *Evidence-Based Health Economics: from effectiveness to efficiency in systematic review*. London: BMJ Books, 2002.

5 Lavis JN, Posada FB, Haines A, Osei E. Use of research to inform public policymaking. *Lancet* 2004; 364(Oct 30): 1615–1621.

6 Petticrew M, Roberts H. Systematic reviews – do they 'work' in informing decision-making around health inequalities? *Health Economics Policy and Law* 2008; 3(2): 197–211.

7 Welsh BC, Farrington DP (eds). *Preventing Crime: What works for children, offenders, victims and places*. Dordrecht: Springer Netherlands, 2005.

8 Gilbody SM, Petticrew M. Rational decision-making in mental health: the role of systematic reviews. *Journal of Mental Health Policy and Economics* 1999; 2(3): 99–106.

9 Shemilt I, Mugford M, Byford S, *et al.* Incorporating economics evidence. In: Higgins JPT, Green S (eds) *Cochrane Handbook for Systematic Reviews of Interventions*. Version 5.0.1 (updated September 2008). Oxford: Cochrane Collaboration, 2008.

10 Shemilt I, Mugford M, Byford S, *et al. Campbell Collaboration Methods Policy Brief: economics methods*. Oslo: Campbell Collaboration, 2008.

11 Cohen MA. Measuring the costs and benefits of crime and justice. In: *Measurement and Analysis of Crime and Justice* (Criminal Justice 2000, Volume 4). Washington DC: National Institute of Justice, 2000.

12 Byford S, McDaid D, Sefton TAJ. *Because It's Worth It. A practical guide to conducting economic evaluations in the social welfare field*. York: Joseph Rowntree Foundation, 2003.

13 Marsh K, Chalfin A, Roman J. What does economic analysis add to decision making? Evidence from the criminal justice literature. *Journal of Experimental Criminology* 2008; 4(2): 117–135.

14 Drummond MF, Sculpher MJ, Torrance GW, O'Brien BJ, Stoddart GL. *Methods for the Economic Evaluation of Health Care Programmes*, 3rd edn. Oxford: Oxford University Press, 2005.

15 National Institute for Health and Clinical Excellence. *Guide to the Methods of Technology Appraisal*. London: National Institute for Health and Clinical Excellence, 2008.

16 HM Treasury. *The Green Book: appraisal and evaluation in central government*. London: The Stationery Office, 2003.

17 Drummond MF, Manca A, Sculpher MJ. Increasing the generalisability of economic evaluations: recommendations for the design, analysis and reporting of studies. *International Journal of Technology Assessment in Health Care* 2005; 21: 165–171.

18 United Nations, European Commission, International Monetary Fund, Organisation for Economic Cooperation and Development, World Bank, *Handbook of National Accounting: integrated environmental and economic accounting 2003* (Studies in Methods, Series F, No.61, Rev.1, Glossary). New York: United Nations, 2005.

19 Marsh K, Fox C. The benefit and cost of prison in the UK. The results of a model of lifetime re-offending. *Journal of Experimental Criminology* 2008; 4(4): 403–423.

20 Welsh B, Farrington DP. Monetary costs and benefits of crime prevention programs. In: Tonry M (ed) *Crime and Justice: a review of research* (Volume 27). Chicago: University of Chicago Press, 2000.

21 Drummond M, Iglesias C, Cooper NJ. Systematic reviews and economic evaluations in technology appraisals conducted for NICE in the UK: a game of two halves? *International Journal of Technology Assessment in Health Care* 2008; 24(2): 146–150.

22 Mugford M. Using systematic reviews for economic evaluation. In: Egger M, Davey Smith G, Altman D (eds) *Systematic Reviews in Health Care: meta-analysis in context*. London: BMJ Publishing Group, 2001.

23 Cooper NJ, Sutton AJ, Ades AE, Paisley S, Jones DR. Use of evidence in economic decision models: practical and methodological issues. *Health Economics* 2007; 16(12): 1277–1286.

24 Philips Z, Ginnelly L, Sculpher M, *et al.* Review of guidelines for good practice in decision-analytic modelling in health technology assessment. *Health Technology Assessment* 2004; 8(36): 1–172.

25 Cooper NJ, Coyle D, Abrams KR, Mugford M, Sutton AJ. Use of evidence in decision models: an appraisal of health technology assessments in the UK to date. *Journal of Health Services Research and Policy* 2005; 10(4): 245–250.

26 Hanratty B, Craig D, Nixon J, Rice S, Christie J, Drummond MF. Are the best available clinical effectiveness data used in economic evaluations of drug therapies? *Journal of Health Services Research and Policy* 2007; 12(3): 138–141.

27 Deeks JJ, Higgins JPT, Altman DG (eds). Analysing data and undertaking meta-analyses. In: Higgins JPT, Green S (eds) *Cochrane Handbook for Systematic Reviews of Interventions*. Version 5.0.1 (updated September 2008). Oxford: Cochrane Collaboration, 2008.

28 Demicheli V, Jefferson T, Vale L. Effectiveness estimates in economic evaluation. In: Donaldson C, Mugford M, Vale L (eds) *Evidence-Based Health Economics: from effectiveness to efficiency in systematic review*. London: BMJ Books, 2002.

29 Sculpher M, Fenwick E, Claxton K. Assessing quality in decision analytic cost-effectiveness models: a suggested framework and example of application. *Pharmacoeconomics* 2000; 17(5): 461–477.

30 Akehurst R, Anderson P, Brazier J, *et al.* Decision analytic modelling in the economic evaluation of health technologies – a consensus statement. *Pharmacoeconomics* 2000; 17(5): 443–444.

31 McCabe C, Dixon S. Testing the validity of cost-effectiveness models. *Pharmacoeconomics* 2000; 17(5): 501–513.

32 Halpern MT, McKenna M, Hutton J. Modeling in economic evaluation: an unavoidable fact of life. *Health Economics* 1998; 7(8): 741–742.

33 Hay JW. Economic modeling and sensitivity analysis. *Value in Health* 1998; 1(3): 187–193.

34 Weinstein MC, O'Brien BJ, Hornberger J, *et al.* Principles of good practice for decision analytic modeling in health-care evaluation: report of the ISPOR Task Force on Good Research Practices – Modeling Studies. *Value in Health* 2003; 6(1): 9–17.

35 Habbema JD, Bossuyt PM, Dippel DW, Marshall S, Hilden J. Analysing clinical decision analyses. *Statistics in Medicine* 1990; 9(11): 1229–1242.

36 Nuijten MJC, Pronk MH, Brorens MJA, *et al.* Reporting format for economic evaluation: Part II: Focus on modelling studies. *Pharmacoeconomics* 1998; 14(3): 259–268.

37 Sendi PP, Craig BA, Pfluger D, Gafni A, Bucher HC. Systematic validation of disease models for pharmacoeconomic evaluations. Swiss HIV Cohort Study. *Journal of Evaluation in Clinical Practice* 1999; 5(3): 283–295.

38 Ramsey SD, Sullivan SD. Weighing the economic evidence: guidelines for critical assessment of cost-effectiveness analyses. *Journal of the American Board of Family Practice* 1999; 12(6): 477–485.

39 Eddy D. Technology assessment: the role of mathematical modelling. In Mosteller F (ed) *Assessing Medical Technologies*. Washington DC: National Academy Press, 1985.

40 Weinstein MC, Toy EL, Sandberg EA, *et al.* Modeling for health care and other policy decisions: uses, roles, and validity. *Value in Health* 2001; 4(5): 348–361.

41 Sonnenberg FA, Roberts MS, Tsevat J, Wong JB, Barry M, Kent DL. Toward a peer review process for medical decision analysis models. *Medical Care* 1994; 32(7 suppl): JS52–JS64.

42 Personal Social Services Research Unit. *Unit Costs of Health and Social Care 2009*. Canterbury: University of Kent, 2009.

43 Pharmaceutical Benefits Advisory Committee. *Manual of Resource Items and Their Associated Costs for Use in Submissions to the Pharmaceutical Benefits Advisory Committee involving Economic Evaluation* (second revision). Canberra: Australian Government Department of Health and Ageing, 2002. Available from: www.health.gov.au/internet/main/publishing. nsf/ Content/health-pbs-general-pubs-manual-content.htm.

44 Castelli A. Guest editorial: National Schedule of Reference Costs data: Community Care Services. In: Personal Social Services Research Unit (ed) *Unit Costs of Health and Social Care 2008*. Canterbury: University of Kent, 2008.

45 British National Formulary. *The British National Formulary*, 57th edn. London: Pharmaceutical Press, 2009.

46 Institut für das Entgeltsystem im Krankenhaus (InEK). *Website des Deutschen DRG-Systems*. Siegburg: InEK, 2010. Available from: www.g-drg.de/cms/index.php.

47 Netten A, Barrett B Brookes N. *Unit Costs in Criminal Justice* (PSSRU Bulletin No. 18). Canterbury: University of Kent, 2008. Available from: www.pssru.ac.uk/pdf/b18/b18_uccj.pdf.

48 Centre for Child and Family Research. Loughborough: Loughborough University, 2010. Available from: www.lboro.ac.uk/research/ccfr.

49 Centre for Reviews and Dissemination. *NHS Economic Evaluation Database*. York: Centre for Reviews and Dissemination, 2010. Available from: www.crd.york.ac.uk/crdweb.

50 Wiley Interscience. *HEED: Health Economics Evaluation Database*. Chichester: Wiley Interscience, 2010. Available from: http://heed.wiley.com.

51 American Economic Association. *Econlit*. Nashville: American Economic Association, 2010. Available from: www.aeaweb.org/econlit/index.php.

52 Hartley RJ, Keen EM, Large JA, Tedd LA. *Online Searching: principles and practice*. London: Bowker-Saur, 1990.

53 Bates MJ. The design of browsing and berrypicking techniques for the online search interface. *Online Review* 1989; 13(5): 407–424.

54 Sculpher M, Claxton K. Establishing the cost-effectiveness of new pharmaceuticals under conditions of uncertainty – when is there sufficient evidence? *Value in Health* 2005; 8(4): 433–446.

55 Coyle D, Lee KM. Evidence-based economic evaluation: how the use of different data sources can impact results. In: Donaldson C, Mugford M, Vale L (eds) *Evidence-Based Health Economics: from effectiveness to efficiency in systematic review*. London: BMJ Books, 2002.

56 Manca A, Willan AR. Lost in translation: accounting for between-country differences in the analysis of multinational cost-effectiveness data. *Pharmacoeconomics* 2006; 24(11): 1101–1119.

57 Sculpher MJ, Pang FS, Manca A, *et al.* Generalisability in economic evaluation studies in healthcare: a review and case studies. *Health Technology Assessment* 2004; 8(49): 1–192.

58 Longworth L. *Guidelines for the reporting of evidence identification and selection in decision models: the NICE perspective*. Presentation at MRC HSRC funded workshops on The Use of Evidence in Economic Decision Models – Workshop 2: Methodology for appropriate use of evidence in decision models. Leicester: University of Leicester, 2005. Available from: www2.le.ac.uk/Members/njc21/mrc-hsrc-workshop.

59 Jadad AR, Moore RA, Carroll D, *et al.* Assessing the quality of reports of randomized clinical trials: is blinding necessary? *Controlled Clinical Trials* 1996; 17(1): 1–12.

60 Wells GA, Shea B, O'Connell D, *et al. The Newcastle-Ottawa Scale (NOS) for Assessing the Quality of Nonrandomised Studies in Meta-analyses*. Ottawa: Ottawa Health Research Institute, 2010. Available from: www.ohri.ca/programs/clinical_epidemiology/oxford.htm.

61 Higgins JPT, Altman DG (eds). Assessing risk of bias in included studies. In: Higgins JPT, Green S (eds) *Cochrane Handbook for Systematic Reviews of Interventions*. Version 5.0.1 (updated September 2008). Oxford: Cochrane Collaboration, 2008.

62 Cochrane Effective Practice and Organisation of Care Group. *The EPOC Risk of Bias Guideline*. Oxford: Cochrane Collaboration, 2009. Available from: www.epoc.cochrane.org/en/ handsearchers.html.

63 Jefferson T, Vale L, Demicheli V. Methodological quality of economic evaluations of health care interventions – evidence from systematic reviews. In: Donaldson C, Mugford M, Vale L (eds) *Evidence-Based Health Economics: from effectiveness to efficiency in systematic review*. London: BMJ Books, 2002.

64 Drummond MF, Jefferson TO, on behalf of the BMJ Economic Evaluation Working Party. Guidelines for authors

and peer reviewers of economic submissions to the BMJ. *British Medical Journal* 1996; 313(7052): 275–283.

65 Chiou C, Hay JW, Wallace JF, *et al.* Development and validation of a grading system for the quality of cost-effectiveness studies. *Medical Care* 2003; 41(1): 32–44.

66 Ofman JJ, Sullivan SD, Neumann PJ, *et al.* Examining the value and quality of health economic analyses: implications of utilizing the QHES. *Journal of Managed Care Pharmacy* 2003; 9(1): 53–61.

67 Evers S, Goossens M, de Vet H, van Tulder M, Ament A. Criteria list for assessment of methodological quality of economic evaluations: Consensus on Health Economic Criteria. *International Journal of Technology Assessment in Health Care* 2005; 21(2): 240–245.

68 Downs SH, Black N. The feasibility of creating a checklist for the assessment of the methodological quality both of randomised and non-randomised studies of health care interventions. *Journal of Epidemiology and Community Health* 1998; 52(6): 377–384.

69 Sefton TAJ, Byford S, McDaid D, Hills J, Knapp M. *Making the Most of It. Economic evaluation in the social welfare field.* York: Joseph Rowntree Foundation, 2002.

70 Marsh K. Economic evaluation of criminal justice interventions: a methodological review of the recent literature. In: Dunworth T, Marsh K, Roman J, Mallender J (eds) *Cost-Benefit Analysis of Criminal Justice Interventions.* Washington DC: Urban Institute Press, in press.

71 Drummond M, Weatherly H, Claxton K, *et al. Assessing the Challenges of Applying Standard Methods of Economic Evaluation to Public Health Interventions.* York: Public Health Research Consortium, 2007.

72 Kelly M, McDaid D, Ludbrook A, Powell J. *Economic Appraisal of Public Health Interventions.* London: Health Development Agency, 2005.

73 Farrington DP, Welsh BC. Randomised experiments in criminology: what have we learned in the last two decades? *Journal of Experimental Criminology* 2005; 1(1): 9–38.

74 Shemilt I, Pössel P, Mugford M, Valentine JC. *Costing program implementation using systematic review: programs to prevent adolescent depression.* Oral paper presentation at the Ninth Annual Colloquium of the Campbell Collaboration, Oslo, 18–20 May, 2009.

75 Claxton K, Sculpher M, Culyer A. *Mark versus Luke? Appropriate methods for the evaluation of public health interventions (CHE Research Paper 31).* York: Centre for Health Economics, University of York, 2007.

76 Rawlins MD, Culyer AJ. National Institute for Clinical Excellence and its value judgements. *British Medical Journal* 2004; 329(7459), 224–227.

77 Brand S, Price R. *The Economic and Social Costs of Crime (Home Office Research Study 217).* London: Home Office, 2000.

78 Dubourg R, Hamed J, Thorns J. *The Economic and Social Costs of Crime Against Individuals and Households 2003/04 (Home Office Online Report 30/05).* London: Home Office. Available from: www.homeoffice.gov.uk/rds/pdfs05/rdsolr3005.pdf.

79 McCormack K, Wake B, Perez J, *et al.* Laparoscopic surgery for inguinal hernia repair: systematic review of effectiveness and economic evaluation. *Health Technology Assessment* 2006; 9(14): 1–203.

80 Dolan P, Metcalfe R, Munro V, Christensen MC. Valuing lives and life years: anomalies, implications and an alternative. *Health Economics, Policy, and Law* 2008; 3(3): 277–300.

81 Dolan P, Peasgood T, White M. Do we really know what makes us happy? A review of the economic literature on the factors associated with subjective well-being. *Journal of Economic Psychology* 2008; 29(1): 93–122.

82 Organisation for Economic Cooperation and Development. *Is happiness measurable and what do those measures mean for policy?* International conference, Rome, 2–3 April 2007. Available from: www.oecd.org/oecdworldforum/happiness.

CHAPTER 3

The role of economic perspectives and evidence in systematic review

Rob Anderson[1], Ian Shemilt[2]

[1]Peninsula Medical School, University of Exeter, Exeter, UK
[2]School of Social Work and Psychosocial Studies, University of East Anglia, Norwich, UK

Introduction

At the heart of evidence-based policy making lies an awkward truth. It is that, for any given policy choice, at a particular time and in a specific country or organisation, there will be no single completed empirical study which generates the ideal and totally applicable evidence for informing that choice. Instead, at best, policy makers must somehow draw upon a number of partially relevant research studies which can inform a given policy choice (see also Chapter 5). It is this inevitable fact which places the need for systematic review methods – or some kind of transparent and credible approach for identifying, integrating and weighing up evidence from different sources – at the heart of evidence-based policy making.

Another truism which complicates matters is that policy makers have multiple objectives. For example, a defensible decision about changing the organisation of a health service will have to consider not only the impact of alternatives on health outcomes but also issues such as accessibility and coverage; possible harms and safety impacts; service responsiveness and patient satisfaction; and of course, the cost and budget impact. In other areas of public policy, such as transport or the environment, the number of different objectives or types of potential impact may be

even greater. However, in many policy processes, the critical information needs of policy makers are often reduced to seeking an answer to two questions: 'What works (best)?' and 'Is it worth the money?'. That is, considerations of cost and cost-effectiveness (or cost-benefit) are paramount alongside consideration of beneficial and adverse effects. Therefore some kind of consideration of economic evidence is often explicitly required or implicitly expected. But how?

This chapter considers the joint implications of these two truisms: that policy makers should consider economic evidence, and that such evidence will typically reside in a number of studies, each of which is only partially relevant to the specific policy choice faced. The chapter opens by briefly identifying some of the main economic perspectives that impinge on evidence-based decision making. This is followed by a section describing the rise in the practice of conducting systematic reviews of economic evidence (most notably in health care), and includes an outline of current guidance and other resources currently available to assist in such reviews (see also, *inter alia*, Chapters 7 and 8).

Next, some of the challenges involved in conducting reviews of economic evidence are described, and a case study profiling one of the rare attempts to conduct a meta-analysis of cost data is presented. This is followed by a section that considers the extent to which systematic reviews of economic studies are (a) feasible and (b) actually conducted, in different applied fields, such as social welfare, education and criminal justice, and in developing countries.

Evidence-Based Decisions and Economics, 2nd edition. Edited by I. Shemilt, M. Mugford, L. Vale, K. Marsh and C. Donaldson. © 2010 Blackwell Publishing.

This section includes a case study of a review of the cost-effectiveness of HIV prevention in developing countries.

The penultimate section questions the widely presumed value of conducting systematic reviews of economic studies, and argues for their use for a more limited range of purposes. Finally, the chapter outlines what we see as the key issues and methodological challenges currently faced in order to make the best use of economic evidence, and of available methods of systematic review and evidence synthesis.[1]

Throughout, although we have endeavoured to draw examples and use sources from a variety of areas of public policy, the authors' backgrounds in health and health economics have inevitably informed many of the arguments made. However, we have tried to make clear distinctions between those arguments and examples which are probably health-specific and those which draw upon knowledge of policy making or the practice of systematic review in other areas.

Economic perspectives in systematic review

The core perspective which underlies much of the discipline of economics also ultimately drives the need for reviewing economic evidence; that is: resources are scarce, therefore choices have to be made and therefore opportunity costs exist (see also, *inter alia*, Chapter 1). Although private-sector decision making is also subject to this logic, it is in the context of public sector organisations, with their more palpable budget constraints and (usually) more stringent processes for public accountability, that the need to justify the cost-effectiveness or 'value for money' of policy decisions is arguably more mandatory.

There are also competing points of view which determine the types of economic study that get commissioned and conducted, and are available to review, in different policy areas. For example, in health care, economic appraisal has evolved to focus almost entirely on health outcomes, rather than monetary valuations of health outcomes. Thus most full economic evaluations in health care – in contrast to those in transport or environmental economics – are cost-effectiveness or cost-utility analyses. These types of full economic evaluation aim to provide a ratio measure

of the incremental costs divided by the incremental effectiveness (e.g. life- years or quality-adjusted life-years). In other areas of policy making, such as transport or the environment, cost-benefit analysis is the more frequently used form of economic appraisal, and so systematic reviews of such studies may be feasible. In criminal justice research, on the other hand, both cost-effectiveness analysis and cost-benefit analysis increasingly have established roles.

Another clear area of overlap between economics and systematic review methods is the use of review methods to appraise numbers of evaluations of so-called 'economic interventions'. For example, in the first edition of this book, Kristiansen and Gosden presented an overview of two systematic reviews of alternative payment methods for primary care doctors.[2] Similarly, the case study presented in Box 3.1 by Aaserud and colleagues draws lessons from a series of Cochrane Collaboration systematic reviews about economics-based policies to alter the use or prescription of pharmaceuticals. This case study clearly illustrates some of the challenges of conducting systematic reviews of policies that are so inherently heterogeneous, and whose implementation and effects will also be so setting specific.

Box 3.1   Case study: heterogeneity of methods and findings in systematic reviews of 'economic interventions'

Background

Pharmaceutical policies may improve rational drug use (i.e. improve health outcomes and save costs without causing adverse health effects). Using three recent reviews on pricing and purchasing policies, financial incentives for prescribers and co-payment and co-payment caps, the challenges and lessons for such reviews and future research are outlined.[3–5]

The approach

The methods for the three reviews were developed from those of the Cochrane Effective Practice and Organisation of Care (EPOC) Group and were published in a protocol which also covered 10 other drug policy reviews.[6,7] The interventions covered by these reviews are often implemented throughout a health system, and randomised controlled trials (RCTs) are not always feasible. Thus, the reviews considered evidence from RCTs, non-randomised controlled trials (CCTs) and studies using quasi-experimental designs, such as interrupted time series (ITS) analyses, repeated measures (RM) designs and controlled before-after studies (CBA).[6]

Key issues and challenges
The search strategy
The search strategy covered all included review topics to gain economies of scale but this, coupled with the poor indexing of studies, resulted in over 25,000 citations and abstracts being identified. Identified studies were conducted by and for a variety of agencies and many are published in the grey literature.

The interventions
The interventions compared within each review were heterogeneous in how they sought to influence practice and the incentives they provided. In the co-payments and co-payment cap review, few data were available on the intensity of the intervention and what data were available were difficult to interpret – how intensive was an increase in co-payment of US $3 in 1995?[5] The answer depends upon the drug price, the original co-payment level, any co-payment ceilings, and so on.

The outcomes
Included studies were limited in terms of both the method used to report outcomes and the outcomes reported. First, standard economic outcomes (e.g. cost per QALY) were not reported in any of the studies. Second, many studies reported only the effects on drug use and drug costs and did not consider the effects on health, health care utilisation or intervention and administrative costs.

Assessment of study quality
The internal validity of included studies was assessed using EPOC criteria.[6] Elements of the BMJ checklist were also used to assess cost data; however, this checklist is a mix of questions addressing internal and external validity and quality of reporting.[8]

Results and conclusions
The results and conclusions of the reviews indicated the potential direction of the effects rather than the size of the effects. This is because it was not possible to explore whether findings were conditional on the design of the policy, the timing, the local health care system, exceptions in the policy, and so on.

Transferability and the usefulness of such reviews
As data were limited, qualitative assessments of the transferability of the results were made by identifying and discussing potential modifying factors, such as incentives, intervention intensity, policy exemptions, political context, and so on. However, since the results of the reviews are tentative and setting specific, careful interpretation is needed. One way such reviews could be used is as part of a stepwise approach to decision making. First, the review could inform whether a specific policy appears promising. If it does, then consideration may be given to obtaining more information to judge the applicability of the policy to a given setting. If the policy still seems promising, this could then be the subject of a new study specific to the setting of interest.

Recommendations for future reviews and methods work
More complete evaluations are required to address all the important strengths and limitations of the policy in a rigorous way. The logistic and analyst resources required to complete these types of reviews are considerable, and development of methods for relatively complex analysis and transferability assessment is needed.

Morten Aaserud and Craig Ramsay

Guidance for conducting systematic reviews of economic studies

In health care, systematic reviews of numbers of economic studies (e.g. of a particular technology or in a particular patient group), have become a common type of journal paper. They have also become a more common requirement within formal processes for evidence-based policy making. An analysis of the NHS Economic Evaluation Database (NHS EED) suggests that between 100 and 200 reviews or systematic reviews of economic studies are published each year, and many national agencies with responsibility for the appraisal of health technologies and public health policies also require systematic reviews of relevant economic studies.[1,9,10]

Since the publication of the first edition of this book in 2002, there has also been considerable expansion in the range of resources available to reviewers of economic evaluations or other economic studies, particularly in the health care field. In 2008 both The Cochrane Collaboration and The Campbell Collaboration published guidance on how authors of reviews working with these organisations could review economic evidence alongside reviews of clinical effects.[11,12] In 2009, the University of York's Centre for Reviews and Dissemination (CRD) published a new edition of its influential guidance on conducting systematic reviews that included a chapter on conducting systematic reviews of economic evaluations.[13] Similar, earlier guidance has also been published by those working for the US Preventive Services Task Force.[14]

There is now also a considerable range of resources available to assist reviewers of economic studies at specific stages of the review process (see Box 3.2 and also Chapters 7 and 8). While many of these are specific to economic evaluations in health care, some may be applicable or adaptable to other forms of economic studies and other policy areas.

Thus, at least in health care, there is both considerable encouragement (e.g. from some national health technology assessment (HTA) agencies) and considerable guidance and support on how to conduct systematic reviews of economic evidence. In general, the stages and processes of conducting a systematic review of economic evaluations are directly comparable with those for reviewing evidence of effects.[11,13,24–31] However, when it comes to methods of synthesis, narrative synthesis dominates; study details are extracted to tables, studies are individually quality assessed (e.g. informed by use of checklists), and studies are summarised and compared according to key similarities and differences in methods and results.[11,12] Those who do consider the possibility of conducting a quantitative synthesis, or meta-analysis (i.e. statistical pooling), of cost data or incremental cost-effectiveness ratios (ICERs) typically dismiss it as either inappropriate or unlikely.[32] Nevertheless, we are currently aware of several examples of reviews or systematic reviews conducted in the health care field in which the authors have pooled either resource use or cost estimates[33–38] or cost-utility ratios.[39] The review by Bower and colleagues[34] is summarised as a case study in Box 3.3.

Challenges to the value of conducting systematic reviews of economic evaluations

Paradoxically, alongside the growth in the practice of reviewing economic evaluations, there has been increasing reflection on the reasons why health economic evidence appears to be used so little in policy making overall.[41–43] Also, in the context of informing technology adoption decisions (such as Health Technology Assessment reports for NICE), use of the variable results of previous economic evaluations is

---

Box 3.2 Tools and resources for conducting reviews of health economic studies

- Bibliographic databases of health economic studies, such as the NHS Economic Evaluation Database (NHS EED) and the Health Economic Evaluation Database (HEED).[15,16]
- Standard search filters to ease the task of identifying health economic evaluations and other health economic studies.[17,18]
- Checklists to facilitate appraisal of the quality of health economic evaluations and checklists specifically to appraise the quality of decision models (see also, *inter alia,* Chapter 10).[8,19,20]
- Graphical tools to summarise the results of numbers of health economic evaluations.[21]
- Indices and charts for assessing and summarising the transferability of health economic evaluations.[22,23]

Box 3.3 Case study: statistical pooling of economic data in a systematic review of counselling in primary care for depression[34]

Background

In the late 1990s, a number of RCTs of counselling versus usual GP care for depression had shown no significant differences in costs. However, since the sample sizes in all these trials were based on expected differences in clinical outcomes, it is likely that they were all statistically underpowered to detect differences in costs.[40]

The response

Although limited methodological guidance existed, Bower and colleagues[34] attempted to pool the cost data from the trials identified in a Cochrane systematic review. They successfully obtained individual patient data from four similar RCTs (total n = 613). Some adjustments were necessary to correct for different analytical perspectives adopted in studies and varying length of study follow-up. However, overall, heterogeneity was judged manageable and the cost data were pooled using fixed-effects meta-analysis.

The outcome

The meta-analysis showed a statistically significantly higher cost of counselling for depression. This finding was in contrast to the results of individual studies. However, the more notable outcome was methodological: the demonstration that, with access to appropriate individual-level data from comparable studies, meta-analysis could be used to overcome sample size limitations in individual economic evaluations.

Reflections

The conduct of the meta-analysis was achieved by adjusting the costs to account for different follow-up periods, narrowing the analytic perspective of the synthesis to a common dataset and applying standardised unit costs to measures of resource use. Arguably, these pragmatic methodological choices may limit the validity of the pooled results. However, if the alternative is funding and awaiting the results of a new larger trial, or perhaps training systematic reviewers to become decision modellers, then meta-analysis of cost data from existing studies may sometimes be a useful (if currently still exploratory) approach.

Sarah Byford

further diminished if a jurisdiction-specific decision model-based analysis is also conducted.

In the health care field, there have also been more systematic examinations of the reasons why the results of single economic evaluations may not be transferable between different places and times (see also, *inter alia*, Chapters 5 and 13).[23,44,45] Building upon these reviews and other arguments made about the generalisability of economic evaluations, it is possible to create a comprehensive picture of the reasons why systematic reviews of economic evaluations may not be considered as useful as their current popularity would imply. This is especially the case when their implied purpose is to discern some average and widely generalisable estimate of intervention cost-effectiveness.

Variation in methods

Clearly, a major reason why the findings of economic evaluations (of the same intervention comparison) vary is that they have used different methods. This is due to both a continuing lack of standardisation of methods and a typical lack of compliance with established standards.[46,47] However, it is also acknowledged that there are a number of methodological considerations that feed into economic evaluations where international variations can be expected and justified.[48] Therefore, even with complete compliance with jurisdiction-specific methods standards, there is considerable scope for methodological variation between economic evaluations included within a review.

Intervention context and intervention costs

Perhaps the most compelling reason for questioning the value of systematic reviews of economic evaluations is that the costs and resource use associated with interventions are highly likely to vary from country to country, in different regional or service settings, as well as over time. Such variations are most commonly attributed to differences in unit costs (e.g. between countries, and over time due to inflation).[45] However, intervention context may also substantially impact on the levels and particular combinations of resources needed for an intervention to be provided in different health or social systems (e.g. with different staff grades or different frequency of client contact or duration of service) or in different service settings (e.g. a different balance between primary and secondary care). Of the many identified factors which impact on the variability of cost-effectiveness estimates in health care, several are explicitly associated with cost (i.e. absolute/relative costs, economies of scale, exchange rates, different combinations of resources, financial incentives, and opportunity costs).[45]

Intervention context and intervention effects

The impact of context on the cost component of the cost-benefit equation is further compounded by all the reasons why the effectiveness of interventions is likely to vary from place to place and over time. These have been well documented elsewhere, so they are not described at length here.[49–51] However, it is worth noting that health economists have contributed to this debate, in terms of an intervention's effectiveness resulting from the interplay of the changes introduced by the intervention and the existing mix of the underlying determinants of health or disease in a population.[52,53]

Birch & Gafni, for example, show that context may impact both on the 'technical component' of economic evaluations (i.e. how an intervention alters the causal relationships between the determinants of health and health outcomes) and the 'subjective component' (i.e. how different states of health are valued and contribute to overall well-being, compared with the mix of other commodities consumed).[53] The health system or service context is also believed to be a major factor in determining the success or failure of using different financial incentives or 'economic interventions'.[2] More recently, health economists have also described the challenges of evaluating public health interventions which intervene in complex systems, and called for greater awareness of the non-linear relationships between resource inputs and the level, types and timing of outcomes (see also Chapters 5 and 13).[54]

Context of the decision

As well as the context of the *intervention*, most economic evaluations will have a particular *decision context* (either explicitly stated or implicit in the chosen perspective of the analysis). At one level, this will determine the current treatment or service comparator(s), which may not be the same as those included in published economic evaluations. However, the decision-making context will also determine what resource use does or does not have an opportunity cost, and indeed what the opportunity cost of a given resource is.[55] In some situations, such as where a hospital operating theatre or another physical resource is being used to full capacity, there

will be an alternative use for any capacity freed up but in other hospitals working under capacity, there may not be any benefits foregone due to theatre slots or beds going unused. Different budgetary constraints would similarly alter the opportunity costs of the consumption of the same resources.[53] Thus, the cost-effectiveness of the same compared interventions in two places and at the same time may be different even in circumstances where the incremental resource use and effects are identical, due to factors relating to the decision context.

The scope and scale of service changes are also often linked to whether new services were primarily intended to expand (i.e. supplement) or relocate (i.e. substitute) existing service capacity, and this can also impact on opportunity costs. The importance of these contextual factors was well illustrated in Coast and colleagues' insightful review of four economic evaluations of hospital at home programmes.[56]

Two main forms of economic evaluation

It is now more fully recognised that there is a key distinction between economic evaluations based on decision models and empirical economic evaluations which collect individual-level data on costs and outcomes. Individual-level data-based economic evaluations and decision models of an intervention will invariably not be comparable for all the same reasons why people advocate using decision models (e.g. the inclusion of the full range of relevant comparators, a representative case-mix of participants, and following participants for a sufficiently long time for all significant cost and outcome differences to be captured).[57,58] At the very least, therefore, in order to retain comparability amongst reviewed studies, any systematic review of economic evaluations should sensibly become two systematic reviews: one of empirical (including trial-based) economic evaluations and one of decision models.

Cost-effectiveness and cost-efficacy

Since most economic evaluations are primarily intended to inform decisions, they are more explicitly concerned with effectiveness than efficacy. In other words, they seek to assess the incremental benefits and incremental costs implied by a 'real-world' choice between a number of interventions *as they would be resourced and implemented in routine practice*. The distinction between effectiveness and efficacy studies is, in fact, further recognition that context matters. Essentially, some commentators argue there is little point in conducting cost-efficacy studies (e.g. in idealised service settings and with highly protocol-driven practice and specially selected participants) because the costs and effectiveness of the 'same treatment' would be different if delivered within routine practice settings and across the whole case-mix of eligible patients. This aspect of generalisability is a key element of the critique of trial-based economic evaluations, and therefore clearly also has implications for the value of conducting systematic reviews of such studies (although it should be noted that not all randomised trials are trials of intervention efficacy).[58]

Other commentators contend that economic evaluations conducted alongside efficacy studies can play a useful role at early stages in the diffusion of new technologies, before they are tested in routine practice. This is because at times when many critical technology adoption decisions need to be made, it is often the case that *only* efficacy (and therefore cost-efficacy) studies are available. In other words, evidence from 'real-world' assessments of cost-effectiveness, comparing alternative interventions used in routine practice, may come too late to inform early decisions about adoption and diffusion of a new technology. It is therefore arguably useful to incorporate economic analysis into the evaluation of new technologies in each phase of their development from the early 'proof of concept' stage, to inform early decisions and to re-evaluate economic findings once the technology is being used in routine practice. Also, in some areas such as the evaluation of pharmaceuticals (i.e. pharmacoeconomics), to rule out consideration of all placebo-controlled trials (for example) would involve ignoring a great deal of the economic evidence available about an intervention, so setting hard and fast preferences for effectiveness rather than efficacy data needs careful thought. Despite the latter considerations, many analysts still argue that all effectiveness and cost-effectiveness research should be conducted in full and heterogeneous populations that are representative of those

in which a technology, programme or policy may ultimately be applied.

Systematic reviews of economic evidence beyond health care and in developing countries

Beyond health care

In health care, since the 1990s, there has been a proliferation of the development and use of economic evaluation methods, making systematic reviews of similar studies feasible. In other areas of policy making, however, economic analyses are a much less common form of applied research. In the policy areas of criminal justice or social care, for example, the relative dearth of economic evaluations inevitably means that systematic reviews of economic studies are similarly scarce.[59]

Nevertheless, there are exceptions, mostly of the 'stock-taking' kind; to establish what economic studies have been conducted and what they tell us. In criminal justice, for example, McDougall and colleagues have conducted a systematic review of the costs and benefits of different sentencing policies, and there have also been systematic reviews of the costs and benefits of more specific and health-related policies such as drug treatment services implemented in criminal justice settings.[60–63] Although such reviews tend to find relatively few relevant economic studies, and those found tend to be of variable and low quality, others have noted increasing numbers of economic evaluations in the field.[64]

For social care policy, the possibilities for systematic reviews of economic evidence are perhaps worse: no or few full economic evaluations that might inform most policy choices, and variable quality of those conducted.[65,66] Again, the exceptions, where systematic reviews of economic studies are feasible and potentially insightful, are often in those areas which overlap with health care (e.g. mental health and social care). Systematic reviews of research evidence are increasingly a required component of social care policy making in the UK.[67,68] Also, the UK Social Care Institute for Excellence (SCIE) has recently published a position paper that includes initial guidance on how analysts might harness the value of the (currently limited) economic evidence base in social care to support decision making.[66] However, some believe it may be some time before there are enough economic evaluations of similar social care interventions for systematic reviews of such studies to regularly produce useful results, beyond serving to highlight a lack of evidence that future research may need to address. The existence of the Campbell & Cochrane Economics Methods Group as a joint endeavour between economists and the systematic review community in health care, social welfare, education and criminal justice will at least mean that standard methods of review and synthesis will be available when this stage is reached, providing stimulus at an international level for policy makers and economists in all fields to use systematic reviews of research evidence.[69,70]

In developing countries

Arguably, the inefficient allocation of scarce resources in developing countries exacts a much higher penalty in terms of foregone benefits than it does in developed nations. Therefore, using evidence about the economics of interventions is clearly relevant to developing countries. But relevance is currently limited by many factors (see also Chapter 5). In health care, most reviews of effectiveness, costs and/or cost-effectiveness produced to date address health conditions that are priorities in the developed world. However, in many developing countries the epidemiology of diseases has shifted substantially so they are now experiencing high burdens of non-communicable disease, as well as continuing high burdens of infectious diseases and injuries; this may improve the relevance of existing reviews somewhat. Also, even though there has been an increase in the number of systematic reviews of economic studies in developing countries – ranging from studies reviewing literature from all developing countries[71,72] to more focused reviews of the evidence base for a particular disease or condition[73,74] to reviews of the cost-effectiveness evidence base for a particular country[75] – there remains a relative dearth of cost-effectiveness studies.

Therefore, as in the non-health areas of public policy, the feasibility and value of systematic reviews of health economic evidence relevant to developing countries must await improvements in the quantity and quality of the cost-effectiveness evidence base on (a) health problems that are priorities in these countries and (b) interventions that are affordable and feasible in low-income and resource-poor settings. Progress may be fairly slow, as there is little formal use of economic evaluations in health care decision making in developing countries. A better understanding of the barriers and enabling conditions that seem to foster the use of economic evaluation in developing countries is therefore first required.[76] This should ideally address both health economic evaluation and factors affecting the perceived need, costs and benefits of producing economic evidence to inform other areas of public policy in developing countries.

The case study by Teerawattananon (see Box 3.4 and Table 3.1) shows, on the one hand, that in some health areas there are sufficient previous economic studies from the developing world to make a systematic review worthwhile. On the other hand, few studies were available from the country whose policies were being informed, and therefore included studies were necessarily drawn from a broad range of countries. This presented challenges in how to present and interpret such heterogeneous results.

Box 3.4   Case study: presenting heterogeneous results of a systematic review of health economic evaluations to inform decisions about HIV prevention in Thailand

Background

This case study illustrates an attempt to present the results from a systematic review of economic evaluations that was conducted to inform decision makers in Thailand about the effectiveness and cost-effectiveness of HIV prevention interventions.[77] This was part of a wider programme of work that aimed to identify and assess the strengths and deficiencies of HIV prevention activities, and to ensure effective policy dialogues with the National AIDS Committee in Thailand.

The review

Researchers from the Health Intervention and Technology Assessment Program (HITAP) conducted a literature review, initially of Thai published and unpublished literature. The review assessed both the effectiveness and cost-effectiveness of HIV prevention interventions in the Thai health care system context. Once Thailand-based studies had been identified, further systematic searches were conducted using international electronic literature databases. Classification and definitions of HIV prevention were adopted from the standard guidelines recommended by UNAIDS, to inform electronic search strategies and screening of studies.[78]

How the results of the review were presented

The final review included 14 Thai studies and 63 studies from other countries (effectiveness and cost-effectiveness). Of these, there were three and 18 relevant economic evaluation studies conducted in Thailand and other settings respectively. The review contained rich information concerning the effectiveness and/or value for money of more than 20 HIV interventions. It was essential to present these findings in a simple manner to help decision makers and other stakeholders, who might have limited knowledge and expertise in health economics, to understand the information. However, the presentation also needed to allow individuals with economic appraisal skills to assess the reliability and heterogeneity of the evidence.

A cost-effectiveness bar chart and matrix table which summarise the reviewed findings were developed and are presented in Table 3.1. Table 3.1 shows results from the review with the aim of prioritising HIV prevention interventions for targeted subgroups of the Thailand populations, including female sex workers, injecting drug users, men who have sex with men and serodiscordant couples. These subgroups are currently the major sources of HIV infection in Thailand. A colour convention – a 'traffic-light system' – was used to simplify both effectiveness and cost-effectiveness evidence within the same table (this system is adapted for presentation in Table 3.1 using symbols and gray-scale shading, where colours were used in the original report).

In the original report a coloured bar chart also compared the incremental cost-effectiveness ratios (ICERs) for each intervention, in terms of 2008 US dollars per HIV infection averted. This diagram clearly suggested that biological/biomedical interventions are likely to be more cost-effective than interventions affecting knowledge, attitudes and beliefs. This provisional finding may not have been discernible if the data had not been presented in this way.

Reflections

When these findings were presented to decision makers in Thailand, it was found that, compared to conventional methods of presentation, the graphical presentation and colour matrix table gave decision makers a better understanding of the results. They could provide informed feedback on the findings and identify areas for further research to improve the evidence base on effectiveness and cost-effectiveness. Effective tools for presenting the results of reviews are needed to support the future use of both clinical and economic evidence in policy and practice decisions.

Yot Teerawattananon

When are systematic reviews of economic studies most valuable?

Given the fairly wide-ranging and commonly present limitations to the generalisability of evidence from economic evaluations discussed above, we suggest that systematic reviews of economic studies is more valuable when they are conducted (1) to inform the development of a new decision model; (2) to identify the most relevant one or two existing studies to inform a particular decision in a specific jurisdiction, or; (3) to identify the key economic (causal) trade-offs implicit in a given policy choice or social problem area. In some circumstances, a review of all economic evaluations relating to a particular policy comparison may provide a fairly consistent 'cost-effectiveness answer' but we suggest that such examples will not be the norm. Of course, it is often also useful to conduct 'mapping reviews' to describe the nature and coverage of economic research in a given policy area, and particularly when the main emphasis is to describe the methods used and their strengths and weaknesses, or to identify gaps in the literature, to inform commissioning and design of full systematic reviews, decision models or primary research.[79,80]

Reviews to justify and inform decision model development

When there is a plan to develop a decision model for estimating the cost and effectiveness of some policy or practice alternatives (see also, *inter alia,*

Table 3.1 Summary of the clinical effectiveness and cost-effectiveness of HIV prevention interventions by targeted subpopulation.

Interventions	FSW	MSM	IDU	SDC	Preg	PI	HCW	Young	G pop
I. Interventions that affect knowledge, attitude and beliefs and influence psychological and social correlates of risk									
Abstinence-only programmes	X	X	X	X	X	X	X	No	X
Abstinence-plus programmes	X	X	X	X	X	X	X	■	X
Community-based education	■	■	No	–	X	–	X	■	■
Mass media campaigns	X	X	X	X	X	X	X	X	■
School-based sex education programs (combined with life skills)	X	X	X	X	X	X	X	■	X
Routine (provider-initiated) voluntary HIV screening at health care settings	–	–	–	–	■	–	–	–	■
Voluntary HIV counselling and testing (VCT) (+ STI clinic and condom distribution)	■	■	■	–	■	■	–	■	■
Workplace-based education (+condom distribution/free STI clinic)	■	X	X	X	X	X	–	X	■
II. Harm reduction interventions that lower the risk of a behaviour, but do not eliminate the behaviour									
Condom use (availability and accessibility)	■	■	■	■	X	–	X	■	■
Introduction of female condoms	■	–	–	–	X	–	X	–	–
Needle and syringe exchange	X	X	■	X	X	X	X	X	X
Needle social marketing	X	X	■	X	X	X	X	X	X
Street outreach	X	X	■	X	X	X	X	X	X
III. Biological/biomedical interventions that strive to reduce HIV infection and transmission risk									
HIV vaccine	–	–	No	–	X	–	–	–	–
Improved STI treatment services	■	■	■	■	X	–	X	■	■
Mass or community treatment of sexually transmitted infections	X	X	X	X	X	X	X	X	No
Male circumcision	X	–	–	–	X	–	X	–	■
Microbicides	No	X	–	–	X	–	X	–	–
Postexposure prophylaxis	–	–	No	–	X	–	No	X	X

Prevention of mother-to-child transmission of HIV	X	X	X	■	X	X	X	X
Screening blood products and donated organs for HIV	X	X	X	X	X	X	X	■
Substitution treatment	X	X	■	X	X	X	X	X
Nucleic acid test screening (NAT) of volunteer blood donations	X	X	X	X	X	X	X	▓

IV. Mitigation of barriers to prevention and negative social outcomes of HIV infection

Increased alcohol tax	X	X	X	X	X	X	X	■
Microfinance	X	X	X	X	X	X	X	No
Microfinance (combined with education)	X	X	X	X	X	X	X	▓

FSW, female sex worker; MSM, men who have sex with men; IDU, injecting drug user; SDC, serodiscordant couples; Preg, pregnant women; PI, prison inmate; HCW, health care worker; Young, people aged 10–24 years old; G pop, general population.

Legend to shading in the table

Colours	Effectiveness	Cost-effectiveness	Description
■	Yes	Yes	The intervention proven to be effective and cost-effective
■	Yes	Data not available	The intervention proven to be effective but no evidence regarding cost-effectiveness
▓	Yes	No	The intervention proven to be effective but not cost-effective
No	No	No, data not available	The intervention proven to be neither effective nor cost-effective
-	Data not available	Data not available	No evidence concerning effectiveness or cost-effectiveness of the intervention
X			The intervention is not relevant or not used for particular target subpopulation

Chapters 2 and 9), some kind of systematic review of previous economic evaluations is at least necessary to determine that there is not already in existence a recent, highly relevant and rigorously conducted economic evaluation of essentially the same decision problem. This is simply the good academic practice of making sure that a piece of research will not be answering a question which has, effectively, already been answered. It may therefore not go much further than a systematic search of the published literature and recent unpublished sources, in order to confirm that there is no recent economic evaluation of the same comparators in similar populations and service settings.

If the development of a new decision model is justified, there are various ways in which reviewing previous economic studies might usefully inform the development of a new decision model (see also, *inter alia*, Chapters 2 and 9).

- Previous analyses with decision models might provide insights into some of the key trade-offs, events and changes in relevant states which are thought to determine how the types and levels of resource use implied by alternative interventions are associated with different outcomes. Previous decision models might not reflect all the important resource–outcome relationships implicit in a given decision problem, but they should provide an initial list of the key ones.
- Previous decision models examining similar decision problems or interventions might also indicate the strengths and weaknesses of different modelling approaches (e.g. simple decision trees versus Markov models versus discrete event simulations).
- Previous empirical economic studies, which have collected and reported resource use and/or effectiveness data in the same types of populations or places, may also usefully inform a new decision model. However, this will largely depend on whether the study is purely descriptive (and exclusively aggregate outcome focused) or has attempted to explain how and why different types of participant or places of implementation are associated with different levels or mixes of resource use, or different levels and patterns of outcomes. Studies which merely report, for example, which types of resource use were measured and valued, but do not provide a breakdown of the cost estimate for each intervention by type of resource use or by participant subgroup, would be less useful for helping decision modellers decide what resource use or participant pathways should be specified in any new model.

This use of reviews of decision models has been encouraged by Pignone and colleagues on the basis of their experience of conducting reviews of economic evaluations for the US Preventive Services Task Force.[81] However, because decision models are themselves syntheses, it makes no sense to consider traditional meta-analysis or the pooling of results from such studies. Instead, Pignone and colleagues suggest that reviews of decision models are 'most useful for comparing and contrasting how different investigators have chosen to structure their models and estimate key variables' and can also 'clarify how results differ between studies based on these different assumptions' (p. 1073).[81] A recent example of such a review, in relation to the impact of structural assumptions in decision models, is that by Drummond and colleagues on models for rheumatoid arthritis[82]; thus in some cases a review of previous models may be regarded as a form of sensitivity analysis, in this case exploring structural uncertainty.

Reviews to identify the most relevant study

In some decision-making situations there may be insufficient resources to develop a new decision model of the specific decision problem being faced. In such situations, rather than not consider any economic evidence at all, it may be better to identify the best-quality study (or few studies) that is most relevant to the decision being faced (see also Chapter 5), and to transfer or adapt those results to the new decision problem. Judging the 'best-quality study' would have to include considerations of both internal validity (i.e. study design and methodological quality) and external validity (e.g. how long ago? similarity of comparators? similarity of health service/system settings?). Only if there happened to be several studies of similar quality and relevance to the current decision context would it be worth examining to what extent and why their cost-effectiveness estimates vary. However, this would be with a view to contextualising the results of the most relevant high-quality study, rather than with the expectation that some 'average result' might emerge.

There may also be the possibility of updating and re-estimating cost-effectiveness using local resource use unit costs, or perhaps by inflating and converting costs from past studies in other countries.[14,23,83] This strategy has parallels with the broad approach of 'best evidence synthesis', in which the threshold for the inclusion of further studies is cumulatively judged according to what the best (most internally valid and most relevant) studies show.[84] Chapter 5 discusses some of the considerations for judging the relevance and transferability of economic evidence to a particular decision context, and Box 3.2 (in this chapter) cites some currently available tools for systematically judging this.

Reviews to understand the key economic trade-offs and causal relationships in a decision problem or treatment area

This reason for conducting systematic reviews of economic studies is currently not often the stated reason for undertaking such reviews; however, such 'explanatory' reviews are increasingly encouraged. The recently published economics methods chapter in the *Cochrane Handbook for Systematic Reviews of Interventions*, for example, recommends that 'Review authors should avoid asking questions of the form "What is the cost-effectiveness of intervention X (compared with Y or Z)?"', since a credible and internationally applicable (or transferable) answer to this question will be unlikely.[11] The chapter suggests a number of possible economic questions, some of which relate to trade-offs between costs and other outcomes or adverse effects and that these questions may link to a description of how the intervention might work (which is a mandatory component of Cochrane review protocols).[85]

Of course, the underlying explanation of why some new interventions or treatments have a particular incremental cost may simply be that the new technology has a much higher per participant price or is more costly to provide and maintain than the comparator. However, more often, explaining why some interventions are more or less resource intensive, costly or cost-effective than others will also be determined by a whole range of other trade-offs to do

with downstream effects, different rates and timing of adverse events, or different levels of participant compliance or valuations of effects. With more complex interventions, it becomes even harder to explain how a specific bundle of intervention components (and their associated resource use), provided in a given context, has generated the levels and types of outcomes measured.[56,86–88]

Therefore, either to inform the structure of a decision model or as an exercise in developing theory, it would often be useful to conduct systematic reviews of economic studies which seek to answer review questions such as: 'How do the level and configuration of resources involved in treatment/service design strategies P, Q and R appear to be related to the levels and types of outcomes observed, and what contextual factors affect these relationships?'. Decision models are, after all, essentially a simplified expression of what these key trade-offs are presumed to be, and we often do not describe clearly where these structural assumptions come from (see also, *inter alia*, Chapters 2, 7 and 9).[89]

Such theory-building or explanatory reviews may need to make more limited use of the intervention-focused and research design (i.e. internal validity)-focused processes typical of conventional systematic reviews of effectiveness evidence, and instead draw upon approaches such as 'realist review' which focus more on intervention theory and the role of the intervention/policy context in order to build up a reliable picture of the key causal relationships at work in a given area of programme design or treatment.[90–92] They would therefore need to make best use of both empirical economic evaluations and decision models, and probably also cost analyses, cost-of-illness studies and other types of economic study. More specific possible questions for a realist review of economic evaluations are suggested in Box 3.5 (although, we should add, to our knowledge no reviews of this kind have yet been completed).

It should also be noted that this type of theory-building or explanatory review of economic studies is complementary to, not incompatible with, the aims and methods of conventional systematic reviews, such as Cochrane or Campbell reviews. This is because reviews aiming to address the question 'How do the level and configuration of resources involved in treatment/service design strategies P, Q and R appear to be related to the levels and types of outcomes observed, and what contextual factors affect these relationships?' alongside those suggested in Box 3.5 still require the analyst to assemble reliable evidence on both the levels of resources and levels and types of outcomes observed.

Finally, in order to summarise this section, Figure 3.1 proposes a potential decision aid to inform considerations of (a) when it is worth conducting a systematic review of economic studies, and (b) which objective of the three broad types described in this section should be the main focus of the review.

Box 3.5 Realist synthesis of economic studies: some possible questions

- What are the hypothesised mechanisms underlying changes in the costs and effects (and therefore cost-effectiveness) of the compared interventions, and how do these relate to existing economic and other conditions?
- What are the conditions (economic or other) necessary for these mechanisms to operate, and how are they distributed within and between programme contexts?
- To what extent do pre-existing conditions within a given system enable or disable the mechanisms underlying the changes in costs and/or effects?

Economic evidence and systematic review methods: making the best of both

Given the widely acknowledged importance of considering economic evidence in policy and practice decisions, and that increasingly varied methods of systematic review and evidence synthesis now exist, where should we go from here? We believe that there are several key challenges, or tensions, which need to be confronted.

First, there needs to be some way of tackling the mismatch between the evidence which decision makers ideally need and that which is actually available. An inevitable aspect of this mismatch is that, for some policy problems in some jurisdictions, there will be no formal, high-quality economic evaluations of the interventions and comparators of interest. In such circumstances, there needs to be clearer strategies for identifying and assessing relevant cost analyses, cost-of-illness studies and studies of effects that contain important resource use data. Ultimately, a review of such studies may provide sufficient evidence on typical levels of resource use and costs, and the key trade-offs involved, for a decision model or other economic analysis to be developed to inform the decision.

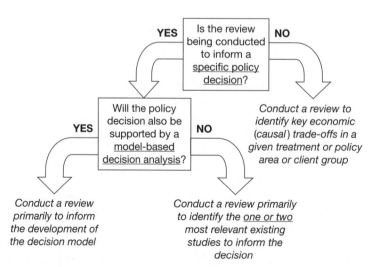

Figure 3.1 Suggested process for deciding whether a review of economic studies is needed and the primary objective of the review.

While clear guidelines now exist for conducting systematic reviews of economic studies in the health care field – where there is an acknowledged abundance of full economic evaluations in many treatment areas, increasingly using standard methods – in other areas of policy making there are so few economic studies of any kind that such methods will currently have limited application.[11–14]

Second, there is a tension between the knowledge-generating and policy-informing purposes of systematic reviews. On one hand, the meta-analysis of studies of the effects of narrowly defined treatments in health care is intended to produce a more powerful and precise estimate of average treatment effect.[28] The 'discovered' empirical regularities of meta-analysis, assuming consistent diagnosis and standardisation of treatments, are often regarded as universally applicable facts or at least (and sometimes, perhaps, spuriously) as a highly predictable and therefore transferrable outcome of that treatment if used elsewhere. In contrast, in other areas of policy and practice there is no expectation that treatments, programmes or policies will consistently either work or not work – or *be* cost-effective. Therefore, the goal of systematic reviews needs to shift towards exploring how and why interventions are more or less effective, resource intensive, costly or cost-effective in different circumstances or when implemented in different ways. Although, in general, economists have not been very clear about the type of evidence synthesis which reviews of economic studies aim to reflect, most examples of such reviews appear to view included studies as 'replications' of the same decision problem (e.g. for alternative approaches, see Hammersley's typology of synthesis strategies in Box 3.6).[93] With such typically mixed patterns of outcomes from different studies of the same policy choice, a different approach to synthesis may be necessary.

Other commentators believe there is an even more fundamental methodological mismatch between the economic evidence available for reviewing and that which is actually needed by policy makers. This point is made most forcefully by Birch & Gafni (and later in this volume by Lessard & Birch – see Chapter 13), who assert that most systematic reviews in health care, including reviews of economic studies, amount to the generation of 'answers in search of questions'

Box 3.6 Hammersley's typology of evidence synthesis strategies

- **Pooling or aggregation.** Each study reviewed is treated as investigating a different sample of cases drawn from the same population. With this type of synthesis, the larger the number of studies, the better, as this allows more reliable prediction of programme effectiveness (or other outcomes).
- **Replication.** Reviewed studies are treated as replications of one another. This type of synthesis applies the logic of experimental research, whereby the strength of conclusions is derived from concordance of findings between studies. It may require a relatively small number of well-conducted studies with very similar aims.
- **Theory developing/testing.** This type of synthesis involves comparative analysis of existing studies with a view to the systematic development and testing of hypotheses (e.g. about how and why interventions work, or not, in different contexts). Ray Pawson's proposal for 'realist review' accords most closely with this notion of synthesis, and has claimed advantages for summarising the evidence base for complex policy interventions.[90,91]
- **Mapping.** This type of synthesis employs the metaphor of a mosaic or map. It uses each included study to add to the complete picture, and studies should ideally cover different aspects of the same phenomenon. Complementarity, not similarity, is valued.
- **Translation of findings between studies (meta-ethnography).** In this type of synthesis, the findings of some studies are 'translated' into the terms of another. This allows the development of key metaphors that give insights into the phenomenon of interest.[94]

Adapted from Hammersley, 2002.[93]

or 'making the problem fit the solution'.[95,96] They argue that if individual economic studies do not address research questions or produce findings that are of relevance to policy makers, then no amount of sophisticated and careful reviewing of numbers of these studies can resolve these deficiences. The key issue is that policy makers' questions are not universal but highly context specific: what will 'work' or be cost-effective in *this* community, with *this* mix of causes of problems, with *this* staff skill mix and *these* levels of resources available (and, critically for deciding the efficiency of alternatives, with *these* alternative uses of those resources), and so on?

These arguments, by health economists, in fact closely echo those of others who have attempted to explain why adopting the 'biomedical model' of systematic review has been so difficult and contentious in other social policy fields. Boaz and colleagues suggest that the adopted 'biomedical model' of systematic review (which actually originated in other areas of the social sciences) is met with scepticism in other public policy areas for three main reasons.[97,98] First, the one-dimensional hierarchy of study designs, with randomised controlled trials at the top as the ideal method, may not be so easily applied in other areas of research where less experimental or simply more eclectic methods tend to be the norm. Second, interventions in other areas are often more complex in operation, and have multiple and highly context-dependent outcomes. And third, researchers in other fields are uncomfortable that the so-called 'biomedical model' of systematic review seems overly intervention and outcome focused, and thereby, they feel, are incapable of refining theories about why certain programmes work (and, conversely why, sometimes, they don't). However, we also acknowledge that the latter arguments are tempered by the observation that use of experimental research designs has long held greater acceptance in other areas of the social sciences in some jurisdictions, perhaps especially in the US.[99-102]

Nevertheless, the challenge to economic evaluators (and, by extension, also to reviewers of economic studies) is to design primary research studies (and develop compatible review methods) which acknowledge that health and other outcomes are jointly produced by both interventions and the multilevel contexts in which they are implemented, such as the underlying characteristics and social dynamics of populations and communities which create or sustain the health and/ or social problems being targeted (see also Chapter 13). As with the approach of realist evaluation and realist review, the key to producing such contextually contingent knowledge is, Birch also argues, greater use theory (see also Chapter 13).[95,96] It is worth noting that although theory-driven evaluation methods have been most advocated and successfully used in relation to effectiveness evaluations, there is, in principle, no

reason why the approach could not be extended to evaluations of cost-effectiveness.[103-106]

The theories in such evaluations might need to include economic theory, as well as psychological or other theories for explaining the production and distribution of health, illness and recovery in populations. Indeed, Ray Pawson's core premise is that programmes are essentially theories about the impact of resources; the basic theory underlying all programmes is some version of: 'if we provide these people with these resources it may change their behaviour [in this way]'.[107]

Interestingly, these conclusions are not so far from what was advocated in the first edition of this book in 2002. In relation to advancing methods and practice in the systematic review of economic valuations, Drummond's conclusion was that:

'… the real contribution of a systematic review of economic evaluations may not be to produce a single authoritative result, but to help decision makers understand the structure of the resource allocation problem they are addressing and the impact, on the overall result, of the main parameters. Thus, the emphasis in such a review is likely to be less on producing a summarised estimate of the cost-effectiveness ratio, and more on demonstrating by how much this varies from setting to setting, and why it varies.'

(Drummond 2002:151)[46]

If this is the goal, then we certainly need to look beyond the established methodological conventions of systematic reviewing which currently dominate evidence-based medicine. These conventions are already being challenged as the techniques are applied in other fields.[108] We should also look beyond purely economic perspectives on the production of programme outcomes, and adopt a broader social science perspective on explaining how programmes and policies produce outcomes of value to society and why such outcomes, including costs, differ from setting to setting and in different populations.

Acknowledgements

Other contributors to this chapter: Miranda Mugford, Professor of Health Economics, University of East Anglia, UK; Damian Walker, Associate Professor, Johns Hopkins School of Public Health, USA;

Yot Teerawattananon, Program Leader of Health Intervention and Technology Assessment Program, Thai Ministry of Public Health, Thailand; Morten Aaserud, Senior Adviser, Norwegian Medicines Agency, Norway; Craig Ramsay, Senior Statistician, University of Aberdeen, UK; Sarah Byford, Senior Lecturer, King's College London, UK.

The contents of some sections of this chapter are the same or similar to sections of an EarlyView paper in the *Health Economics* journal: see reference 1, below.

How this chapter should be cited

Anderson R, Shemilt I. Chapter 3: The role of economic perspectives and evidence in systematic review. In: Shemilt I, Mugford M, Vale L, Marsh K, Donaldson C (editors). *Evidence-based decisions and economics: health care, social welfare, education and criminal justice.* Oxford: Wiley-Blackwell, 2010.

References

1 Anderson R. Systematic reviews of economic evaluations: utility or futility? *Health Economics* 2009; DOI: 10.1002/nec.1486; published online as EarlyView at: www3.inter-science.wiley.com/journal/122326496/abstract

2 Kristiansen I, Gosden T. Evaluating economic interventions: a role for non-randomised designs? In: Donaldson C, Mugford M, Vale L (eds) *Evidence-Based Health Economics: from effectiveness to efficiency in systematic review.* London: BMJ Books, 2002.

3 Aaserud M, Austvoll-Dahlgren A, Kösters J, Oxman A, Ramsay C, Sturm H. Pharmaceutical policies: effects of reference pricing, other pricing, and purchasing policies. *Cochrane Database of Systematic Reviews* 2006, Issue 2.

4 Sturm H, Austvoll-Dahlgren A, Aaserud M, *et al.* Pharmaceutical policies: effects of financial incentives for prescribers. *Cochrane Database of Systematic Reviews* 2007, Issue 3.

5 Austvoll-Dahlgren A, Aaserud M, Vist G, *et al.* Pharmaceutical policies: effects of cap and co-payment on rational drug use. *Cochrane Database of Systematic Reviews* 2008, Issue 1.

6 Bero L, Eccles M, Grimshaw J, *et al.* Cochrane effective practice and organisation of care group. *About The Cochrane Collaboration (Cochrane Review Groups (CRGs))* 2009, Issue 3.

7 Aaserud M, Austvoll-Dahlgren A, Sturm H, *et al.* Pharmaceutical policies: effects on rational drug use, an overview of 13 reviews (Protocol). *Cochrane Database of Systematic Reviews* 2006, Issue 2.

8 Drummond MF, Jefferson TO, on behalf of the BMJ Economic Evaluation Working Party. Guidelines for authors and peer reviewers of economic submissions to the BMJ. *British Medical Journal* 1996; 313(7052): 275–283.

9 National Institute for Health and Clinical Excellence. *Guide to the Methods of Technology Appraisal.* London: National Institute for Health and Clinical Excellence, 2008.

10 National Institute for Health and Clinical Excellence. *Methods for the Development of NICE Public Health Guidance,* 2nd edn. London: National Institute for Health and Clinical Excellence, 2009.

11 Shemilt I, Mugford M, Byford S, *et al.* Incorporating economics evidence. In: Higgins JPT, Green S (eds) *Cochrane Handbook for Systematic Reviews of Interventions.* Version 5.0.1 (updated September 2008). Oxford: Cochrane Collaboration, 2008.

12 Shemilt I, Mugford M, Byford S, *et al. Campbell Collaboration Methods Policy Brief: economics methods.* Oslo: Campbell Collaboration, 2008.

13 Centre for Reviews and Dissemination. *Systematic Reviews: CRD's guidance for undertaking reviews in health care,* 3rd edn. York: Centre for Reviews and Dissemination, 2009.

14 Carande-Kulis V, Maciosek M, Briss P, *et al.* Methods for systematic reviews of economic evaluations for the Guide to Community Preventive Services. *American Journal of Preventive Medicine* 2000; 18(1S): 75–91.

15 Centre for Reviews and Dissemination. *NHS Economic Evaluation Database.* York: Centre for Reviews and Dissemination, 2010. Available from: www.crd.york.ac.uk/crdweb.

16 Wiley Interscience. *HEED: health economics evaluation database.* Chichester: Wiley Interscience, 2010. Available from: http://heed.wiley.com.

17 Craig D, Rice S. *CRD Report 6: NHS economic evaluation database handbook,* 3rd edn. York: Centre for Reviews and Dissemination, 2007.

18 InterTASC Information Specialists Subgroup. *Search Filter Resource: economic evaluations.* InterTASC Information Specialists Subgroup, 2010. Available from: www.york.ac.uk/inst/crd/ intertasc/econ.htm.

19 Evers S, Goossens M, de Vet H, van Tulder M, Ament A. Criteria list for assessment of methodological quality of economic evaluations: Consensus on Health Economic Criteria. *International Journal of Technology Assessment in Health Care* 2005; 21(2): 240–245.

20 Philips Z, Ginnelly L, Sculpher M, *et al.* Review of guidelines for good practice in decision-analytic modelling in health technology assessment. *Health Technology Assessment* 2004; 8(36): 1–172.

21 Nixon J, Khan KS, Kleijnen J. Summarising economic evaluations in systematic reviews: a new approach. *British Medical Journal* 2001; 322(7302): 1596–1598.

22 Antonanzas F, Rodríguez-Ibeas R, Juárez C, Hutter F, Lorente R, Pinillos M. Transferability indices for health economic evaluations: methods and applications. *Health Economics* 2009; 18(6): 629–643.

23 Welte R, Feenstra T, Jager H, Leidl R. A decision chart for assessing and improving the transferability of economic evaluation results between countries. *Pharmacoeconomics* 2004; 22(13): 857–876.

24 O'Connor D, Green S, Higgins JPT. Defining the review question and developing criteria for including studies. In: Higgins JPT, Green S (eds) *Cochrane Handbook of Systematic Reviews of Intervention.* Version 5.0.1 (updated September 2008). Oxford: Cochrane Collaboration, 2008.

25 Lefebvre C, Manheimer E, Glanville J. Searching for studies. In: Higgins JPT, Green S (eds) *Cochrane Handbook for Systematic Reviews of Interventions.* Version 5.0.1 (updated September 2008). Oxford: Cochrane Collaboration, 2008.

26 Higgins JPT, Deeks JJ. Selecting studies and collecting data. In: Higgins JPT, Green S (eds) *Cochrane Handbook for Systematic Reviews of Interventions.* Version 5.0.1 (updated September 2008). Oxford: Cochrane Collaboration, 2008.

27 Higgins JPT, Altman DG. Assessing risk of bias in included studies. In: Higgins JPT, Green S (eds) *Cochrane Handbook for Systematic Reviews of Interventions.* Version 5.0.1 (updated September 2008). Oxford: Cochrane Collaboration, 2008.

28 Deeks JJ, Higgins JPT, Altman DG. Analysing data and undertaking meta-analyses. In: Higgins JPT, Green S (eds) *Cochrane Handbook for Systematic Reviews of Interventions.* Version 5.0.1 (updated September 2008). Oxford: Cochrane Collaboration, 2008.

29 Sterne JAC, Egger M, Moher D. Addressing reporting biases. In: Higgins JPT, Green S (eds) *Cochrane Handbook for Systematic Reviews of Intervention.* Version 5.0.1 (updated September 2008). Oxford: Cochrane Collaboration, 2008.

30 Schünemann HJ, Oxman AD, Higgins JPT, Vist GE, Glasziou P, Guyatt GH. Presenting results and 'summary of findings' tables. In: Higgins JPT, Green S (eds) *Cochrane Handbook for Systematic Reviews of Interventions.* Version 5.0.1 (updated September 2008). Oxford: Cochrane Collaboration, 2008.

31 Schünemann HJ, Oxman AD, Vist GE, *et al.* Interpreting results and drawing conclusions. In: Higgins JPT, Green S (eds) *Cochrane Handbook for Systematic Reviews of Interventions.* Version 5.0.1 (updated September 2008). Oxford: Cochrane Collaboration, 2008.

32 Glasziou P, Irwig L, Bain C, Colditz G. *Systematic Reviews in Health Care: a practical guide.* Cambridge: Cambridge University Press, 2001.

33 Birks J, Harvey RJ. Donepezil for dementia due to Alzheimer's disease. *Cochrane Database of Systematic Reviews* 2006, Issue 1.

34 Bower P, Byford S, Barber J, *et al.* Meta-analysis of data on costs from trials of counselling in primary care: using individual patient data to overcome sample size limitations in economic analyses. *British Medical Journal* 2003; 326(7401): 1247–1252.

35 Crystal E, Garfinkle MS, Connolly SS, Ginger TT, Sleik K, Yusuf SS. Interventions for preventing post-operative atrial fibrillation in patients undergoing heart surgery. *Cochrane Database of Systematic Reviews* 2004, Issue 4.

36 Halpern MT, Khan ZM, Stanford R, Spayde KM, Golubiewski M. Asthma: resource use and costs for inhaled corticosteroid vs leukotriene modifier treatment – a meta-analysis. *Journal of Family Practice* 2003; 52(5): 382–389.

37 Linden A, Adams J. Determining if disease management saves money: an introduction to meta-analysis. *Journal of Evaluation in Clinical Practice* 2007; 13(3): 400–407.

38 Rivetti D, Jefferson T, Thomas R, *et al.* Vaccines for preventing influenza in the elderly. *Cochrane Database of Systematic Reviews* 2006, Issue 3.

39 Cheng AK, Niparko JK. Cost-utility of the cochlear implant in adults: a meta-analysis. *Archives of Otolaryngology - Head & Neck Surgery* 1999; 125(11): 1214–1218.

40 Briggs A. Economic evaluation and clinical trials: size matters. *British Medical Journal* 2000; 321(7273): 1362–1363.

41 Drummond M. Economic evaluation in health care: is it really useful or are we just kidding ourselves? *Australian Economic Review* 2004; 37(1): 3–11.

42 Hoffman C, Graf von der Schulenburg JM, on behalf of the EUROMET Group. The influence of economic evaluation studies on decision making. A European survey. *Health Policy* 2000; 52(3): 179–192.

43 Jan S. Why does economic analysis in health care not get implemented more? Towards a greater understanding of the rules of the game and the costs of decision making. *Applied Health Economics and Health Policy* 2003; 2(1): 17–24.

44 Drummond M, Pang F. Transferability of economic evaluation results. In: Drummond M, McGuire A (eds) *Economic Evaluation in Health Care: merging theory with practice.* Oxford: Oxford University Press, 2001.

45 Sculpher MJ, Pang FS, Manca A, *et al.* Generalisability in economic evaluation studies in health care: a review and case studies. *Health Technology Assessment* 2004; 8(49): 1–192.

46 Drummond M. Evidence-based medicine meets economic evaluation – an agenda for research. In: Donaldson C, Mugford M, Vale L (eds) *Evidence-Based Health Economics: from effectiveness to efficiency in systematic review.* London: BMJ Books, 2002.

47 Jefferson T, Vale L, Demicheli V. Methodological quality of economic evaluations of health care interventions – evidence from systematic reviews. In: Donaldson C, Mugford M, Vale L (eds) *Evidence-Based Health Economics: from effectiveness to efficiency in systematic review.* London: BMJ Books, 2002.

48 Sculpher M, Drummond M. Analysis sans frontieres: can we ever make economic evaluations generalisable across jurisdictions? *Pharmacoeconomics* 2006; 24(11): 1087–1099.

49 Jackson N, Waters E, for the Guidelines for Systematic Reviews in Health Promotion and Public Health Taskforce. Criteria for the systematic review of health promotion and public health interventions. *Health Promotion International* 2005; 20(4): 367–374.

50 Kraemer HC, Frank E, Kupfer DJ. Moderators of treatment outcomes: clinical, research, and policy importance. *Journal of the American Medical Association* 2006; 296(10): 1286–1289.

51 Kravitz R, Duan N, Braslow J. Evidence-based medicine, heterogeneity of treatment effects, and the trouble with averages. *Milbank Quarterly* 2004; 82(4): 661–687.

52 Birch S. As a matter of fact: evidence-based decision-making unplugged. *Health Economics* 1997; 6(6): 547–559.

53 Birch S, Gafni A. Economics and the evaluation of health care programmes: generalisability of methods and implications for generalisability of results. *Health Policy* 2003; 64(2): 207–219.

54 Shiell A, Hawe P, Gold L. Complex interventions or complex systems? Implications for health economic evaluation. *British Medical Journal* 2008; 336(7656): 1281–1283.

55 Craig N, Sutton M. Opportunity costs on trial: new options for encouraging implementation of results from economic evaluations. In: Donald A, Haines A (eds) *Getting Research Findings into Practice*. London: BMJ Books, 1998.

56 Coast J, Hensher M, Mulligan JA, Sheppard S, Jones J. Conceptual and practical difficulties with the economic evaluation of health services developments. *Journal of Health Services Research and Policy* 2000; 5(1): 42–48.

57 Buxton MJ, Drummond MF, van Hout BA, *et al.* Modelling in economic evaluation: an unavoidable fact of life. *Health Economics* 1997; 6(3): 217–227.

58 Sculpher M, Claxton K, Drummond M, McCabe C. Whither trial-based economic evaluation for health care decision making? *Health Economics* 2006; 15(7): 677–687.

59 Marsh K. Economic evaluation of criminal justice interventions: a methodological review of the recent literature. In: Dunworth T, Marsh K, Roman J, Mallender J (eds) *Cost-Benefit Analysis of Criminal Justice Interventions*. Washington DC: Urban Institute Press, in press.

60 McDougall C, Cohen MA, Swaray AP. The costs and benefits of sentencing: a systematic review. *Annals of the American Academy of Political and Social Science* 2003; 587(1): 160–177.

61 Cartwright W. Cost-benefit analysis of drug treatment services: review of the literature. *Journal of Mental Health Policy and Economics* 2000; 3(1): 11–26.

62 Cartwright WS. Economic costs of drug abuse: financial, cost of illness and services. *Journal of Substance Abuse Treatment* 2008; 34(2): 224–233.

63 Simoens S, Ludbrook A, Matheson C, Bond C. Pharmacoeconomics of community maintenance for opiate dependence: a review of evidence and methodology. *Drug and Alcohol Dependence* 2006; 84(1): 28–39.

64 Welsh B, Farrington DP. Monetary costs and benefits of crime prevention programs. In: Tonry M (ed) *Crime and Justice: a review of research (Volume 27)*. Chicago: University of Chicago Press, 2000.

65 Sefton TAJ, Byford S, McDaid D, Hills J, Knapp M. *Making the Most of It. Economic evaluation in the social welfare field*. York: Joseph Rowntree Foundation, 2002.

66 Francis J. *SCIE's Approach to Economic Evaluation in Social Care*. London: Social Care Institute for Excellence, in press.

67 Coren E, Fisher M. *The Conduct of Systematic Research Reviews for SCIE Knowledge Reviews*. London: Social Care Institute for Excellence, 2006.

68 Macdonald G. *Using Systematic Reviews to Improve Social Care (SCIE Report No.4)*. London: Social Care Institute for Excellence, 2002.

69 Shemilt I. Campbell and Cochrane Economics Methods Group. *About The Cochrane Collaboration (Methods Groups)* 2010, Issue 2.

70 Campbell and Cochrane Economics Methods Group website. Available from: www.c-cemg.org.

71 Mulligan JA, Walker D, Fox-Rushby J. Economic evaluations of non-communicable disease interventions in developing countries: a critical review of the evidence base. *Cost-Effectiveness and Resource Allocation* 2006; 4(7).

72 Walker D, Fox-Rushby J. Economic evaluation of communicable disease interventions in developing countries: a critical review of the published literature. *Health Economics* 2000; 9(8): 681–698.

73 Creese A, Floyd K, Alban A, Guinness L. Cost-effectiveness of HIV/AIDS interventions in Africa: a systematic review of the evidence. *Lancet* 2002; 359(9318): 1635–1643.

74 Goodman CA, Mills AJ. The evidence base on the cost-effectiveness of malaria control measures in Africa. *Health Policy and Planning* 1999; 14(4): 301–312.

75 Teerawattananon Y, Russell S, Mugford M. A systematic review of economic evaluation literature in Thailand: are the data good enough to be used by policy-makers? *Pharmacoeconomics* 2007; 25 (6): 467–479.

76 Iglesias CP, Drummond MF, Rovira J. Health-care decision-making processes in Latin America: problems and prospects for the use of economic evaluation. *International Journal of Technology Assessment in Health Care* 2005; 21(1): 1–14.

77 Pattanaphesuj J, Teerawattananon Y. *Identifying Information Regarding Effectiveness and Cost-Effectiveness of Policies and Strategies for Reorientation to Mitigate the Impact of HIV/AIDS in Thailand. Revitalizing HIV prevention and impact mitigation in Thailand*. Nonthaburi: Health Intervention and Technology Assessment Program, 2008.

78 Sweat MD. *A Framework for Classifying HIV Prevention Interventions*. Geneva: Joint United Nations Programme on HIV/AIDS (UNAIDS), 2008.

79 Clapton J, Rutter D, Sharif N. *SCIE Systematic Mapping Guidance (SCIE Research Resource 03)*. London: Social Care Institute for Excellence. Available from: www.scie.org.uk/publications/researchresources/rr03.asp.

80 Evidence for Policy and Practice Information and Co-ordinating Centre. Mapping and refining the review's scope. London: Evidence for Policy and Practice Information and Co-ordinating Centre. Available from: http://eppi.ioe.ac.uk/cms/Default.aspx?tabid=175.

81 Pignone M, Saha S, Hoerger T, Lohr K, Teutsch S, Mandelblatt J. Challenges in systematic reviews of economic evaluations. *Annals of Internal Medicine* 2005; 142(12): 1073–1079.

82 Drummond MF, Barbieri M, Wong JB. Analytic choices in economic models of treatments for rheumatoid arthritis. What makes a difference? *Medical Decision Making* 2005; 25(5): 520–533.

83 Shemilt I, Thomas J, Morciano M. A new web-based tool for adjusting costs to a common currency and price year. *Evidence and Policy*, submitted.

84 Slavin RE. Best evidence synthesis: an intelligent alternative to meta-analysis. *Journal of Clinical Epidemiology* 1995 48(1): 9–18.

85 Higgins JPT, Green S (eds). Guide to the contents of a Cochrane protocol and review. In: Higgins JPT, Green S (eds) *Cochrane Handbook for Systematic Reviews of Interventions.* Version 5.0.1 (updated September 2008). Oxford: Cochrane Collaboration, 2008.

86 Byford S, Sefton T. Economic evaluation of complex health and social care interventions. *National Institute Economic Review* 2003; 186(1): 98–108.

87 Godber E, Robinson R, Steiner A. Economic evaluation and the shifting balance towards primary care: definitions, evidence and methodological issues. *Health Economics* 1997; 6(3): 275–294.

88 Kelly M, McDaid D, Ludbrook A, Powell J. *Economic Appraisal of Public Health Interventions (HDA Briefing Paper).* London: Health Development Agency, 2005.

89 Cooper N, Coyle D, Abrams K, Mugford M, Sutton A. Use of evidence in decision models : an appraisal of health technology assessments in the UK to date. *Journal of Health Services Research and Policy* 2005; 10: 245–250.

90 Pawson R. *Evidence-Based Policy: a realist perspective.* London: Sage Publications, 2006.

91 Pawson R, Greenhalgh T, Harvey G, Walshe K. Realist review – a new method of systematic review designed for complex policy interventions. *Journal of Health Services Research and Policy* 2005; 10(suppl 1): S1:21-S1:34.

92 Pawson R. Evidence-based policy: the promise of 'realist synthesis'. *Evaluation* 2002; 8(3): 340–358.

93 Hammersley M. *Systematic or Unsystematic, Is That The Question? Some reflections on the science, art and politics of reviewing research evidence.* London: Health Development Agency Public Health Steering Group, 2002. Available from: www.nice.org.uk/nicemedia/pdf/sys-unsys-phesg-hammersley.pdf

94 Noblit G, Hare R. *Meta-Ethnography: synthesizing qualitative evidence.* Newbury Park: Sage, 1988.

95 Birch S. Making the problem fit the solution: evidence-based decision making and 'Dolly' economics. In: Donaldson C, Mugford M, Vale L (eds) *Evidence-Based Health Economics: from effectiveness to efficiency in systematic review.* London: BMJ Books, 2002.

96 Birch S, Gafni A. Evidence-based health economics. Answers in search of questions? In: Kristiansen I, Mooney G (eds) *Evidence-Based Medicine in Its Place.* London: Routledge, 2002.

97 Boaz A, Ashby D, Young K. *Systematic Reviews: what have they got to offer evidence based policy and practice? (Working Paper No. 2).* London: ESRC UK Centre for Evidence Based Policy and Practice, 2002.

98 Glass GV, McGaw B, Smith ML. *Meta-Analysis in Social Research.* Beverly Hills: Sage, 1981.

99 Cronbach LJ. *Designing Evaluations of Education and Social Programs.* San Francisco: Jossey-Bass, 1983.

100 Cronbach LJ. Functional evaluation design for a world of political accommodation. In: Shadish W, Cook TD, Leviton L (eds) *Foundations of Program Evaluation.* Newbury Park: Sage Publications, 1991.

101 Campbell DT, Russo MJ. *Social Experimentation.* Thousand Oaks: Sage, 1999.

102 Oakley A. *Experiments in Knowing: gender and method in the social sciences.* Oxford: Polity Books, 2000.

103 Berwick DM. The science of improvement. *Journal of the American Medical Association* 2008; 229(10): 1182–1184.

104 Byng R, Norman I, Redfern S. Using realistic evaluation to evaluate a practice level intervention to improve primary health care for patients with long-term mental illness. *Evaluation* 2005; 11(1): 69–93.

105 Judge K, Mackenzie M. Theory-based approaches to evaluation: complex community-based initiatives. In: Mackenbach J, Bakker M (eds) *Reducing Inequalities in Health: a European perspective.* London: Routledge, 2002.

106 Anderson R. New MRC guidance on evaluating complex interventions: clarifying what interventions work by researching how and why they are effective. *British Medical Journal* 2008; 337(a1937): 944–945.

107 Pawson R. Nothing as practical as good theory. *Evaluation* 2003; 9(4): 471–490.

108 Konnerup M, Kongsted H. *There is More to Seeing than Meets the Eye: observational studies, research synthesis and the social sciences (Contingency and Dissent in Science Technical Report 06/09).* London: Centre for the Philosophy of Natural and Social Science, 2009.

The role of economic evidence in formulation of public policy and practice

Sarah Byford[1], Barbara Barrett[1], Richard Dubourg[2], Jennifer Francis[3], Jane Sisk[4]

[1]King's College London, London, UK
[2]Home Office, London, UK
[3]Social Care Institute for Excellence, London, UK
[4]National Center for Health Statistics, US Center for Disease Control and Prevention, Hyattsville, MD, USA

Introduction

The value of economic evidence has been increasingly recognised as an important constituent in the formulation of public policies and practices, with economic evaluation being widely applied in government appraisals of public projects and policies.[1,2] In the health care sector in particular, many countries now require or encourage the use of economic evaluation techniques to support reimbursement decisions, principally of pharmaceuticals but also in the evaluation of new and existing health technologies.[3] However, the contribution of economics to policy formulation in other social policy areas has been more limited. This chapter compares and contrasts the role of economic evidence in formulating public policy and practice in three policy areas – health care, social care and criminal justice – and explores the issues from the perspective of both high-income and low- and middle-income countries. The availability of economic evidence capable of supporting systematic review and decision models is explored and the policy systems and initiatives that encourage the inclusion of economic evidence in decision making are

Evidence-Based Decisions and Economics, 2nd edition. Edited by I. Shemilt, M. Mugford, L. Vale, K. Marsh and C. Donaldson. © 2010 Blackwell Publishing.

described in order to explore incentives and barriers to the production and use of economic evidence.

The role of economic evidence in health care

The health care sector has a relatively well-developed and established history of economics research, with substantial investments worldwide in the development of appropriate methodological frameworks, training of health economists and the application of health economic techniques to the evaluation of health technologies. The NHS Economic Evaluation Database currently contains 24,000 abstracts of health economics papers published worldwide, including 7000 full economic evaluations.[4] However, the application of economic methods to the evaluation of health technologies has been inconsistent between different disease classifications and thus the ability to systematically review and synthesise economic evidence in the health care field is highly variable.[5,6]

Guidelines for the economic evaluation of health technologies are commonly applied in health policy making in a number of European countries, Canada, Australia and New Zealand, and increasingly in health insurance and managed care organisations in the United States.[3] The first mandatory set of guidelines for economic evaluations was issued by Australia in 1992.[7] These focused specifically on the evaluation of pharmaceuticals for reimbursement purposes and many of the guidelines that followed had a similarly narrow focus. However, some guidelines are broader in scope, covering health promotion, disease prevention and treatment interventions, both pharmaceutical and non-pharmaceutical.[8,9]

Although mandatory guidelines did not begin to emerge until the 1990s, less formal guidelines have been widely available since the 1980s. Whilst perhaps the earliest consideration of the cost-effectiveness of public health policies was of the great plague in London in the 17th century,[10] Drummond & Jefferson note that in the UK the essential components of health economic evaluation were first published in 1974.[11,12] A more detailed exposition of the methods of health economic evaluation was published a few years later[13] and more formalised criteria for the critical appraisal of published economic evaluations were published in 1987,[14] which later formed the basis for guidelines for authors and peer reviewers of economic submissions to the *British Medical Journal*.[11] Similar criteria have been developed and applied in other countries, including the United States, Canada and Spain.[15]

A review of 25 available guidelines from 17 different countries found substantial variation in the levels of agreement between the guidelines for some methodological components, such as cost perspective and measures of effectiveness.[3] However, there was a relatively consistent preference for controlled experimental study designs capable of producing unbiased estimates of the effectiveness and cost implications of health care interventions, particularly randomised controlled trials (RCTs) or systematic reviews of RCTs. This 'gold standard' is consistent with the preferences found in the field of clinical evaluation,[16] which has made the incorporation of economic evaluation into clinical trials relatively straightforward.

There is also a preference amongst economists, derived from the theoretical principles of welfare economics and utilitarianism, to measure effectiveness in terms of utility, variously defined as the satisfaction, well-being, happiness or fulfilment of needs derived from consuming a good or service.[17,18] Although the measurement of utility is complex and can conflict with clinical preferences for disease-specific measures of outcome, there is growing academic and policy support for the use of preference-based, single-index measures of health-related quality of life capable of supporting comparisons between diverse health care technologies, in particular the quality-adjusted life-year (QALY).[19] Generating QALYs is not without its methodological challenges.[20] Perhaps as a result, international support for the QALY is variable, with some guidelines requiring outcome measures capable of producing QALYs, whilst others allow greater flexibility in the choice of measure.[3] However, substantial investment has been and continues to be made in the development and advancement of outcome measures capable of generating QALYs (see also Chapter 8).

The National Institute for Health and Clinical Excellence (NICE) in the UK, perhaps the most visible indication of central UK government support for the inclusion of economic evidence in health care decision making, is a strong proponent of the measurement of effectiveness in terms of QALYs. Established in 1999, NICE is charged with providing national guidance on the promotion of good health and the prevention and treatment of ill health and in making its recommendations, NICE is required to consider the best available evidence of both effectiveness and cost-effectiveness.[21] Systematic review and synthesis of clinical and economic evidence are thus standard practice in the work that NICE undertakes and commissions, including decision modelling to explore cost-effectiveness.

NICE provides specific directions on the framework required for estimating clinical and cost-effectiveness in the assessment of health technologies, including the cost perspective that should be taken (national health and personal social services), the method of economic evaluation to be used (cost-effectiveness analysis) and the measure of the value of health effects to be employed (QALYs).[22] NICE does, however, allow greater flexibility in the development of public health guidance, acknowledging the more complex and multidimensional nature of public health interventions, the more limited economic evidence available and the greater variability in study designs used.[23] In particular, a wider societal perspective, alternative methods of economic evaluation (such as cost-consequences or cost-benefit analyses) and alternative measures of effectiveness (such as disease-specific outcomes) may be employed, where appropriate or necessary due to lack of data.

In contrast to the UK, the United States, with its decentralised mix of multiple public and private health care payers and providers, as yet has no consistent policy for the use of economic evidence in health care decision making, despite having the highest per capita level of health care expenditure in the world[24] and leading the field in the application of experimental methods to the evaluation of public policies.[25] In the Medicare health insurance programme, a government programme that provides health insurance coverage for people aged 65 and over and some disabled people, attempts over the last 20 years to include cost or cost-effectiveness as a criterion for deciding which interventions are included in the scheme's coverage have been consistently rejected as a result of strong opposition to explicit consideration of cost and rationing of health service resources.[84] In addition, despite support for the QALY by the US Panel on Cost-Effectiveness in Health and Medicine and inclusion of preference-based measures of health-related quality of life in a number of major US health surveys, there is limited application of the QALY in economic evaluations, with commentators suggesting that maximisation of the health of the nation, whilst a clear objective in centralised health care systems, may be less obvious in decentralised systems, such as that in the United States.[26,27]

A major obstacle to the efficient use of resources in the United States is the lack of incentives to control costs. For clinicians, the predominance of payment per item of service supplied does little to encourage cost-conscious behaviour or to support moves towards evidence-based economic policies. In fact, incentives typically encourage provision of additional services if revenue exceeds costs. Medicare and some other insurers pay hospitals a fixed amount per discharge, dependent on diagnosis-related group classification. Although this arrangement contains incentives for hospitals to be cost-conscious and to reduce lengths of stay, it also rewards cost shifting from inpatient facilities to other settings. For patients, co-payments and deductibles in the insurance-based system provide some incentives to curb demand for health care, but may be blunt instruments that also reduce access to and use of cost-effective interventions.

The picture differs somewhat for providers and insurers responsible for providing comprehensive care within fixed annual budgets. The Kaiser-Permanente Medical Care Program, a private organisation, and the Department of Veterans Affairs fall into this category. The latter, for example, has used information on cost and effectiveness to establish a drug formulary. In addition, economic evidence is increasingly being incorporated into guidelines developed by the Centers for Disease Control and Prevention, the lead US public health agency. For example, cost-effectiveness evidence is included in national-level recommendations for new immunisations that will soon be introduced to the market. The national Guide to Community Preventive Services, whilst basing recommendations on evidence of effectiveness, additionally reports evidence of cost-effectiveness.[28]

More widespread changes are also taking place in US health care. The private plans that administer the Medicare drug budget are considering use of evidence on cost or cost-effectiveness to set formularies or reimbursement conditions. Federal policy makers are also emphasising the need to control Medicare expenditures to ensure long-term control of the federal budget deficit.[29] As part of legislation in early 2009 designed to stimulate the US economy and help develop the infrastructure for future universal health insurance coverage and reform of health care delivery, funding for comparative effectiveness research was greatly increased. Though silent about cost-effectiveness, the legislation intended to stimulate the development of better evidence to guide health care decision making.

The contrasting examples of the UK and US highlight clear inconsistencies in policy preferences for economic evidence to support decisions relating to health care. Thus, although economic evidence is relatively plentiful and health economic evaluation methods well developed, not all health policy bodies support their application on a consistent basis. In addition, concerns have been raised regarding the limited impact evidence from economic evaluations has on policy making. Williams & Bryan describe a number of barriers to the utilisation of economic evidence to inform policy decisions, including issues of accessibility (availability of relevant evidence, difficulties commissioning new research in a timely manner and difficulties understanding and interpreting the studies) and acceptability (inflexible financial structures, conflicting values and competing objectives).[30] They suggest a number of methods for improving implementation that may be of value to all policy sectors, such as efforts to improve the communication of evaluations to decision makers, a better understanding of the local contexts and competing priorities involved in decision making, closer relationships between researchers and decision makers and training and work-based experience of researchers. Thus, there continues to be room for improvement in the health sector.

The role of economic evidence in social care

Social care, and its close analogues social services and social pedagogy, are defined here as the planning and delivery of services to care for and support those who are vulnerable, dependent, marginalised or disadvantaged. In comparison to health care, the economic evaluation of social care programmes is rare but the demand for such evaluation, particularly from research funding bodies, is rising.

Internationally, we are aware of only limited evidence of any substantial or sustained policy support for commissioning or undertaking economic evaluations or utilising available economic evidence in decision making in the social care sector. A systematic review of economic evaluations in the broader social welfare field, encompassing social care, early intervention schemes, housing, regeneration, community development, work with children, young people and families, and welfare to work was undertaken between 1996 and 2000.[31] The authors located only 131 economic evaluations worldwide, approximately 30 studies per annum, and contrasted this with an average of 500 health economic evaluations published each year over the same time period. This shortage of economic evaluations greatly restricts the ability of researchers and service providers to synthesise economic evidence, and in areas such as social care, attention may need to be paid to the development of consistent economics methods and incentives to undertake economic evaluations, as enabling conditions for the more widespread use of economic evidence in policy and practice decisions.

To encourage greater use of economic evaluation, social care researchers need to gain a better understanding of the philosophy behind such evaluation and the methodologies necessary to carry out economic analyses in practice. However, there is also a need for economists to better understand the nature and context of social care in order to ensure that economics methods are appropriate and feasible in practice. In some senses, social care may not lend itself to economic evaluation as readily as health care. In particular, there is less of a focus on experimental methods of evaluation which are common to clinical evaluation. Whilst the 1960s and 1970s were witness to a 'golden era' of public sector randomised experimentation, particularly in the United States, disappointing results from these experiments were greeted with scepticism towards the methods of evaluation used, rather than towards the policies under evaluation. As a result, such designs fell out of favour and a corresponding rise in qualitative methods followed.[25] This scepticism towards quantitative methods of evaluation is in part responsible for the relative scarcity of economic evaluations in the social care field.

Despite differences between the health and social care fields, initiatives to encourage the application of economic methods to the evaluation of social care programmes have generally taken health economic methods as a starting point upon which to build an appropriate framework. In the UK, one early attempt to encourage greater application of economic techniques to social care research came from the Joseph Rowntree Foundation, an independent charity that aims to identify and overcome social problems.[32] In 1999, the Foundation funded an initiative to develop the infrastructure for economic evaluation in order to promote better understanding and use of economic evaluation in the social care field. The primary outputs included guidance on the practical application of economic evaluation techniques in a social care context,[31,33] which were largely based on the adaptation of health economic methods to the context of social care.[34]

Around the same time, the UK Department of Health announced an initiative to explore costs and outcomes in children's social care. This focused on understanding and explaining how resources are distributed between different services and exploring the relationship between costs and outcomes, rather than on estimating the relative cost-effectiveness of alternative resource distributions.[35] The funders understood that development of economic techniques was not well advanced in social care at the time the initiative was launched and thus efforts needed to be directed at capacity building to support future economics research and to encourage collaboration between economists and social care researchers and professionals. One example of the success of this initiative in developing enduring alliances is the development of the Cost Calculator, a computer software application and costing methodology designed to help local authorities monitor the costs of services for children in order to support their planning and commissioning functions.[36]

In drawing conclusions from the Joseph Rowntree Foundation and the Department of Health initiatives, Sefton and colleagues and Beecham & Sinclair made a number of recommendations that help to highlight the context within which social care research takes place and the challenges that economists and systematic reviewers face in this sector.[31,35] As discussed above, few experimental interventions are undertaken, requiring economists to consider how to work alongside and synthesise different kinds of research evidence, including that generated by qualitative, observational and quasi-experimental designs. In addition, there has been a historical focus in social care research on measures of the performance of services or indicators of service user needs, with less attention paid to the effectiveness of services in improving well-being. Economists who strongly support the application of preference-based measures of quality of life, such as the QALY, must recognise the limitations of this approach in the social care field, which is characterised by multiple and diverse objectives and outcomes, greater reliance on qualitative assessment of outcomes and a lack of appropriately validated and reliable quantitative outcome scales.[37] Current research into the development of a preference-based measure of social care outcomes for adults, being carried out by the Personal Social Services Research Unit at the University of Kent in the UK, may improve this situation in the future.

Some of these challenges are currently being explored by the Social Care Institute for Excellence (SCIE), an independent charity which aims to identify and disseminate good practice in social care in the UK. Set up in 2001 and funded by the Department of Health in England and the devolved administrations in Wales and Northern Ireland, SCIE aims to raise standards of practice across the social care sector, through the better use of knowledge and research.[38] To this end, SCIE recently developed methodologies to incorporate economic evidence into its knowledge production process, including systematic reviews. SCIE is also developing strategies for estimating the economic implications of their practice recommendations. A number of factors have driven this move towards the inclusion of economic evidence in the research undertaken and commissioned by SCIE, including pressure on local governing bodies to make efficiency savings,[39] concern that despite considerable social care investments, the rate of improvement among care services has stalled in recent years[40] and a growing awareness that existing social care systems are making poor use of limited resources.[41]

In addition to its methodological developments, SCIE has produced a statement of its position on economic evaluation in social care.[42] Reflecting the particular characteristics of the sector and recognising the often complex interaction between social care policies and health and other public services, SCIE's statement calls for a tailored approach to the application of economic evaluation methods in social care research. For example, SCIE supports a multisector perspective to examine intersectoral costs and benefits and to enable the impact on different stakeholders involved in the delivery of social services to be clearly assessed. Stakeholders in the commissioning and delivery of social care include service users and their families, and their centrality is increasing with the advent of personalisation, whereby people will be supported to become commissioners of their own services.[43] It is therefore important that economic evaluation of social care services should include the costs to service users and their families, including the costs of informal care,[44] and that the benefits generated should be defined from the perspective of service users. This broad focus is in contrast to the narrower health service and personal social services perspective preferred by NICE.[22]

Although SCIE's costing methodology represents an attempt to overcome the dearth of available evidence from economic evaluations, it is limited in its narrow focus on the financial implications of implementing its practice recommendations. The methodology does not yet encompass consideration of the impact of these recommendations on other parts of the social care system, such as the health service (albeit this is recognised in SCIE's position statement).[42] In this sense, the position statement can be seen as an aspiration, or goal, for the social care sector and the development of SCIE's methodologies as building the necessary infrastructure to support economic evaluation in the social care field. This does not negate the value of the costing evidence SCIE hopes to produce, since there is a growing recognition of the importance of economic evidence synthesis and decision modelling early in the stages of technology appraisal, to explore the appropriate research question, to support research prioritisation processes and to assess the need for additional information.[45]

Whilst the social care sector may be suffering from a shortage of economic evidence to support policy making, evidence of policy initiatives directed towards increasing the capacity for producing economic evidence in the future would suggest that this situation is likely to change over time. Although the methodological framework that is developing in the social care field was initially based on the principles of health economic evaluation, there is reason to believe that the methods that emerge will diverge from this path in some important respects, as the architects strive for approaches that better suit the context of social care. Thus far, efforts more closely resemble the methods guiding the NICE appraisal of public health interventions than those prescribed for health technology appraisals.[22,23] A recently published government Green Paper on the care and support system in the UK, which recognises the worldwide shortage of robust evidence about what works and the need for service provision to consider value for money, hints at the need for a social care equivalent to NICE by calling for an independent body to provide advice to support service provision that is both evidence based and cost-effective.[41] Such a body would further advance the development of a divergent framework for economic evaluations that are sensitive to the current capabilities of the social care sector and the different preferences for perspective, outcome measurement and study design that exist within it.

The role of economic evidence in crime and justice

The issues for the crime and justice system overlap greatly with those found in social care, although with a few notable differences. In some senses, there has been more of a history of applying economic techniques to the evaluation of criminal justice interventions, with microeconomic methods being applied to theories of crime and justice as early as the 1960s.[46] Since then there has been considerable investment in the application of economics to the criminal justice field, dominated by research in the US.[47–49] However, in common with the social care sector, experimental study designs are rare, the number of economic evaluations that have been undertaken is small and their methodological grounding limited.[50,51] As a result, systematic reviews of existing economic analyses in a given topic area are likely to identify little useful research-based material.

Whilst in social care there has been a tendency to learn from and adapt health economic methods,[34] criminal justice is less amenable to the direct application of standard health economic techniques, for a number of reasons. First, although societal well-being generally, and the well-being of victims of crime more specifically, might be the ultimate objectives of criminal justice policy, these cannot easily be observed or measured. This means that direct measures of well-being analogous to QALYs are unlikely to be the most appropriate metric for evaluations in this sector, and instead evaluations will generally need to rely on intermediate or surrogate outcomes that can be shown to be correlated with measures of well-being.

In practice, the majority of evaluations in the criminal justice field focus on the impact of interventions on measures of crime, such as recorded offences, self-reported offending, arrests, convictions and incarcerations.[52] The wide range of crime measures available limits the ability to compare results between studies, and reflects variation in the goals of policy interventions and the availability and accessibility of data. For example, data on crimes reported to the police are available in most countries but not all crimes are reported; of those that are, not all are associated with arrests, charges or convictions. The difficulties associated with crime and offending as measures of outcome are compounded by variation in the severity of crimes. Burglary is not the same as murder, thus evaluations that are limited to counts of offences fail to provide an accurate valuation of outcomes. For these reasons, attempts are increasingly being made to value outcomes in monetary terms so that volume and severity, and indeed other impacts of crime, can be combined into a single measure.[53]

Second, and closely related, the focus on crime as the primary outcome of many criminal justice evaluations has had an inevitable impact on the economic evaluation methodologies adopted. Cost-effectiveness analyses, where applied, tend to adopt intermediate measures of crime, with no attempt to establish a link with well-being. The main exceptions are evaluations of health care interventions delivered within criminal justice settings, such as services for mental health and substance misuse problems.[54] Cost-offset methods have been used but these often take a limited cost and outcome perspective, as do the small number of cost-benefit analyses that exist.[55,56] Attention has tended to focus on the taxpayer perspective, which limits the evaluation to the question of whether a publicly funded intervention pays for itself (i.e. costs are offset) through reductions in other public sector costs, principally cost savings as a result of crime reduction. However, consideration of the benefits of crime reduction has tended to be limited to direct victim costs such as the value of lost property,[56] ignoring the more intangible losses associated with being a victim of crime, which research suggests constitute the greatest proportion of the total costs of personal victimisation.[53,57]

In their original estimates of the costs of crime in England and Wales, Brand & Price set out a costing methodology comprising a number of components: costs in anticipation of crime (defensive expenditure such as burglar alarms, crime safety information and insurance administration); costs as a consequence of crime (the physical and emotional impact on victims, victim services, lost or damaged property, medical treatments and lost productivity); and costs in response to crime (police and prison services, courts, probation and legal aid).[58] Dubourg & Hamed's more recent estimates suggest that intangible costs are around 20% of the total costs of acquisitive crime (theft and robbery, business, retail and vehicle crime) and at least 50% of the total for violent crime.[53] Thus, omitting these intangible costs might be expected to produce substantially misleading results. Internationally, there is a need for data of this type but there is some debate about the best methodologies for estimating the costs of crimes.[51] The need for futher development was recently recognised by the European Commission, which funds a research consortium concerned with estimating the costs of crime in Europe, including a review of the methods applied in different countries.[59]

Third, unit costs of criminal justice interventions are difficult to calculate or locate, and data needed to calculate them are not often published routinely. In secure settings, such as prisons, average costs per prisoner per year are available for some countries but these give no indication of variations in costs between different regimes within individual prisons.[60] Currently, for example, it would be impossible to separate out the cost of a prisoner who attended an intensive treatment service from that of a prisoner who received no such service, thus making individual-level costing for the purpose of economic evaluation extremely difficult. In the community, few unit costs are available and there has been little centralised support or incentive for criminal justice services to calculate such unit costs or make any estimates that are produced publicly available. This has begun to change with, for example, UK Ministry of Justice investment in a programme of work to develop unit costs in criminal justice settings.[61]

Finally, experimental study designs can be difficult to implement in the criminal justice sector. The use of RCTs in crime and justice was not uncommon in the 1960s and 1970s, but such studies fell out of favour in the 1980s and remain rare today.[62,63] Key difficulties include resistance by frontline service providers to the denial of services to individuals whom they consider appropriate for intervention, the challenging circumstances of some participants (e.g. problem drug users), which can make follow-up difficult and attrition rates high, the complex nature of many criminal justice interventions, and a lack of adequate research funding.[64–66] Commentators have also pointed to the separation of the roles of service provider and researcher, which is in contrast to health care evaluation where the two groups are often one and the same, thus ensuring the service provider has a stake in the research enterprise and an engaged interest in the integration of research evidence into practice. However, there is some evidence of an increase in the number of RCTs in recent years[67,68] and there is increasing interest in quasi-experimental designs[69,70] and decision modelling.[71] The latter is particularly useful in the criminal justice field because of its flexibility where data are limited or where outcomes occur long into the future, such as reconvictions (see also, *inter alia*, Chapters 2, 3 and 9).

The development of economics methods in the crime and justice field is hindered by a lack of co-ordinated strategies at the policy level. In the UK, for example, there have been a number of indications of policy-level interest in utilising economic evidence to support criminal justice policy making, including estimations of the unit costs of crime,[53,58] guidance for the analysis of costs and benefits of specific interventions[72] and evaluations incorporating economic analysis components.[66,73] However, there has been no long-term co-ordinated strategy between the many stakeholders in the criminal justice system to support a consistent and systematic approach to economic evaluation, and one significant attempt to do so had only limited sucess.[74] The Crime Reduction Programme was a large central government initiative to reduce crime in England and Wales, which included independent evaluations of the effectiveness and cost-effectiveness of the supported interventions. Of the many problems encountered during the evaluation component of this initiative, unrealistically short timescales for research project design and resulting weaknesses in the quality of the evaluations undertaken have been suggested.[74] In addition, requirements laid down for the collection of economic data proved impossible to apply consistently across the diverse range of evaluations.

The lack of centralised strategies to incorporate economic evidence into criminal justice policy-making processes is due in part to the methodological complexities encountered in evaluations conducted in this field. However, an additional contributing factor is the lack of independent research capacity in many countries, particularly in criminal justice economics. Whilst central governments in many countries financially support various training courses in health economics, such centralised support for economists working in other sectors of public policy has been more limited. This situation suggests a lack of demand for economic evidence, since it is the demand for evidence that drives the funding, which in turn encourages the supply of training courses, independent research capacity and methodological development. Whilst demand may be on the increase, it may be some time yet before enough economic data are available to stimulate the more routine use of systematic review methods in crime and justice, at least in relation to evidence from existing economic evaluations. Instead, use of decision models to synthesise the available evidence from disparate sources and variable study designs should continue to prove useful.

The role of economic evidence in low and middle income countries

This chapter has so far focused on the role of economic evidence in the development of public policy and practice in high-income countries. Whilst wealthier countries are, to varying degrees, employing economic evidence to promote cost-consciousness in relatively well-resourced public systems faced with rising costs and rising demands, the issues for low- and middle-income countries (LMICs) are more complex. Questions of which service to provide for which social problem can be too simplistic in societies that may not be able to afford to fund any intervention, and often economic evidence is used in such settings to highlight the substantial burden of failing to provide support, particularly the burden that falls on individuals, their families and the wider communities.

Resource constraints also greatly limit the ability of LMICs to undertake local evaluations of either effectiveness or cost-effectiveness, and those economic evaluations that do exist tend to be of poor quality, as a result of a scarcity in research expertise as well as research funding.[75] Instead LMICs must rely to a large degree on evidence produced by high-income countries, or other developing countries where available. As a result, systematic review and evidence synthesis can be extremely valuable tools for LMICs faced with significant gaps in local knowledge. The relevance of evidence from high-income countries to the developing world, and indeed the relevance of evidence from one LMIC to another, is highly context dependent and subject to significant limitations (see Chapter 5). The focus here is on the extent to which economic evidence is considered in policy formulation in LMICs.

Apart from a few notable exceptions in the health care sector, such as Thailand and South Korea,[76] few LMICs have developed centralised policy strategies for the use of economic evidence to support decision making. In South Korea, which has a primarily insurance-based health care system with private provision, the Ministry of Health and the National Health Insurance Corporation are considering the use of economic evidence to support reimbursement decisions for pharmaceuticals in the first instance, but also for other technologies.[76]

To this end, pharmacoeconomic guidelines have been developed to provide pharmaceutical companies with instructions on how economic analyses are to be prepared before a drug is submitted for reimbursement and pricing. In Thailand, which has a mixed system of health care provision and financing, although the public sector dominates, the use of economic evidence to inform policy and practice in the health sector is more advanced. The Thai government has established the Health Intervention and Technology Assessment Program (HITAP) to support health policy decision making, has endorsed the development of national guidelines for conducting economic evaluations and supports the production of national reimbursement lists containing health technologies that are likely to be effective and cost-effective in the Thai context.[76,77] Systematic review of the international literature is central to this process, with higher priority given to studies conducted in Thailand.

Although more generally, few national strategies of this kind yet exist within LMICs, public policy making in LMICs is also influenced by external multinational organisations, such as the World Bank and the World Health Organization. The World Bank is one of the world's largest sources of funding and technical support for LMICs, investing in various sectors, including health care, education, agriculture and the environment. By disseminating both resources and expertise, the World Bank is in a strong position to influence the infrastructure and public policies of many of the world's poorest countries. From a research perspective, the World Bank considers evaluation of the initiatives it funds to be essential to their success and is heavily involved in research and development to promote effective policies that produce value for money.[78]

Similarly, the World Health Organization (WHO), which produces health guidelines and standards for the international community, aims to support and promote health research to inform evidence-based and cost-effective policy making. Since 1998, the WHO has funded a programme of work on choosing interventions that are cost-effective (WHO-CHOICE), which includes applied research (in particular the development of regional cost databases and undertaking economic evaluations of key health interventions) and methodological development of a framework for economic evaluation, known as generalised cost-effectiveness analysis, which includes methods to adapt regional results to the context of individual countries.[1] International pharmaceutical companies have also played a role in encouraging the use of economics methods as applied to the health sector, with applications for drug reimbursement in LMICs increasingly including economic evidence to support submissions and pricing decisions, despite no formal requirement to do so.[76]

Whilst a gradual proliferation of health economics methods may be evident in some LMICs, a number of obstacles to the use of economic evidence to support policy decisions in the health care sectors of LMICs have been highlighted in previous research. These include a lack of infrastructure and expertise, a lack of knowledge and understanding, a lack of appropriate training, inadequate access to existing literature, a lack of clearly defined criteria to facilitate decision making, and scepticism on the part of a range of key actors.[76,79–81] These obstacles are as relevant to the social care and criminal justice sectors (and likely also the education sector) as to health care, and continued efforts to support infrastructure development and knowledge transfer would help to reduce the constraints imposed by these obstacles over time. The current global financial crisis and the perennial problem of rising costs of public services are likely to see LMICs show an increasing interest in the cost-effectiveness of the policies they support. As the strategies set in place by countries such as Thailand and South Korea continue to develop, their usefulness as exemplars to guide developments in other LMICs will grow.

Conclusion

Although this chapter has predominantly focused on UK systems, the patterns described for the different public sectors are arguably as relevant to other countries as to the UK. International reviews highlight the limited availability and quality of economic evaluations worldwide in both the social care and criminal justice fields.[31,51] In contrast, the relative abundance of health economic studies is clear from international databases of abstracts such as the NHS EED, albeit with some concerns that such studies are less prominent within particular disease classifications, such as mental health and paediatrics.[6,82,83]

The evidence presented here suggests considerable variation in the development of infrastructure to support and promote the use of economic evidence in policy making between sectors, between countries and between high- and low- and middle-income countries. However, there is a clear and growing appreciation of the need for such evidence, with investment from many parts of the public policy arena in the advancement of methods for the economic evaluation of public sector services and technologies and the commissioning of economic analyses. All areas of public policy are concerned with scarcity of resources and budgetary constraint, increasingly so given the current global financial crisis, and the need to make policy decisions that ensure the provision of quality services that are also value for money. Whilst the social care and criminal justice sectors are only beginning to formulate consistent, sustainable and context-relevant methodological frameworks, the health care sector, having benefited from three decades of investment in the discipline of health economics, is grappling with methodological refinements and methods to improve the impact of the economic evidence that is available.

Social care and criminal justice have learnt much (and will continue to learn) from the frameworks already in place in the health care field (and the health care sector can learn from the experiences of other fields too). Similarly, LMICs have learnt much (and will continue to learn) from the frameworks already in place in high-income countries. However, clear differences in the nature of the social problems tackled, the philosophical stance taken, the study designs employed, the perspectives of interest and the questions posed mean that blind transfer of health economic methods is inappropriate. Instead, variations in the methods of economic evaluation are emerging, with the social care sector prioritising a broad, multisector perspective and a more user-focused view of outcomes, the criminal justice sector increasingly employing decision modelling techniques to synthesise disparate sources of evidence and focusing more on monetary valuations of intermediate outcomes than 'QALY analogue' measures, and LMICs relying heavily on evidence synthesised from high-income countries. There is also reason to believe that the dominant method of economic evaluation that emerges will differ between sectors, with the health care sector having a preference for cost-effectiveness and cost-utility analyses, social care perhaps requiring the flexibility of cost-consequences analysis, criminal justice moving towards cost-benefit analysis and LMICs applying generalised cost-effectiveness methods.

Barriers to the synthesis of economic evidence exist in all sectors. There is evidence of scepticism in some countries, such as the United States, and in sectors that are less familiar with a quantitative research culture, such as social care, which hinders the implementation of economics methods and the impact of the evidence that is available. There are methodological difficulties with the measurement of outcomes in all sectors and in all regions around the world, which are particularly stark in the social care and criminal justice fields, and in the more complex areas of health, such as public health and mental health. In addition, a lack of unit cost data is a problem, particularly for LMICs, but also for certain sectors within high-income countries, such as criminal justice and to a lesser extent social care. However, a number of initiatives have been highlighted that are supporting the development of economics methods to overcome some of these limitations and thus the validity and usefulness of economic evidence should continue to improve over time.

The capacity to undertake economic analysis, including evidence synthesis, is less clear. Whilst there is substantial investment in the training of health economists, in high-income countries at least, there is limited evidence of similar moves in other public sectors, and the problem is particularly acute in LMICs. Improvements in the ability to apply economics methods must go hand in hand with increases in the capacity to do so. Only then will it be possible to bridge the gap between the demand for good quality economic evidence and its availability.

Disclaimer

The views expressed in this chapter are those of the authors and do not necessarily represent the views of the employing institutions.

How this chapter should be cited

Byford S, Barrett B, Dubourg R, Francis J, Sisk J. Chapter 4: The role of economic evidence in formulation of public policy and practice. In: Shemilt I,

Mugford M, Vale L, Marsh K, Donaldson C (editors). *Evidence-based decisions and economics: health care, social welfare, education and criminal justice.* Oxford: Wiley-Blackwell, 2010.

References

1 Tan-Torres Edejer T, Baltussen RMPM, Adam T, *et al.* (eds). *Making Choices in Health: WHO guide to cost-effectiveness analysis.* Geneva: World Health Organization, 2003.

2 H.M. Treasury. *The Green Book: appraisal and evaluation in central government.* London: The Stationery Office, 2003.

3 Hjelmgren J, Berggren F, Andersson F. Health economic guidelines – similarities, differences and some implications. *Value in Health* 2001; 4(3): 225–250.

4 Centre for Reviews and Dissemination. *NHS Economic Evaluation Database.* York: Centre for Reviews and Dissemination, 2010. Available from: www.crd.york. ac.uk/crdweb.

5 Pritchard C. *Trends in Economic Evaluation.* London: Office of Health Economics, 1998.

6 Ungar WJ, Santos MT. Trends in paediatric health economic evaluation: 1980 to 1999. *Archives of Disease in Childhood* 2004; 89(1): 26–29.

7 Australian Commonwealth Department of Health HaCS. *Guidelines for the Pharmaceutical Industry on Preparation of Submissions to the Pharmaceutical Benefits Advisory Committee.* Canberra: Australian Commonwealth Department, 1995.

8 National Institute for Clinical Excellence. *Revised Guidelines for Manufacturers, Sponsors of Technologies: making submissions to the Institute.* London: National Institute for Clinical Excellence, 2001.

9 Lopez Bastida J. *Propuesta de Guia para La Evaluacion Economica Aplicada a Las Tecnologias Sanitarias (Report No. 22).* Tenerife, Canary Islands: Servicio de Evaluacion del Servico Canario de la Salud (SESCS), 2006.

10 Banta JE. Sir William Petty: modern epidemiologist (1623–1687). *Journal of Community Health* 1987; 12(2–3): 185–198.

11 Drummond MF, Jefferson TO, on behalf of the BMJ Economic Evaluation Working Party. Guidelines for authors and peer reviewers of economic submissions to the BMJ. *British Medical Journal* 1996; 313(7052): 275–283.

12 Williams A. The cost-benefit approach. *British Medical Bulletin* 1974; 30(3): 252–256.

13 Drummond MF. *Principles of Economic Appraisal in Health care.* Oxford: Oxford Medical Publications, 1980.

14 Drummond MF, Sculpher MJ, Torrance GW, O'Brien BJ, Stoddart GL. *Methods for the Economic Evaluation of Health care Programmes,* 3rd edn. Oxford: Oxford University Press, 2005.

15 Ungar WJ, Santos MT. The paediatric quality appraisal questionnaire: an instrument for evaluation of the paediatric health economics literature. *Value in Health* 2003; 6(5): 584–594.

16 Sheldon T, Oakley T. Why we need randomised controlled trials. In: Duley L, Farrell B (eds) *Clinical Trials.* London: BMJ Books, 2002.

17 Bannock G, Baxter RE, Rees R. *Dictionary of Economics.* London: Penguin Books, 1984.

18 Barr N. *The Economics of the Welfare State.* London: Weidenfeld and Nicolson, 1987.

19 Loomes G, McKenzie L. The use of QALYs in health care decision making. *Social Science and Medicine* 1989; 28(4): 299–308.

20 Nord E, Daniels N, Kamlet M. QALYs: some challenges. *Value in Health* 2009; 12(S1): S10–S15.

21 Rawlins MD, Culyer AJ. National Institute for Clinical Excellence and its value judgements. *British Medical Journal* 2004; 329(7459): 224–227.

22 National Institute for Health and Clinical Excellence. *Guide to the Methods of Technology Appraisal.* London: National Institute for Health and Clinical Excellence, 2008.

23 National Institute for Health and Clinical Excellence. *Methods for the Development of NICE Public Health Guidance,* 2nd edn. London: National Institute for Health and Clinical Excellence, 2009.

24 Anderson GF, Frogner BK. Health spending in OECD countries: obtaining value per dollar. *Health Affairs* 2008; 27(6): 1718–1727.

25 Oakley A. *Experiments in Knowing: gender and method in the social sciences.* Oxford: Polity Books, 2000.

26 Lipscomb J, Drummond M, Fryback D, Gold M, Revicki D. Retaining, and enhancing, the QALY. *Value in Health* 2009; 12(S1): S18–S26.

27 Drummond M, Brixner D, Gold M, Kind P, McGuire A, Nord E. Toward a consensus on the QALY. *Value in Health* 2009; 12(S1): S31–S35.

28 Guide to Community Preventive Services. *The Community Guide: what works to promote health.* Atlanta: National Center for Health Marketing (NCHM), Centers for Disease Control and Prevention, 2010. Available from: www.thecommunityguide.org.

29 Sisko A, Truffer C, Smith S, *et al.* Health spending projections through 2018: recession effects add uncertainty to the outlook. *Health Affairs* 2009; 28(2): w346–w357.

30 Williams I, Bryan S. Understanding the limited impact of economic evaluation in health care resource allocation: a conceptual framework. *Health Policy* 2007; 80(1): 135–143.

31 Sefton TAJ, Byford S, McDaid D, Hills J, Knapp M. *Making the Most of It. Economic evaluation in the social welfare field.* York: Joseph Rowntree Foundation, 2002.

32 Joseph Rowntree Foundation. *About us.* York: Joseph Rowntree Foundation, 2010. Available from: www.jrf.org. uk/about-us.

33 Byford S, McDaid D, Sefton TAJ. *Because It's Worth It. A practical guide to conducting economic evaluations in the social welfare field.* York: Joseph Rowntree Foundation, 2003.

34 Byford S, Sefton T. *First Aid: lessons from health economics for economic evaluation in social welfare (LSE Health and Social Care Discussion Paper).* London: LSE Health and Social Care, 2002.

35 Beecham J, Sinclair I. *Costs and Outcomes in Children's Social Care: messages from research.* London: Jessica Kingsley Publishers, 2007.

36 Centre for Child and Family Research. Loughborough: Loughborough University, 2010. Available from: www.lboro.ac.uk/research/ccfr.

37 Byford S, Sefton T. Economic evaluation of complex health and social care interventions. *National Institute Economic Review* 2003; 186(1): 98–108.

38 Social Care Institute for Excellence. *Research into the Impact of SCIE.* London: Social Care Institute for Excellence, 2007.

39 HM Treasury. *Pre Budget Report and Comprehensive Spending Review.* London: The Stationery Office, 2007.

40 Commission for Social Care Inspection. *The State of Social Care in England 2006–07.* London: Commission for Social Care Inspection, 2008.

41 HM Government. *Shaping the Future of Care Together (Green Paper).* London: The Stationery Office, 2009.

42 Francis J. *SCIE's Approach to Economic Evaluation in Social Care.* London: Social Care Institute for Excellence, in press.

43 HM Government. *Putting People First: a shared vision and commitment to the transformation of adult social care.* London: HM Government, 2007.

44 Netten A, Beecham J. *Costing Community Care: theory and practice.* Aldershot: Ashgate, 1993.

45 Sculpher MJ, Claxton K, Drummond M, McCabe C. Whither trial-based economic evaluation for health care decision making? *Health Economics* 2006; 15(7): 677–687.

46 Becker GS. Crime and punishment: an economic approach. *Journal of Political Economy* 1968; 76(2):169–217.

47 Cohen MA. Pain, suffering, and jury awards: a study of the cost of crime to victims. *Law and Society* 1988; 22(3): 537–555.

48 McDougall C, Cohen MA, Swaray R, Perry A. The costs and benefits of sentencing: a systematic review. *Annals of the American Academy of Political and Social Science* 2003; 587(1): 160–177.

49 Cohen MA. Measuring the costs and benefits of crime and justice. *Criminal Justice* 2000; 4: 263–315.

50 Roman J. Can cost-benefit analysis answer criminal justice policy questions, and if so, how? *Journal of Contemporary Criminal Justice* 2004; 20(3): 257–275.

51 Swaray RB, Bowles R, Pradiptyo R. The application of economic analysis to criminal justice interventions: a review of the literature. *Criminal Justice and Policy Review* 2005; 16(2): 141–163.

52 Chambers J, Yiend J, Barrett B, *et al.* Outcome measures used in forensic mental health research: a structured review. *Criminal Behaviour and Mental Health*, 2009; 19(1): 9–27.

53 Dubourg R, Hamed J. *The Economic and Social Costs of Crime Against Individuals and Households 2003-4.* London: Home Office, 2005.

54 Daley M, Love CT, Shepard DS, Petersen CB, White KL, Hall FB. Cost-effectiveness of Connecticut's in-prison substance abuse treatment. *Journal of Offender Rehabilitation* 2004; 39(3): 69–92.

55 Welsh BC, Farrington DP. Correctional intervention programs and cost-benefit analysis. *Criminal Justice and Behavior* 2000; 27(1): 115–133.

56 Welsh BC, Farrington DP, Sherman LW. *Costs and Benefits of Preventing Crime.* Boulder: Westview Press, 2001.

57 Cohen MA. *The Crime Victim's Perspective in Cost-Benefit Analysis: the importance of monetizing tangible and intangible crime costs.* Boulder: Westview Press, 2001.

58 Brand S, Price R. *The Economic and Social Costs of Crime.* London: Home Office, 2000.

59 European Commission. *Estimating the costs of crime.* European Commission, 2010. Available from: http://www.costsofcrime.org

60 HM Prison Service. *Prison Service Annual Report and Accounts.* London: The Stationery Office, 2006.

61 Netten A, Barrett B, Brookes N. *Unit Costs in Criminal Justice (PSSRU Bulletin No. 18).* Canterbury: University of Kent, 2008. Available from: www.pssru.ac.uk/pdf/b18/b18_uccj.pdf.

62 Nuttall C. The Home Office and random allocation experiments. *Evaluation Review* 2003; 27(3): 267–289.

63 Palmer T, Petrosino A. The 'experimenting agency'. The California Youth Authority research division. *Evaluation Review* 2003; 27(3): 228–266.

64 Farrington DP. A short history of randomized experiments in criminology: a meagre feast. *Evaluation Review* 2003; 27(3): 218–227.

65 Shepherd JP. Explaining feast or famine in randomized field trials: medical science and criminology compared. *Evaluation Review* 2003; 27(3): 290–315.

66 Tyrer P, Barrett B, Cooper S, *et al.* The assessment of dangerous and severe personality disorder: lessons from a randomised controlled trial linked to qualitative analysis. *Journal of Forensic Psychology and Psychiatry* 2009; 20(1): 132–146.

67 Shapland J, Atkinson A, Colledge E, *et al. Implementing Restorative Justice Schemes (Crime Reduction Programme): a report on the first year (Home Office Online report 32/04).* London: Home Office, 2004. Available from: www.homeoffice.gov.uk/rds/pdfs04/rdsolr3204.pdf.

68 McDougall C, Perry AE, Clarbour J, Bowles R, Worthy G. *Evaluation of HM Prison Service Enhanced Thinking Skills Programme. Report on the outcomes from a randomised controlled trial (Ministry of Justice Research Series 3/09).* London: Ministry of Justice, 2009.

69 Kessler DP, Levitt SD. Using sentence enhancements to distinguish between deterrence and incapacitation. *Journal of Law and Economics* 1999; 42(1): 343–363.

70 Levitt SD. Using electoral cycles in police hiring to estimate the effect of police on crime. *American Economic Review* 1997; 87(3): 270–290.

71 Sutton AJ, Edmunds WJ, Gill ON. Estimating the cost-effectiveness of detecting cases of chronic hepatitis C infection on reception in to prison. *BMC Public Health* 2006; 6(170).

72 Dhiri A, Brand S. *Analysis of Costs and Benefits: guidance for evaluators.* London: Home Office, 1999.

73 Barrett B, Byford S, Seivewright H, Cooper S, Tyrer P. Economic evaluation of assessment for dangerous

and severe personality disorder in an English prison. *Journal of Forensic Psychology and Psychiatry* 2009; 20(1): 120–131.

74 Maguire M. The Crime Reduction Programme in England and Wales: reflections on the vision and the reality. *Criminal Justice* 2004; 4(3): 213–237.

75 Walker D, Fox-Rushby JA. Economic evaluation of communicable disease interventions in developing countries: a critical review of the published literature. *Health Economics* 2000; 9(8): 681–698.

76 Tarn Y-H, Hu S, Kamae I, *et al*. Health care systems and pharmacoeconomic research in Asia-Pacific region. *Value in Health* 2008; 11(suppl 1): S137–S155.

77 Teerawattananon Y, Chaikledkaew U. Thai health technology assessment guideline development. *Journal of the Medical Association of Thailand* 2008; 91(suppl 2): 11–15.

78 World Bank. *World Bank Group: working for a world free of poverty*. Washington DC: World Bank, 2007.

79 Teerawattananon Y, Russell S. A difficult balancing act: policy actors' perspectives on using economic evaluation to inform health care coverage decisions under the Universal Health Insurance Coverage Scheme in Thailand. *Value in Health* 2008; 11(suppl 1): S52–S60.

80 Teerawattananon Y, Russell S. The greatest happiness of the greatest number? Policy actors' perspectives on the limits of economic evaluation as a tool for informing health care coverage decisions in Thailand. *BMC Health Services Research* 2008; 8(197).

81 Iglesias CP, Drummond MF. Health care decision-making processes in Latin America: problems and prospects for the use of economic evaluation. *International Journal of Health Technology Assessment in Health care* 2005; 21(1): 1–14.

82 Evers SMAA, van Wijk AS, Ament AJHA. Economic evaluation of mental health care interventions: a review. *Health Economics* 1997; 6(2): 161–177.

83 Romeo R, Byford S, Knapp M. Annotation: economic evaluations of child and adolescent mental health interventions: a systematic review. *Journal of Child Psychology and Psychiatry and Allied Disciplines* 2005; 46(9): 919–930.

84 Bryan S, Sofaer S, Siegelberg T, Gold M. Has the time come for cost-effectiveness analysis in US health care? *Health Economics, Policy and Law* 2009; 4: 423–425.

CHAPTER 5

Generalisability, transferability, complexity and relevance

Damian G. Walker[1], Yot Teerawattananon[2], Rob Anderson[3], Gerry Richardson[4]

[1]Johns Hopkins University, Bloomberg School of Public Health, Baltimore, MD, USA
[2]Health Intervention and Technology Assessment Program (HITAP), Thai Ministry of Public Health, Nonthaburi, Thailand
[3]Peninsula Medical School, University of Exeter, Exeter, UK
[4]Centre for Health Economics, University of York, York, UK

Introduction

The value of economic evaluation as an aid to decision making is often limited by concerns about the generalisability and transferability of cost-effectiveness data. Concerns about the generalisability of cost-effectiveness data are in turn predicated on concerns about the generalisability of all the different components of data that feed into evaluations of cost-effectiveness (i.e. effects, resource use, unit costs, epidemiology, utilities or other outcome values).

Most concerns about the generalisability of cost-effectiveness data have to date focused on the generalisability of unit costs and resource use data. However, issues of context, generalisability and transferability arguably apply equally to effects data. For example, it is generally supposed that the effects obtained from administering a drug to a sample population in the UK will generally be similar to administering a drug to a sample population in, say, the Middle East. However, as we increasingly understand diversity in the physiological context within which drugs are administered, issues regarding DNA and genetic profiling, and so on (are we really as homogeneous as we think we are?), the issues of

context, generalisability and transferability may be increasingly recognised to apply to the effects of pharmaceutical interventions. As one moves away from pharmaceutical interventions on a continuum through surgical interventions and into more complex interventions, both within health care and also into those implemented within and across other applied fields, such as social welfare, education and criminal justice, the importance of context and its impact on (variations in) effects (and hence the effectiveness component of the cost-effectiveness equation) are likely to apply even more strongly.

Essentially, context matters. If economic, epidemiological and behavioural factors were the same everywhere there would be no need to consider the generalisability and transferability of results; one could simply apply the same findings to different settings. However, differences in these factors do exist, across time and space. It is the principal reason why resource use and cost data relating to specific target populations and jurisdictions of interest are widely regarded as the best available source of data for use in economic evaluations, including decision models, to inform resource allocation decisions in a specific setting (see Chapter 9).[1]

However, the question of generalisability is also important in the context of multinational economic evaluations. Multinational economic evaluations have become an important method for measuring the relative cost-effectiveness of different interventions.

Evidence-Based Decisions and Economics, 2nd edition. Edited by I. Shemilt, M. Mugford, L. Vale, K. Marsh and C. Donaldson. © 2010 Blackwell Publishing.

The appeal of these studies comes from the possibility of combining efficacy data from multinational clinical trials with cost estimates to give an overall incremental cost-effectiveness ratio (ICER). Also, the perspective of these studies is multinational and the authors sometimes imply that the results may be generalisable to many other health care settings. Yet the use of these studies raises important questions concerning the extent to which estimates of costs and the effects they produce are in fact generalisable. In addition, in the developing world, limited local capacity for undertaking economic evaluations, and the prohibitive cost of performing many, has also generated interest in pooling data and results of previously published studies.[2] Over the past decade, the World Health Organization (WHO) has been building an evidence-base that can be used for 'generalised cost-effectiveness analysis' (see also Chapter 4): 'The purpose is . . . to provide broader guidance to policy makers about cost-effectiveness. They should be able to re-examine existing interventions as well as new ones'.[2–4]

Hence, the purpose of this chapter is to critically examine why it is important to consider the notions of generalisability and transferability with respect to economic analysis, the factors that affect generalisability and transferability, and approaches used to examine the generalisability and transferability of resource use, cost and cost-effectiveness data. The chapter also considers two specific issues: complex interventions and the relevance of economic evidence, with particular reference to generalising and transferring data from developed to developing countries. Finally, the majority of the material presented originates from health economic research, although many of the concepts and methods should have broader applicability beyond the health care field.

Terminology

The first edition of this book defined the concept of generalisability of results as being 'similar to external validity in that it refers to the extent to which information (both clinical and economic) can be extrapolated to either a patient group with different characteristics or to a similar patient group treated in a different geographic, political or time structure'.[5] Transferability was defined as 'the ability to extrapolate results obtained from one setting or context to another'.[5] We use the same definitions in this chapter.

However, there is an important difference, not often distinguished, between what might be called the potential (or generic) transferability of a study and its actual (or specific) transferability to another policy or practice decision context at another time and place.[6] Potential transferability hinges especially on how fully the intervention has been described, how comprehensively the implementation context is described and which patient or participant groups were selected for exposure to the intervention. This allows practitioners or policy makers elsewhere to assess whether the choice of options they face, and their target populations and organisational contexts, are similar. The important thing to note is that this type of transferability is a property of the particular study, what it has evaluated and how fully it has been described. In contrast, actual transferability assesses the same things as described above but in relation to a particular decision or policy choice in a particular jurisdiction, population and health system. This is a property of the original programme, study and setting, and the population, setting and potential constraints on programme design and funding in the place where the same programme may be applied. This cannot be a property of an individual study and evaluated programme, but will change depending on where you want to transfer the evidence to and when.

Complex interventions are usually described as interventions that contain several interacting components, but they also have other characteristics that researchers should take into account.[7] The components usually include behaviours, parameters of behaviours (e.g. frequency, timing) and methods of organising and delivering those behaviours (e.g. type(s) of practitioner, setting and location); the number of groups or organisational levels targeted by the intervention; and the number and variability of outcomes.

We define 'relevant' evidence as evidence that may be useful in addressing the decision problem, and we assume that the local decision maker is the appropriate person to determine relevance. While it is important that economic evaluations incorporate 'relevant' evidence, there is not a simple dichotomy between relevant and irrelevant evidence.

And finally, a brief word on the concept of exchangeability in economic evaluation. Exchangeability encompasses both the likely exchangeability of the relative treatment effect on costs and the relative treatment effect on outcome data. The assumption of exchangeability between two trials requires that there are no *a priori* reasons for expecting a systematically different (higher or lower) estimate of the relative treatment effect on costs and/or effects between the two trials.[8,9] As with relevance, exchangeability can be represented on a continuum ranging from 'not exchangeable' to 'totally exchangeable' via 'partially exchangeable'.[10]

Why is generalisability important?

A greater understanding of generalisability in economic evaluation has potential benefits for three main groups: producers, users and funders. From a producer's perspective, there is value in understanding which components of data that feed into economic evaluations are likely to vary across time and space in such a way as to alter the conclusions of a particular study. Producers will also benefit from the identification and development of methods to assess the extent of variability in cost-effectiveness between settings.

It is understandable that decision makers prefer to use local economic evaluation information for making coverage decisions about health technology.[11] It is, however, also important that they know about the factors that make economic results of particular studies vary from place to place because these factors can be useful not only for decision makers outside the study setting, but also for decision makers in the study setting to use for future monitoring and evaluation

of programmes. For example, an analysis of the cost-effectiveness of six strategies consisting of single or double voluntary counselling and testing (VCT) and three choices of drug regimens for the prevention of mother-to-child HIV transmission in Thailand found that the higher the HIV prevalence among pregnant women, the lower the incremental cost-effectiveness ratio (see Figure 5.1).[12] In addition, the difference in cost-effectiveness between single VCT and double VCT in each of the three drug regimens is greatest at lower seroprevalence levels. Hence, if a change of HIV prevalence is observed in Thailand, Thai decision makers can identify the best policy option given the new situation.

But probably the main reason why users of economic evaluations benefit from a greater understanding of generalisability is that resources and expertise to conduct economic evaluation studies are scarce and it is, therefore, not possible to perform a specific study for each local setting. Therefore, decision makers need to consider whether the results of a study that was performed elsewhere can be applied to their setting, and how to adapt results if this is not the case.

Finally, funders, especially international organisations such as the World Health Organization, the World Bank or multinational pharmaceutical companies, should be well aware of transferability issues when they commission economic evaluation studies, since they are likely to use the results to inform

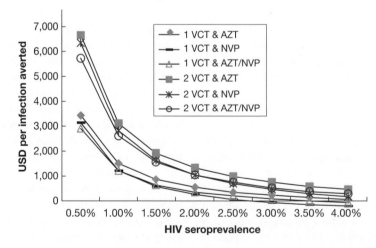

Figure 5.1 Analysis of cost per infection averted of interventions as a function of HIV seroprevalence. VCT, voluntary counseling and testing; AZT, zidovudine regimen; NVP, nevirapine regimen; AZT/NVP, a combination of AZT for early antenatal attenders and NVP for late arrivals. Data from Teerawattananon *et al.*, 2005.[12]

policy decisions in more than one setting. As a result, they may request the use of multinational trials for estimating the clinical efficacy of an intervention, not only for faster recruitment of the necessary numbers of patients, and to introduce the product into clinical practice more widely, but also to provide for the collection of local data on factors affecting transferability.

Factors affecting generalisability

Since the first edition of this book was published in 2002, there have been important contributions from a number of researchers on the issues of generalisability and transferability of economic evaluations.[13-16] Specifically, much work has been done itemising the potential factors affecting the generalisability of economic evaluations, which are summarised below.

Population factors

Age, gender, race, education, socio-economic status and risk behaviours of populations and subpopulations eligible for an intervention will typically vary across settings. These variations may affect not only clinical outcomes but also resources used and this will eventually influence the results of economic evaluation studies. A population's attitude towards health care and interventions, compliance and adherence, preferences for and valuations of health states, and incentives, such as level of co-payment, are also important components that can have a significant impact on cost-effectiveness.

Disease characteristics

Because there are differences in population demographic and socio-economic status between locations, it is likely that the prevalence and incidence of particular diseases and/or their co-morbidities are different across settings. Such differences will inevitably impact costs and/or the effectiveness of health care interventions, especially diagnostic and preventive interventions. Disease characteristics also include disease progression. Moreover, it is important to note that the spread of disease can vary from one setting to another because of the differences in populations' lifestyles and density, environment and disease control systems.

Provider and system factors

Although it is difficult to quantify the differences in skills, experience and efficiency of the clinical practice of health professionals across jurisdictions, these factors can influence the effectiveness, resources used and cost-effectiveness of health care interventions. For example, Teerawattananon & Mugford found a higher cost of laparoscopic surgery for gallstone disease compared to open cholecystectomy in Thailand while laparoscopic surgery was a cost-saving intervention in most Western countries.[17] This different conclusion was explained in two ways. First, a higher wage rate for health professionals and patients in developed countries caused both significantly higher hospital admission costs and also a higher opportunity cost of taking leave from work for sickness, compared to Thailand. Second, there was a difference in the employment rate of patients undertaking cholecystectomy between the two settings. In Thailand, only 50% of cholecystectomy patients were active workforce members, which contrasts with employment rates in Western countries.

Similarly, the personal skills of clinicians can greatly influence the process of care and treatment outcome of patients. This is particularly dominant in the case of labour-intensive procedures such as surgical interventions and social care services. Dissimilarities in liability and incentives of remuneration systems observed across health care settings can also have a clear effect on the performance of health personnel. Furthermore, availability of social and health service infrastructures may differ among locations, due to differences in public resources or differences in the way such resources are allocated; these differences are likely to affect both the costs and outcomes of an intervention.

Methodological factors

It has been well documented that there is a degree of diversity regarding methodological requirements for conducting economic evaluation across jurisdictions.[18] Variations exist in terms of the perspective of the analysis, the choice of comparators, measurement of costs and clinical outcomes, choice of discount rates, and so on. Such variation can be overcome by using a reference case to produce a standard set of results that are presented in a standard manner.[19]

Given different decision-making contexts and a wide range of methodological choices, it is inevitable that variations of methodological recommendations exist. However, although some variation is reasonable (e.g. perspective of the study), some may be much

Table 5.1 Variability among guidelines on discount rate.

Recommended discount rates (%)	No. of guidelines
3–3.5	3
4	1
5	9
6	3
10	1
0–5	2
2.5–5	2
3 & 5	2
Not specific	5

n = 28. Data from Tarn and Smith, 2004.[18]

more arbitrary (e.g. choice of discount rate).[20] Table 5.1 provides an overview of the range in discount rates used in economic evaluations recommended by 28 methodological guidelines from around the world.[18] These variations can affect the results of economic evaluation studies and their transferability across settings unless more uniform methodological guidelines from different jurisdictions are observed.

Methods used for transferring economic evaluation data

The simplest practice of transferring the results of economic evaluation across settings is to use the original outcomes but to convert costs of an intervention from the local currency unit of the original setting into the local currency unit of the targeted setting using foreign exchange rates.[21] However, using market exchange rates to compare countries' costs of social and health care services can be misleading since the rates do not necessarily reflect the relative purchasing power of different currencies. An improved approach is to employ exchange rates based on purchasing power parities (PPPs), which take into account the relative cost of living and the inflation rates of different settings, and international dollars are the most frequently used currency in this approach.[22–25] However, this approach completely ignores any variations in the aforementioned factors that affect generalisability within and between settings.

Methods for decision models

Because decision models allow for researchers to examine the effects of varying key input parameters on economic evaluation results, modelling by substituting setting-specific characteristics into aggregate summary results from the original setting tends to be used more frequently to deal with transferability issues. Relative clinical efficacy, resource utilisation and unit costs are three key parameters often cited as the most important determinants of economic evaluation results when the transferability issue is of special interest. The original data related to these parameters used in the original economic evaluation can be replaced with local information from the target setting to quantify the value for money of the intervention in the target health care setting.

A systematic review of literature to identify approaches for transferring economic evaluation data across locations found that the most common approach for the decision model was to use the original setting's relative clinical efficacy but to substitute target setting-specific resource utilisation and unit costs into the analysis.[14] The second most common approach was to use relative clinical efficacy established in the original setting, but to use a mixture of original and target setting resource utilisation and target setting unit costs. This may reflect the fact that, rightly or wrongly, many researchers believe that clinical effects of the interventions are transferable across health care systems, whilst resource use and unit costs are more jurisdiction specific (see the 'Introduction' to this chapter).

Methods for empirical economic evaluations that utilise individual-level data

Since there has been a growing concern in economic evaluations conducted alongside multicentre randomised controlled trials (RCTs) that the pooled or average cost-effectiveness results using trial-wide costs and outcomes may not be reflective of the results that would have been observed individually in each participating centre's setting, several researchers have proposed approaches for analysing economic evaluation using patient-level information. For example, both Menzin and colleagues and Jonsson & Weinstein have proposed the use of location-specific resource utilisation and unit costs but trial-wide clinical results.[26,27] However, this approach ignores the fact that clinical and economic variables may influence one another; for example, outcomes such as survival (effectiveness outcome) and quantity of use of hospital care (economic outcome) may be correlated.

There are currently no agreed-upon methods for pooling estimates of cost-effectiveness (e.g. incremental cost-effectiveness, cost-utility or cost-benefit ratios), extracted from multiple economic evaluations, using meta-analysis or other quantitative synthesis methods.[28] However, if estimates of measures of resource use and costs are available in a common metric (with associated measures of uncertainty) from two or more included studies, for an intervention and its comparator, these can, in principle, be pooled using a meta-analysis (see also Chapter 3). Cook and colleagues offer an approach to examine the homogeneity of the results of economic evaluations across different settings.[29] If there is no evidence of meaningful differences in treatment effects and costs between locations, then it is sensible to apply the pooled results to all settings that participated in the trial. However, the appropriate approach if evidence of heterogeneity is observed is less clear.

In practice, extreme caution is advised when considering whether to undertake a meta-analysis of resource use or cost data. Prior to any decision to pool estimates using a meta-analysis, particular attention should be paid to whether the metric in question has equivalent meaning across studies. Furthermore, these issues have also generated debate on whether meta-analysis of measures of resource use or costs across wider geographical and political boundaries is likely to generate meaningful results, how the results of such meta-analyses should be interpreted (e.g. do you just end up with a pooled estimate that is not applicable in any setting?), and what additional value the results may have for end-users.[28]

A recent development using multilevel modelling for a cost-effectiveness analysis alongside multicentre trials is recommended by Sculpher and colleagues in order to take into account the between location variability concerning cost-effectiveness.[13] This variability occurs if there is close association between costs and outcomes among samples recruited in particular locations. As a result, the patient-level information is clustered by location and the model estimates local-specific uncertainty around an intervention's cost and effectiveness data.[30]

Multinational economic evaluations often calculate a single measure of cost-effectiveness using cost data pooled across several countries. To assess the validity of pooling international cost data, the reasons for cost variation across countries need to be assessed. Previously, ordinary least-squares (OLS) regression models have been used to identify factors associated with variability in resource use and total costs. However, multilevel models (MLMs), which accommodate the hierarchical structure of the data, may be more appropriate. A study by Grieve and colleagues compared these different techniques using a multinational dataset comprising case-mix, resource use and cost data on 1757 stroke admissions from 13 centres in 10 European countries.[9] OLS and MLMs were used to estimate the effect of patient-level covariates, including patient characteristics (sex, age, prestroke living conditions), stroke severity measures (incontinence during the first week after stroke, dysphasia, paralysis at hospital admission), stroke subtype (cerebral infarction, intracerebral haemorrhage or unspecified stroke), centre-level co-variates (the level of health spending; the reimbursement system for acute hospital costs; the level of patient co-payment for acute care), the total length of hospital stay (LOS), and total cost. MLMs with normal and gamma distributions for the data within centres were compared. The results from the OLS model showed that both patient- and centre-level co-variates were associated with LOS and total cost. However, the results for the effects of patient-level variables from OLS regression models were incorrect because differences between centres are not accounted for in OLS regression. Therefore, the estimates from the MLMs showed that none of the centre-level characteristics were associated with LOS, and the level of spending on health was the centre-level variable most highly associated with total cost. The authors concluded that using OLS models for assessing international variation can lead to incorrect inferences, and that MLMs are more appropriate for assessing why resource use and costs vary across centres.

Checklists for assessing the generalisability of economic evaluations

Boxes 5.1 and 5.2 present checklists for assessing the generalisability of economic evaluations for empirical trial-based and decision-modelling studies, respectively.[20,31] The checklists are intended to be useful for decision makers using economic evaluations, but may also be useful for those planning or undertaking economic evaluations. If the principles suggested in the

Box 5.1 Checklist for assessing the generalisability of trial-based studies

- Are study sites representative of the jurisdiction(s) for which data are required?
- Are study sites (centres) randomly selected?
- Can data on centre characteristics be collected (e.g. bed occupancy levels)?
- Does the trial include a high proportion of the normal clinical caseload?
- Does the comparator therapy (to the technology of interest) represent current practice in the settings concerned?
- Is a wide range of user perspectives represented in the study?
- Are prices (unit costs) being collected separately from resource use data?
- Is a widely used generic instrument being used for quality of life (e.g. utility) measurement?
- Can regression-based techniques be used to obtain centre-specific measures of cost-effectiveness?

Adapted from Drummond et al,, 2005[31] and Sculpher & Drummond, 2006.[20,]

Box 5.2 Checklist for assessing the generalisability of decision-modelling studies

- Are the decision problem, the relevant settings and audiences (i.e. decision makers) clearly specified?
- Does the overall analytical approach incorporate the relevant perspectives (e.g. health service or societal) and relevant objective functions (e.g. maximizing health gain)?
- Are the data used to populate the model relevant to the target audiences (i.e. decision-makers) and settings?
- Where data from different sources are pooled, is this done in a way that the uncertainty relating to their precision and possible heterogeneity is adequately reflected?
- If data from other settings are used, have these been assessed for relevance in the settings of interest?
- Is uncertainty (i.e. parameter uncertainty and heterogeneity) adequately reflected in the model?
- Are results reported in a way that allows the assessment of the appropriateness of each parameter input and each assumption in the target settings?

Adapted from Drummond et al., 2005[31] and Sculpher & Drummond, 2006.[20]

checklists are followed by those conducting studies, it is likely that, over time, more economic evaluations will produce generalisable results.

In contrast to the body of work summarised above, some commentators have made the case that the generalisability of current economic evaluation methods is inherently flawed by the 'intervention-focused' approach of the methods, ignoring both the decision context and the epidemiological context, whereby the effectiveness of interventions is actually jointly produced by the combination of the underlying social determinants of health with the intervention (see also Chapters 3 and 13).[32–34]

Complexity and economic evidence

Since the publication of the 2000 UK Medical Research Council (MRC) guidance on developing and evaluating complex interventions, there has been a major ongoing debate on issues around methods to address complexity.[35–39] However, this debate has focused almost exclusively on evaluating the effectiveness of

complex interventions, with only two contributions by health economists on the implications for assessing their cost-effectiveness.[40,41]

Despite these contributions, the revised MRC guidance on complex interventions published in 2008 made very little mention of the implications for conducting (or synthesising) economic evaluations; it merely stated that evaluations of complex interventions should include an economic evaluation.[42] Crucially, the guidance does not indicate how the different dimensions of intervention complexity challenge existing methods for conducting an economic evaluation. Also, by repeating the conventional view that 'the main purpose of an economic evaluation is estimation rather than hypothesis testing', the guidance may unwittingly encourage the status quo. While disappointing, this is perhaps unsurprising. With the exception of the recent article by Shiell and colleagues, few attempts have been made to bridge the gap between methods of economic evaluation and the broader methodological debates about the definition and evaluation of complex interventions.[41]

Shiell and colleagues paper argues that 'As long as one can specify the inputs and outcomes with sufficient clarity to ensure that changes in resource use and benefits can be measured and valued, it is not necessary to understand the workings inside the box. This is important for describing what works and why, but not for evaluating cost-effectiveness'.[41] Yet if one acknowledges that evaluating effectiveness requires some (causal) understanding of *how* and *why* interventions are effective, this necessarily extends to evaluating and understanding cost-effectiveness (see Chapter 3). Furthermore, the argument that in order to estimate cost-effectiveness, we only need estimate 'what goes in' (resources) and 'what comes out' (outcomes) would only be valid if the sole purpose is to estimate the cost-effectiveness of an intervention *in a specific situation*. However, most evaluation has (or should have) the dual purpose of serving both the needs of the immediate programme managers/funders and aiming to add to the cumulative evidence base for others who might implement similar programmes in the future.

With more complex interventions, it becomes even harder to explain how a specific bundle of intervention components (and their associated resource use), provided in a given context, has generated the levels and types of outcomes measured. In areas of health care such as public health, where effectiveness is recognised as inherently more complex and contingent, it has become increasingly accepted that asking whether an intervention is 'effective' is of limited value; there is very rarely a clear answer to this question. It can confidently be predicted that complex interventions will work in some instances and not others, that it makes much more sense to ask from the beginning 'how and why' an intervention is or is not effective in different contexts, or when its components are configured or implemented in different ways.[43,44] These same insights need to be extended to the consideration of economic evidence more generally, as this book aims to do.

Relevance of evidence

When conducting an evidence synthesis, it is necessary to define what constitutes relevant evidence. Relevant evidence may vary not only across geographical regions and different conditions, but also according to who is making the decision on behalf of whom, and when. Using the example of a UK decision maker, a single UK-based economic evaluation conducted alongside an RCT may be the most relevant evidence. However, it is unlikely to be the only evidence; there may be estimates of treatment effect on surrogate outcomes, evidence from non-randomised studies, and so on, and inclusion of these different sources and types of evidence may lead to different results. Box 5.3 provides an example of how findings can be affected dramatically by the definition of relevance.[45]

But how are we to judge what evidence is relevant in making a decision in a given context? As highlighted at the outset of this chapter, context

---

Box 5.3 Example of the importance of defining relevance

Background

Chronic conditions account for around two-thirds of the global burden of disease, with 32% of the adult UK population suffering from a long-standing condition. Therefore policy makers wish to address the management of these conditions. In the UK, the National Health Service (NHS) policy for patients with chronic conditions who are at 'low risk' has been to encourage and support these individuals to 'self-care'.

However, until recently, the cost-effectiveness of interventions to support self-care was based on poorly conducted studies generating unreliable conclusions. In the last few years one particular intervention to support self-care, the Expert Patients Programme (EPP), has been rolled out across England and Wales, largely on the basis of studies conducted in the USA, and prior to evaluation in UK populations.

A single trial-based economic evaluation was subsequently conducted alongside a UK-based RCT. While this evaluation demonstrated that the EPP intervention was very likely to be cost-effective, this single trial-based analysis was not the only evidence addressing the decision problem nor did it incorporate all 'relevant' evidence. In this instance, data from other RCTs (one UK based) and other weaker experimental designs were available that could provide evidence relevant to the decision problem and the value of future research.

Aims

To assess the cost-effectiveness of one intervention designed to support self-care, the EPP, using a variety of alternative data sources. Also, to assess impact on the adoption decision, the uncertainty around the decision and the value of further research when evidence from alternative sources is included.

Methods

As some sources used an intermediate endpoint (self-efficacy) while others used final decision endpoints (cost and QALYs), it was necessary to use novel techniques to synthesise these data. The impact of considering alternative datasets as 'relevant' on the cost-effectiveness of the EPP intervention, the uncertainty around this decision and the value of future research were assessed using incremental cost-effectiveness ratios (ICERs), cost-effectiveness acceptability curves (CEACs) and value of information methods respectively.

Results

The single trial-based analysis concluded that the EPP was likely to be cost-effective with reduced costs and increased QALYs and a 97% probability of being cost-effective at a threshold QALY value of £30,000. However, synthesising these data with the other UK-based RCT increased both the ICER and the uncertainty around the decision (ICER £30,300 and probability of being cost-effective about 50% at £30K per QALY). Introducing additional data from non-UK, including non-randomised, studies reduced the ICER to £23,400 per QALY with a probability of the intervention being cost-effective of 68%.

Conclusions

The adoption decision, the uncertainty around that decision, and the value of conducting further research can be affected dramatically by the definition of relevance. Decision makers and analysts need to state *a priori* what evidence is considered to be relevant in the analysis

Adapted from Richardson, 2008.[45]

matters. But how are we to judge which aspects of context matter or not in a given set of circumstances? Decision makers are the appropriate people to decide what weight or importance to ascribe to each piece of evidence and which aspects of context matter.

The role of the analyst is to support the decision maker by providing scenarios that examine the impact of pivotal variables or data upon results. Therefore, the analyst has influence over the analyses presented but the decision as to which analysis influences policy is left to the legitimate decision maker. The point is that there is a decision maker with a role to judge these various aspects and, whilst researchers can contribute by making analyses explicit and identifying crucial variables, economic evaluation should be viewed as a part of the decision-making process rather than something that dictates which decision is to be made.

The relevance of systematic reviews previously published and unpublished health economic analyses (and those in other social sectors) remains limited in developing countries because most systematic reviews of evidence on effectiveness, cost and/or cost-effectiveness produced to date address health conditions that are priorities in the developed world.[46] Accordingly, the available reviews of this type focus on more recent, (generally) more expensive, 'higher-tech' technologies. One implication is that, within the Cochrane Collaboration, whose reviews are intended for audiences in both developed and developing countries, it is important to strengthen links between Cochrane Review Groups, the Cochrane Developing Countries Network and the Campbell and Cochrane Economics Methods Group. However, it should also be noted that the epidemiology of diseases has shifted substantially over recent years, with the result that many developing countries are now experiencing high burdens of non-communicable disease, as well as continuing high burdens of infectious diseases and injuries. Thus, the relevance of existing reviews may become greater, although not out of design.

The relevance of systematic reviews of evidence on effectiveness, cost and/or cost-effectiveness to developing countries is further limited by the relative dearth of primary research on relevant topics and settings, which is also of variable quality (see also Chapter 4). As such, there is clearly an overarching need to perform more primary empirical studies. However, even when relevant research is conducted in developing country settings, it might not be published or indexed. To address this situation with respect to economic analyses, ideally a database with a focus on analyses relevant to developing countries should be prepared, and made accessible to researchers and policy makers, that is akin to the Cost-Effectiveness Analysis Registry.[47]

Conclusion

Not only effectiveness but also the costs of (complex) interventions are strongly determined by contextual factors, the exact combination and 'dose' of intervention components, and the behavioural predispositions of participants or providers. We cannot generalise or transfer the results to other places unless we can explain what causes particular relationships between opportunity costs and outcomes in each setting. There are serious challenges to the potential to generalise results if all we have are evaluations that are essentially 'black-box': those which diligently measure and value the inputs and outcomes associated with an intervention, but do not address (or collect data on!) the reasons why particular combinations and amounts of resources produce particular patterns and levels of outcomes.

In conclusion, we need to develop and evaluate theories about how these relationships arise, and it is the tested theories that would become transferable across decision-making contexts rather than the results of economic analyses *per se.*

Acknowledgements

Other contributors to this chapter: Juntana Pattanaphesuj, Researcher, Health Intervention and Technology Assessment Program (HITAP), Ministry of Public Health, Thailand.

How this chapter should be cited

Walker DG, Teerawattananon Y, Anderson R, Richardson G. Chapter 5: Generalisability, transferability, complexity and relevance. In: Shemilt I, Mugford M, Vale L, Marsh K, Donaldson C (editors). *Evidence-based decisions and economics: health care, social welfare, education and criminal justice.* Oxford: Wiley-Blackwell, 2010.

References

1 Cooper N, Coyle D, Abrams K, Mugford M, Sutton A. Use of evidence in decision models: an appraisal of health technology assessments in the UK to date. *Journal of Health Services Research and Policy* 2005; 10: 245–250.

2 Murray CJL, Evans DB, Acharya A, Baltussen RMPM. Development of WHO guidelines on generalized cost-effectiveness analysis. *Health Economics* 2000; 9(3): 235–251.

3 World Health Organization. *CHOosing Interventions that are Cost Effective (WHO-CHOICE).* Geneva: World Health Organization, 2010. Available from: www.who.int/choice/en/.

4 Tan-Torres Edejer T, Baltussen RMPM, Adam T, *et al.* (eds). *Making Choices in Health: WHO guide to cost-effectiveness analysis.* Geneva: World Health Organization, 2003.

5 Currie G, Manns B. Glossary of terms for health economics and systematic review. In: Donaldson C, Mugford M, Vale L (eds) *Evidence-Based Health Economics: from effectiveness to efficiency in systematic review.* London: BMJ Books, 2002.

6 Antonanzas F, Rodríguez-Ibeas R, Juárez C, Hutter F, Lorente R, Pinillos M. Transferability indices for health economic evaluations: methods and applications. *Health Economics* 2009; 18(6): 629–643.

7 Anderson R. New MRC guidance on evaluating complex interventions: clarifying what interventions work by researching how and why they are effective. *British Medical Journal* 2008; 337(a1937): 944–945.

8 Spiegelhalter DJ, Best NG. Bayesian approaches to multiple sources of evidence and uncertainty in complex cost-effectiveness modelling. *Statistics in Medicine* 2003; 22(23): 3687–3709.

9 Grieve R, Nixon R, Thompson S, Cairns J. Multilevel models for estimating incremental net benefit in multinational studies. *Health Economics* 2007; 16(8): 815–826.

10 Manca A, Willan AR. Lost in translation: accounting for between-country differences in the analysis of multinational cost-effectiveness data. *Pharmacoeconomics* 2006; 24(11): 1101–1119.

11 Teerawattananon Y, Russell S. A difficult balancing act: policy actors' perspectives on using economic evaluation to inform health-care coverage decisions under the Universal Health Insurance Coverage Scheme in Thailand. *Value in Health* 2008; 11(suppl 1): S52–S60.

12 Teerawattananon Y, Vos T, Tangcharoensathien V, Mugford M. Cost-effectiveness of models for prevention of vertical HIV transmission – voluntary counseling and testing and choices of drug regimen. *Cost Effectiveness and Resource Allocation* 2005; 3: 7.

13 Sculpher MJ, Pang FS, Manca A, *et al.* Generalisability in economic evaluation studies in health care: a review and case studies. *Health Technology Assessment* 2004; 8(49): 1–192.

14 Goeree R, Burke N, O'Reilly D, Blackhouse G, Tarride J-E. Transferability of economic evaluations: approaches and factors to consider when using results from one geographic area for another. *Current Medical Research and Opinion* 2007; 23(4): 671–682.

15 Welte R, Feenstra T, Jager H, Leidl R. A decision chart for assessing and improving the transferability of economic evaluation results between countries. *Pharmacoeconomics* 2004; 22(13): 857–876.

16 Boulenger S, Nixon J, Drummond M, Ulmann P, Rice S, de Pouvourville G. Can economic evaluations be made more transferable? *European Journal of Health Economics* 2005; 6(4): 334–346.

17 Teerawattananon Y, Mugford M. Is it worth offering a routine laparoscopic cholecystectomy in developing countries? A Thailand case study. *Cost Effectiveness and Resource Allocation* 2005; 3: 10.

18 Tarn TY, Smith MD. Pharmacoeconomic guidelines around the world. *ISPOR Connections* 2004; 10: 5–15.

19 Gold MR, Siegel JE, Russell LB, Weinstein MC (eds). *Cost-Effectiveness in Health and Medicine*. New York: Oxford University Press, 1996.

20 Sculpher MJ, Drummond MF. Analysis sans frontieres: can we ever make economic evaluations generalisable across jurisdictions? *Pharmacoeconomics* 2006; 24(11): 1087–1099.

21 Kumaranayake L. The real and the nominal? Making inflationary adjustments to cost and other economic data. *Health Policy and Planning* 2000;15(2): 230–234.

22 Wordsworth S, Ludbrook A. Comparing costing results in across country economic evaluations: the use of technology specific purchasing power parities. *Health Economics* 2005; 14(1): 93–99.

23 Busse R, Schreyögg J, Smith PC. Variability in health care treatment costs amongst nine EU countries – results from the HealthBASKET project. *Health Economics* 2008; 17(suppl 1): S1–S8.

24 Schreyögg J, Tiemann O, Stargardt T, Busse R. Cross-country comparisons of costs: the use of episode-specific transitive purchasing power parities with standardised cost categories. *Health Economics* 2008; 17(suppl 1): S95–S103.

25 Shemilt I, Thomas J, Morciano M. A new web-based tool for adjusting costs to a common currency and price year. *Evidence and Policy*, in press.

26 Menzin J, Oster G, Davies L, *et al*. A multinational economic evaluation of rhDNase in the treatment of cystic fibrosis. *International Journal of Technology Assessment in Health care* 1996; 12(1): 52–61.

27 Jonsson B, Weinstein MC. Economic evaluation alongside multinational clinical trials. Study considerations for GUSTO IIb. *International Journal of Technology Assessment in Health care* 1997; 13(1): 49–58.

28 Shemilt I, Mugford M, Byford S, *et al*. Incorporating economics evidence. In: Higgins JPT, Green S (eds) *Cochrane Handbook for Systematic Reviews of Interventions*. Version 5.0.1 (updated September 2008). Oxford: Cochrane Collaboration, 2008.

29 Cook JR, Drummond M, Glick H, Heyse JF. Assessing the appropriateness of combining economic data from multinational clinical trials. *Statistics in Medicine* 2003; 22(12): 1955–1976.

30 Manca A, Rice N, Sculpher MJ, Briggs AH. Assessing generalisability by location in trial-based cost-effectiveness analysis: the use of multilevel models. *Health Economics* 2005;1 4(5): 471–485.

31 Drummond M, Manca A, Sculpher M. Increasing the generalizability of economic evaluations: recommendations for the design, analysis, and reporting of studies. *International Journal of Technology Assessment in Health care* 2005; 21(2): 165–171.

32 Birch S. As a matter of fact: evidence-based decision-making unplugged. *Health Economics* 1997; 6(6): 547–559.

33 Birch S, Gafni A. Evidence-based health economics. Answers in search of questions? In: Kristiansen IS, Mooney G (eds) *Evidence-Based Medicine in Its Place*. Adington: Routledge, 2004.

34 Birch S, Gafni A. Economics and the evaluation of health care programmes: generalisability of methods and implications for generalisability of results. *Health Policy* 2003; 64(2): 207–219.

35 MRC Health Services and Public Health Research Board. *A Framework for the Development and Evaluation of RCTs for Complex Interventions to Improve Health*. London: Medical Research Council, 2000.

36 Hawe P, Shiell A, Riley T. Complex interventions: how far 'out of control' should a randomised controlled trial be? *British Medical Journal* 2004; 328(7455): 1562–1563.

37 Hawe P, Shiell A, Riley T, Gold L. Methods for exploring implementation variation and local context within a cluster-randomised community intervention trial. *Journal of Epidemiology and Community Health* 2004; 58(9): 788–793.

38 Oakley A, Strange V, Bonell C, Allen E, Stephenson J. Process evaluation in randomised controlled trials of complex interventions. *British Medical Journal* 2007; 332(7538): 413–416.

39 Pawson R, Greenhalgh T, Harvey G, Walshe K. Realist review – a new method of systematic review designed for complex policy interventions. *Journal of Health Services Research and Policy* 2005; 10(suppl 1): S1:21–S1:34.

40 Byford S, Sefton T. Economic evaluation of complex health and social care interventions. *National Institute Economic Review* 2003; 186(1): 98–108.

41 Shiell A, Hawe P, Gold L. Complex interventions or complex systems? Implications for health economic evaluations. *British Medical Journal* 2008; 336(7656): 1281–1283.

42 Medical Research Council. *Developing and Evaluating Complex Interventions: new guidance*. London: Medical Research Council, 2008.

43 Jackson N, Waters E, for the Guidelines for Systematic Reviews in Health Promotion and Public Health Taskforce. Criteria for the systematic review of health promotion and public health interventions. *Health Promotion International* 2005; 20(4): 367–374.

44 Petticrew M, Roberts H. *Systematic Reviews in the Social Sciences: a practical guide*. Malden: Blackwell Publishing, 2006.

45 Richardson G. *Cost-effectiveness of interventions to support self care*. PhD thesis. York: University of York, 2008.

46 Chinnock P, Siegfried N, Clarke M. Is evidence-based medicine relevant to the developing world? *PLoS Medicine* 2005; 2(5): e107.

47 Centre for the Evaluation of Value and Risk in Health. *CEA Registry*. Boston: Tufts Medical Center, 2010. Available from: https://research.tufts-nemc.org/cear/Default.aspx.

CHAPTER 6

Equity, efficiency and research synthesis

David McDaid[1], Franco Sassi[2]

[1]LSE Health and Social Care and European Observatory on Health Systems and Policies, London School of Economics and Political Science, London, UK

[2]Directorate for Employment, Labour and Social Affairs, OECD – Organisation for Economic Co-operation and Development, Paris, France

Introduction

As described elsewhere in this volume, it is insufficient in a situation where resources are finite for evidence-informed practice and policy making simply to consider what works (see, *inter alia*, Chapters 1 to 4). We also need to be mindful of the context and costs. In a situation of limited resources, each decision to invest in an intervention or programme represents an opportunity foregone to invest these resources elsewhere. If our objective is to maximise health and/or other outcomes, such as educational attainment, crime reduction, social cohesion and so on, then it is clearly important that we take account of both the costs and consequences of different potential investment decisions.

This is where economic evaluation comes in. Economic evaluation can be used by decision makers to help assess the merits of such investment decisions. It is concerned with the opportunity costs of different actions, where opportunity costs represent the 'foregone benefits of the next best alternative use of the set of resources used to implement that action'.[1] Although many different approaches are available, in essence they all involve the comparison of the costs and outcomes of two or more interventions. The focus is on maximising efficiency, by allocating resources to different interventions in such a way

as to improve overall health or other social welfare benefits to society.

Of course, in policy making, such information on potential welfare gains is not considered in isolation; policy makers will always be interested in issues such as budgetary impact, acceptability to the local population, local political concerns, the need to safeguard human rights and, last but not least, the distributional impacts of investment decisions. It is this latter additional concern, which might also be thought of as the impact of resource allocation decisions on dimensions of equity within society, which is the focus of this chapter.

Inequalities in health status and other outcomes are widespread, persistent and, in many cases, increasing. A course of action that may appear to be a sensible strategy because of its effectiveness and cost-effectiveness may also have the consequence of increasing inequalities. Such trade-offs between equity and efficiency concerns require specific consideration as part of policy design and implementation processes. Thus it may be of great importance to address equity concerns within systematic reviews and economic evaluations of interventions in health care, social welfare, education and criminal justice.

After briefly describing what is meant by equity and illustrating how different interventions can have different distributional consequences, this chapter explores how the issue of equity has been addressed within economic evaluation and reflects on how equity concerns may be considered within systematic reviews and syntheses related to economic evaluations in different areas of health and social policy and practice.

Evidence-Based Decisions and Economics, 2nd edition. Edited by I. Shemilt, M. Mugford, L. Vale, K. Marsh and C. Donaldson. © 2010 Blackwell Publishing.

What do we mean by equity?

There are many different definitions of equity in the health care field alone.[2] In this chapter, we focus predominantly on inequalities in final health, social welfare, education or crime-related outcomes. Overall improvements in such outcomes for a whole population may mask significant variations between population subgroups. These variations may be indicated by socio-economic status, age, educational attainment, gender, ethnicity or a range of other co-variates.

Some individuals (or groups of individuals) may be more adept at benefiting from interventions than others, even where there are no obvious barriers to access to be overcome. This has been observed in studies which indicate that higher socio-economic groups are typically more likely to respond to health awareness messages compared to disadvantaged groups.[3] Factors such as perceived or real stigmatisation and discrimination can also play their part in reducing the use of services that may help to promote better final outcomes. For example, people with mental health problems may be reluctant to access services due to a fear of being identified with a mental health problem.[4] Geographical location may be influential too. For instance, whilst there is some evidence to suggest that restrictions on smoking may be effective in reducing smoking prevalence and tobacco consumption, health inequalities may be at risk of increasing if such restrictions were variably enforced in different geographical localities.[5]

However, not all inequalities in final outcomes may be viewed as unfair or inappropriate. For example, differences in educational status that may emerge as a result of a policy of selection and streaming may be seen as acceptable in some circumstances. It is therefore argued that efforts to ameliorate equity should focus on identifying and tackling what Dahlgren & Whitehead have viewed as avoidable inequalities in outcomes that society deems as being significant and unjust.[6]

Examples of policy actions aiming to tackle such inequalities in outcomes can be found in many different jurisdictions. For instance, the English government is pursuing initiatives to tackle health inequalities across the population following the publication of the report of the WHO Commission on the Social Determinants of Health.[7,8] The development of some criminal justice policies has also included goals to reduce inequalities in the rates of crime across a country.[9] In education, work has been undertaken to examine the impact of streaming and selection on long-term educational attainment, with one recent analysis suggesting that academic ability streaming reinforces educational attainment inequalities.[10] Another education-related example found in US research indicates that financial incentives provided to families to help them to relocate to better neighbourhoods have no demonstrable impact on inequalities in academic achievement.[11] Other recent educational research (a systematic review) has focused on the impact of early childhood education and care on social and cultural inequalities.[12] Indeed, many actions that include a focus on reducing inequalities may be intersectoral in nature; the prime objectives of early years education and childcare interventions may focus not only on equity in educational outcomes, but also on reducing childhood health inequalities and inequalities in rates of contact with the criminal justice system in later life.[13,14]

Therefore, when work is undertaken to determine whether interventions are effective, it may also be important to consider the equity impacts of investment in these interventions. If inequalities in outcomes such as health or education status are likely to arise, this may merit additional consideration of the costs and effectiveness of investing in mechanisms that help promote uptake of those interventions by disadvantaged segments of the population. Policy makers and practitioners, and those who support them, may also need to be mindful of the impact of inequalities in access to and/or utilisation of services. This may especially be the case when there is likely to be a long time lag between implementation of an intervention and its impact on social welfare outcomes. For example, in the field of public health, reductions in inequalities in the utilisation of services or in behaviour change across different population subgroups may be proxies for a reduction of inequalities in final health outcomes.

Examples of equity considerations

Social, financial and environmental factors may lead to considerable differences in both final outcomes and in access to services among different socio-economic groups and geographical communities.[8] This may indicate a need to examine upstream interventions (i.e. interventions that target the circumstances that produce adverse health behaviours or outcomes) in terms of planning and local infrastructures. But in general, the evidence base on the effectiveness of such upstream interventions in reducing inequalities remains limited, at least in the health care field.[15,16]

To date, research has tended to focus on more downstream interventions (i.e. interventions that aim to change adverse health behaviours or outcomes). For example, much work has been undertaken on the factors leading to differential rates of cancer by socio-economic and demographic characteristics, as well as the effectiveness of screening programmes in early diagnosis and treatment.[17,18] Differences in both the utilisation of screening programmes and outcomes may vary significantly according to ethnicity. For example, research in the US has reported inequalities in mortality rates from breast cancer for African American women compared to their white compatriots, despite the fact that their rates of screening, adjusted for socio-economic status, are now higher than those of white women.[18] Whilst rates of early diagnosis for breast cancer are also relatively low amongst African American women, another study suggests this may be attributable to these women perceiving their risks of cancer to be low, lower rates of contact with doctors, participation in more restrictive health insurance plans, a lack of cultural sensitivity by physicians, and the results of borderline screening tests being more often assumed to be negative compared to white women due to the lower prevalence rate for breast cancer in African American women.[19] Equally, studies which have investigated the uptake of universal cervical cancer screening programmes in Britain indicate that a greater level of benefits is attained by those in higher socio-economic groups and/or with higher levels of educational attainment.[20–22] Uptake rates of cervical screening can again be lower for some minority groups.[23]

For more complex actions, including those that require behavioural change, there may be significant equity concerns. Take, for instance, the example of interventions to increase participation in sporting activities as a way of improving health and well-being. Although assessments of cost-effectiveness have been conducted, there has been little attempt to gauge the equity concerns of these programmes.[24] Geographical areas of socio-economic deprivation may be less likely to have sports facilities and individuals living in such areas may have low levels of physical activity compared with the general population.[25] If access to gymnasiums and sports centres is associated with improved health outcomes for all the population, rather than predominantly for those already engaged in physical activity, questions to be considered may include geographical location, means-tested subsidies and investment in local transport infrastructure.

Thus, while economic evaluations may suggest that investing in an intervention is efficient and will increase overall social welfare, the distribution of gains in social welfare across society is not homogeneous. Some groups will gain more than others, while some may even see a decrease in welfare following implementation of an intervention that is deemed to be, overall, cost-effective. It therefore follows that even if a strategy appears cost-effective, if policy and practice also propose to address equity considerations, it is important to examine local contextual factors and to investigate the extent to which interventions need to be adapted to reach key population subgroups. In the case of the example of variations in US breast cancer diagnosis and mortality rates described above, this suggests it may be important to focus less on the aim of increasing overall rates of screening and more on identifying mechanisms to tailor screening programmes to increase uptake by high-risk women (such as those with a familial history of cancer), as well as improving the extent to which physicians follow guidance and ensure that diagnosis is undertaken in a timely fashion for minority groups.

Equity versus efficiency

In many cases, investing in actions intended to tackle inequalities across a population may be a cost-effective strategy. Indeed, as Sassi and colleagues have suggested, the national cervical cancer screening programme in England could have been at least as cost-effective if it had adopted a less extensive approach and focused instead on achieving a more equitable increase in cervical cancer screening rates across socio-economic groups.[26] This example demonstrates that the aims of equity and efficiency need not necessarily be at odds with each other. However, conversely, it does not follow that an intervention that appears cost-effective for the population as a whole will be as cost-effective for different population sub-groups. For example, recent work on interventions for smoking cessation suggests that these are more cost-effective for high socio-economic groups than those in low socio-economic groups.[27]

Let us consider the case of a hypothetical intervention that aims to improve health status by getting more people to swim regularly. In this illustration, the incremental cost per quality-adjusted life-year (QALY) gained of a nationally funded universal swimming programme (i.e. available to the whole population) is £20,000. In a country where a cost-effectiveness threshold of £30,000 per QALY gained is applied, this intervention would be considered to be a cost-effective use of resources and (subject to budgetary constraints) would be recommended for implementation. However, we are also interested in assessing the incremental cost-effectiveness of the same intervention in a specific population subgroup (e.g. a female ethnic minority population). When cost-effectiveness analysis is conducted for this subgroup alone, we find that the incremental cost per QALY gained is now £35,000. This figure is above our cost-effectiveness threshold and the intervention would not generally be considered to be a cost effective use of resources. However, if society wishes to avoid increasing inequalities in health outcomes, policy makers may be willing to trade off some loss in efficiency in order to invest more resources in ensuring that the intervention reaches the specific population subgroup. In such cases, it is important that the analyst is able to present potential differences in uptake, outcomes and cost-effectiveness for different population subgroups, in order to inform any policy and practice decisions.

What use has been made of equity within economic evaluations?

Despite its importance to policy makers, and much debate over the 'equity/efficiency trade-off' over many years (see, for example, Wagstaff, 1991[28]), there has been relatively little work to incorporate formal considerations of equity into health economic evaluations. Indeed, one review of health economic evaluations, albeit on studies published in between 1987 and 1997, reported 'a complete neglect for the equity dimension within studies surveyed'.[26] Moreover, the authors reported that these studies 'did not even provide enough information for decision makers to make their own judgments about the distributional impact of given policies – for example, on the characteristics of the population affected by the policy or on the policy's effectiveness and cost effectiveness in subgroups'.[26]

One implicit example of an equity judgement in health economic evaluation is the view that 'a QALY is a QALY is a QALY', which implies that each QALY carries the same weight regardless of the age, gender, health status or capacity to benefit of the individual to whom it accrues.[29] Explicit considerations of equity in health include disability weightings attached to an alternative measure of the value of health outcome, the disability-adjusted life-year (DALY), as well as the application of the 'rule of rescue', whereby in some settings there is positive discrimination in the use of resources towards individuals who need life-saving treatments regardless of whether the treatments are considered to be conventionally cost-effective (e.g. provision of renal dialysis).[30,31]

Research is ongoing (albeit dominated by health equity concerns) to investigate methods to explicitly value whether it is worth sacrificing some efficiency in order to promote equity gains.[32] It has been proposed for some time that equity weights could be incorporated into health economic evaluation.[33] Such weights could, for example, be constructed on the basis of information elicited from members of the public presented with a series of questions in respect of different equity/efficiency trade-offs.[27] Lindholm and colleagues were able to calculate the implicit relative weights assigned by Swedish policy makers to blue- and white-collar workers with regard to policies aimed at improving health: they pointed, on average, to a willingness to sacrifice about 15% of possible overall health gain to achieve a more equitable distribution of health gain.[34]

Formally addressing equity concerns within economic evaluations does not necessarily mean providing a quantitative synthesis between efficiency and equity indicators. Few weighting examples are available (especially outside health) and some commentators argue that such weights may make the results of economic evaluation less transparent and are undesirable.[35] For example, although some ethnic minorities may be among the most disadvantaged in society, the relevance of ethnicity as an equity dimension appears to vary by country in relation to cultural attitudes. Concerns may also be expressed in some societies over public attitudes towards other segments of the population, for instance in respect of sexual orientation, lifestyle, mental health status or religion.

Less sophisticated approaches that can be used include ensuring that information on current levels of inequality in respect of interventions under consideration is presented to decision makers, or that an analysis of incremental cost-effectiveness is undertaken for various population subgroups. Such an approach has been advocated by Sassi and colleagues, who have argued that it is unlikely that a robust health equity weighting system will be developed,[35] whilst Culyer has argued that equity concerns are best left to informed debate and consultation.[36]

Indeed, the agency responsible for producing guidance on the effectiveness and cost-effectiveness of health-related interventions in England and Wales, the National Institute for Health and Clinical Excellence (NICE), has developed recommendations in respect of social value judgements, following consultation with its layperson Citizen Council.[37] These recommendations recognise that NICE has a duty to take into account the impact of its guidance on health inequalities, and that its advisory bodies should seek to ensure that implementing NICE guidance will not widen existing inequalities.[37]

Increased interest in the evaluation of public health and health-promoting interventions, whose effectiveness will by nature often be dependent on individual changes in behaviour, also provides impetus for a more explicit consideration of the impacts of interventions on health inequalities. Although, to date, few economic evaluations of public health interventions have explicitly considered equity concerns, decision models constructed to aid in the public health intervention appraisal process at NICE can, to some extent, present outcomes for different population subgroups.[38,39] They can also take account of outcomes and costs other than health status; for example, in the case of smoking cessation in the workplace, the impact on workplace productivity was one additional outcome of interest.[40]

Outside the health and social care sector, economic evaluations may be more reliant on the cost-benefit analysis (CBA) approach, whereby measures of both costs and benefits are valued in monetary terms (see also Chapter 2). Traditionally, there have been only limited attempts to build equity concerns into CBAs.[41] One implicit way in which analysts have suggested that equity can be considered is through the use of techniques that adjust willingness to pay or willingness to accept values for specific interventions so as to avoid a situation in which those with lower incomes or budgets record lower values. Other approaches proposed by Pearce and colleagues are similar to those seen within the health arena: documenting and calculating how different intervention-related costs and benefits are distributed; making use of an implicit weighting system (e.g. if an intervention overall had net losses but net gains for a specific population target subgroup, what weight would have to be attached to the benefits so that the project overall had a net social benefit?); or calculating the net benefits of interventions based on explicit weights assigned to the costs and benefits incurred by different population subgroups.[41]

What does this mean for economic considerations in research synthesis?

As introduced in Chapters 2 and 3 of this volume, there are several ways in which systematic reviews may be conducted to inform a new economic analysis. In essence, these involve either explicit attempts to identify relevant economic evaluations for the interventions being evaluated as part of a systematic review and/or extracting relevant data on costs, resource utilisation, effects and values from relevant studies of effects, economic analyses and other sources to inform a secondary economic analysis (e.g. decision model).

As discussed above, there have been relatively few attempts to formally consider equity within and/or alongside economic evaluation, although methodological work (primarily in the health sector) continues. Of course, the primary focus of many interventions (e.g. housing improvements) is not primarily on reducing inequalities in outcomes and therefore collecting appropriate data may be challenging. This raises a fundamental issue, beyond the scope of this chapter, that there is the need for more primary research to be undertaken to evaluate the extent to which a range of policy interventions, such as improvements in the environment, housing and poverty alleviation, can help tackle underlying causes of inequality and thus address some of the social determinants of inequalities in social welfare outcomes.[15,42] However, notwithstanding these limitations of primary research to date, what are our requirements if we also wish to include equity considerations within systematic reviews and syntheses of research conducted to inform deliberations on the economic case for investment?

Information retrieval

An immediate challenge concerns information retrieval. If we are considering equity issues across several sectors, we may need to contend with large numbers of bibliographic databases and sources of grey literature. Comparatively few full economic evaluations are to be found in the applied fields of social welfare, education and criminal justice (see also Chapter 2).[43–47] Moreover, currently we are not aware of any specialist electronic literature databases of economic evaluations outside the field of health, which also cover some areas of social care (see also Chapter 7). Many bibliographic databases, perhaps especially (but not only) in non-health fields, do not provide structured keywords closely related to equity, economics or costs, making searches for relevant studies and data challenging.

Study participants in randomised controlled trials (RCTs) that typically form the mainstay of systematic reviews of effects may often exclude some of the target population groups that are potentially most vulnerable to widening inequalities. Identification of information on equity concerns is thus likely to require a broader search of the literature than might typically be used within a Cochrane or Campbell review. It has been argued that searches restricted to RCTs have the potential to exclude a proportion of relevant economic analyses (i.e. formal economic analyses not conducted alongside RCTs).[48] Intervention selection bias towards experimental studies has also been noted in reviews of complex upstream health-related interventions.[16] It is therefore important that searches

conducted for systematic reviews that include an aim to focus an 'equity lens' on interventions are sufficiently broad to retrieve a diverse range of qualitative, quantitative, geographical and epidemiological studies that may contain important information on the impact of interventions in tackling inequalities. One medium-term objective might be to establish a 'knowledge hub', perhaps within the Cochrane and Campbell Collaborations, to begin to compile a database of primary and secondary research relevant to equity in different health care, social welfare, education and criminal justice outcomes.

Data collection

To date, equity impact has rarely been documented in systematic reviews of studies of effects or in clinical guidelines.[15,49] This does not mean that equity-relevant information is not available, but rather that authors of reviews have failed to foresee the value of recording information on the distributional impacts of interventions. An analysis of Cochrane Musculoskeletal Group systematic reviews found that they have so far failed to document basic differences in health equity in terms of demographic and socio-economic factors, even when such information was available in primary studies.[50] Another review of smoking cessation studies, which found some evidence that smoking bans and youth access restrictions reduce social inequalities in smoking, was nevertheless restricted by differing contexts, leading to a recommendation for more explicit incorporation of equity in future reviews.[51]

Such limitations have provided the impetus for explicit discussion of equity within the Cochrane and Campbell Collaborations.[52] Subsequently, work has started on development of an international, systematic evidence base of the effectiveness of interventions in reducing socio-economic inequalities in health, as well as on conducting methodological research aiming to develop ways of better incorporating considerations of equity into systematic reviews.[53] There is a parallel need to build on recent moves towards collaborative work on considerations of both equity and economic aspects of systematic reviews.[54]

Augmenting existing equity checklists

Initial sources of evolving guidance on when and how to incorporate evidence on economic aspects of interventions into Cochrane and Campbell systematic reviews are already available.[55,56] This guidance does not yet specifically address equity concerns. However, as a basic minimum, the resource use and cost impacts of an intervention should be documented for specific population subgroups of interest (subject to the availability of such data in included studies), and not just the effect for the population as a whole. Sassi and colleagues list a number of basic items of information that should be provided if such a descriptive approach is adopted alongside a cost-effectiveness analysis (e.g. characteristics of the beneficiaries of a health intervention, costs and health impacts in different population groups, etc.).[35] Although economic evaluation is never value free, presenting a table of such information would avoid the analyst implicitly introducing their own social value judgements into assessment of the value of effects to different population subgroups.

If techniques that explicitly consider equity considerations are used, it will also be important not only to document their use within systematic reviews, but also to identify their features and limitations to aid judgement of the quality of such approaches. One starting point for methods research in this area, at least from a health perspective, may be to harness existing work on health utility estimation checklists (see also Chapter 8).[57] Detailed information from individual studies would also help with any proposed attempts to calculate equity impacts or potential equity/efficiency opportunity cost trade-offs.[38]

In addition, a pragmatic approach that could be adopted when undertaking research synthesis within the context of systematic reviews would be to make use of a context and equity checklist for data collection and assessment of published and unpublished economic evaluations. Such a checklist would at least provide end-users of reviews with information on the extent to which equity issues are explicitly considered within included studies. Documenting contextual information may also aid in the consideration of issues of generalisability and transferability (see also, *inter alia*, Chapters 3, 5 and 13). This could include documentation of any weighting methods used and might potentially be complemented by subsequent modelling of the cost-effectiveness of an intervention for different population subgroups (see the next section of this chapter).

Within the Cochrane and Campbell Collaborations, a joint equity group has already adapted the PROGRESS framework (PROGRESS refers to various groups vulnerable to inequity by virtue of Place of residence, Race, Occupation, Gender, Religion, Education, Socio-economic status, and Social network and capital) to make available a 14-item equity checklist for systematic review authors (see Box 6.1).[58,59]

Box 6.1 Equity checklist for systematic review authors[59]

Title registration
Objectives
Eq-1. Is there potential for differences in relative effects between advantaged and disadvantaged populations?

Eq-2. Are interventions likely to be aimed at the disadvantages?

Protocol
Search strategy
Eq-3. Will your search include databases relevant for health equity?

Eq-4. Will your search strategy include terms and concepts relevant for health equity?

Eq-5. Will your search strategy avoid using limits (such as language, age) that could miss relevant literature for health equity?

Methods
Eq-6. Will inclusion/exclusion criteria and data extraction use structured methods to access dimensions of disadvantage (e.g. socio-economic status, gender, race, etc.)?

Eq-7. Will you conduct a process evaluation that considers the disadvantaged?

Eq-8. Will you conduct subgroup analyses across dimensions of disadvantage where appropriate?

Review
Description of studies; characteristics of included studies/characteristics of excluded studies
Eq-9. Could the included studies bias the generalisability to disadvantaged populations (e.g. restrictive exclusion criteria)?

Continued on p.74

Eq-10. Did you appropriately describe sociodemographics (e.g. socio-economic status, gender, race, etc.), given the details in the included studies?

Eq-11. Did you describe the social context in each study?

Methodological quality of included studies
Eq-12. Did you describe the sociodemographic characteristics of withdrawals and dropouts?

The results
Eq-13. Did you conduct subgroup analyses across categories of disadvantage where appropriate?

Eq-14. If subgroups were analysed, did you interpret the results appropriately, given statistical power?

Reviewers' conclusions
Implications for practice
Eq-15. Did you consider potential implications for health equity?

Implications for research
Eq-16. Did you identify whether there are research needs specific to promoting health equity?

Whilst this checklist focuses solely on variations in health outcomes, it could be further adapted to take account of additional issues relevant to economic analysis, and for primary and economic outcomes in other applied fields, such as social welfare, education and criminal justice. In addition to documenting whether equity issues can be identified within a systematic review, Box 6.2 provides some examples of additional questions that might be built into such a checklist to aid in economic analysis. There may also be scope for the adaptation of established economic evaluation checklists to include explicit consideration of the quality of approaches used to elicit equity weights and other distributional issues.[60,61]

Making use of contextual analysis to inform decision modelling
Economic methods guidance already notes that 'review authors should avoid attempting to draw definitive conclusions regarding the cost-effectiveness of interventions on the basis of a critical review of

Box 6.2 Examples of economic considerations that could potentially be incorporated into an equity checklist

- Are distributional issues discussed appropriately?[61]
- Where cost-effectiveness is reported, is this reported for different population subgroups? Is there any discussion of equity versus efficiency issues?
- Are differences in resource utilisation and/or costs reported separately for different population subgroups?
- Are the costs and/or resource use of any specific mechanisms used to promote increased uptake of the interventions documented?
- Is there an assessment of the resources required and/or costs of adapting interventions for implementation in different contexts?
- Are the costs and consequences of unintended effects of interventions documented?
- If equity weights are used in the analysis, what specific methods were used to derive these weights?
- In eliciting information for equity weights:
  - What framing effects can be identified?
  - What are the characteristics of the population sample?
  - Were study participants blinded to knowledge of whether they would or would not be in future need of intervention?
- Where feasible, estimate the potential incremental cost-effectiveness of targeting intervention at specific subgroups of interest. What potential outcome gains may be sacrificed if a more equitable approach (e.g. targeting versus universal provision) were implemented?

economics studies'.[55] This is important since the circumstances in which evidence have been generated may be very different from the settings in which an intervention is to be implemented. As highlighted elsewhere in this volume, understanding context is another key issue for systematic reviews (see, *inter alia*, Chapters 3–5, 10 and 13). The extent to which the context in which an intervention is delivered will impact on the generalisability and transferability of evidence on its costs, effects and distributional impacts will clearly vary from intervention to intervention. However, the delivery context is likely to be of greater importance as levels of intervention complexity and reliance on behaviour change increase. Thus, by incorporating contextual concerns into economic analysis, we can better understand some of the equity implications of interventions.

Approaches such as decision modelling might be used to help explore the impact of different contexts on both the equity of outcomes and cost-effectiveness. A checklist that helps capture some of the principal contextual factors might be used by those creating decision models to estimate potential differential equity and economic impacts. Recent work on the development checklists for the critical appraisal of public health interventions may be one tool to adapt for use in assessing the importance of contextual factors in other applied fields.[62]

Decision models developed using information identified from such checklists could help to identify whether significant adaptations will be needed (e.g. when implementing education-based interventions in England that may have been developed in the very different US educational system) or, in situations where there is insufficient training and capacity within a country to implement a new intervention, what the costs of scaling this up might be. Information from an equity audit on the extent to which inequalities exist and/or interventions are targeted at reducing inequalities can also help determine whether it may be necessary to invest additional time and resources in building decision models that take equity issues into consideration.

For interventions where context and equity considerations make an important difference, decision models might then be constructed to assess cost-effectiveness to different population subgroups. For example, a decision model developed using a simple decision tree structure (see Chapter 2) might include scenario pathways that investigate different approaches to adapting interventions for implementation in different settings. Such models could also examine how uptake and use of an intervention might be influenced by the use of additional mechanisms, such as financial incentives or media campaigns, and so on. Decision models could also provide some projections of the costs and consequences of scaling up an intervention from a pilot initiative to a nationwide programme.

Conclusions

Equity concerns, alongside efficiency, can be key factors to consider in both systematic reviews of economic analyses and those of studies of effects, which may also be used to help inform the development of decision models. Policy actions intended to help reduce inequalities between different subgroups in society can be identified in the health care, social welfare, education and criminal justice sectors alike. However, to date, systematic reviews and economic evaluations have largely avoided analysis of the implications of interventions on equity in outcomes between different subgroups.

Some cost-effective interventions will help promote equity and may indeed be designed to target specific population subgroups, but others may widen inequalities because of differential rates of uptake or capacity to benefit between different subgroups. Different societies may be willing to give up some levels of efficiency gains in order to target more resources at specific population subgroups, with the explicit aim of seeking to reduce (or at least not widen) health inequalities.

The interest shown in equity concerns by contributors to the Cochrane and Campbell Collaborations is one recognition of the need to think about the distributional impacts of interventions. This should also be of concern to those interested in undertaking economic analysis as part of, or building upon, the systematic review process. One area for action is to conduct more reviews of the effectiveness and potential cost-effectiveness of interventions, both within specific sectors as well as in respect of complex interventions further upstream, which may have subsequent impacts on inequalities in different outcomes, such as health status and level of educational attainment. Work in respect of the latter group of interventions remains limited, perhaps in part because evidence of effects is required from a range of study designs that go beyond comparative effectiveness research.

A second step is to systematically develop procedures to build considerations of equity into existing methods that critically appraise economic evidence identified in studies within systematic reviews. The importance of equity issues will vary between reviews depending on the nature of the interventions being assessed. Reviewers may need to make a pragmatic judgement as to whether equity issues thus merit concern. One pragmatic means of achieving this would be to make use of the current equity checklist highlighted in this chapter. This could be augmented to include some questions with a specific economic focus. Information might then be presented to decision makers on the equity implications of interventions and also used to inform new decision models.

Methodological work to develop equity weights within economic evaluations continues but caution is required here. Research appears to focus largely on health inequalities rather than other social welfare, education or criminal justice outcomes, no accepted weighting mechanism is as yet available, and not all public preferences may be socially desirable. However, should such techniques become more accepted, quality assessment tools for economic evaluation may also need to be modified to include more in-depth appraisal of methods used in economic evaluations to address distributional issues, including details of methods used to elicit equity weights.

Context checklists may also help in identifying the need for local adaptation of interventions in different settings. Collating information in this way might then allow economists, working in partnership with colleagues more conversant with contextual issues, to create decision models on the basis of material derived from reviews that take account of some equity-related concerns, such as the need for investment in different engagement mechanisms to increase uptake of interventions to reach different population subgroups.

Tackling inequalities is a complex business and many factors contribute to such inequalities. Whilst the appraisal of equity implications within reviews may necessarily be limited by resources and methodological developments, it is nonetheless essential to more routinely highlight their importance alongside efficiency issues in analysis of systematic reviews.

Acknowledgements
Other contributors to this chapter: Francesca Borgonovi, Analyst, Organisation for Economic Co- operation and Development, Paris, France.

How this chapter should be cited
McDaid D, Sassi F. Chapter 6: Equity, efficiency and research synthesis. In: Shemilt I, Mugford M, Vale L, Marsh K, Donaldson C (editors). *Evidence-based decisions and economics: health care, social welfare, education and criminal justice*. Oxford: Wiley-Blackwell, 2010.

References

1 Drummond MF, Sculpher MJ, Torrance GW, O'Brien BJ, Stoddart GL. *Methods for the Economic Evaluation of Health care Programmes*, 3rd edn. Oxford: Oxford University Press, 2005.

2 Macinko JA, Starfield B. Annotated bibliography on equity in health, 1980–2001. *International Journal for Equity in Health* 2002; 1(1): 1–20.

3 Sassi F, Hurst J. *The Prevention of Lifestyle-Related Chronic Diseases: an economic framework (OECD Health Working Papers No. 32)*. Paris: Organisation for Economic Co- operation and Development, 2008.

4 Demyttenaere K, Bruffaerts R, Posada-Villa J, *et al.,* for the WHO World Mental Health Survey Consortium. Prevalence, severity, and unmet need for treatment of mental disorders in the World Health Organization World Mental Health Surveys. *Journal of the American Medical Association* 2004; 291(21): 2581–2590.

5 Tocque K, Edwards R, Fullard B. The impact of partial smokefree legislation on health inequalities: evidence from a survey of 1150 pubs in North West England. *BMC Public Health* 2005; 5(91).

6 Dahlgren G, Whitehead, M. *Policies and Strategies to Promote Social Equity in Health*. Stockholm: Institute of Futures Studies, 1991.

7 Department of Health. *Post-2010 Strategic Review of Health Inequalities (Marmot Review)*. London: Department of Health, 2009.

8 Commission on Social Determinants of Health. *Closing the Gap in a Generation: health equity through actions on the social determinants of health*. Geneva: World Health Organization, 2008.

9 Grover C. *Crime and Inequality*. Uffculme: Willan Publishing, 2008.

10 Kirabo-Jackson C. *Ability-Grouping and Academic Inequality: evidence from rule-based student assignments*. Cambridge, MA: National Bureau of Economic Research, 2009.

11 DeLuca S. All over the map: explaining educational outcomes of the Moving to Opportunity program. *Education Next* 2007; 4: 29–36.

12 Leseman P. The impact of high quality education and care on the development of young children: review of the literature. In: Eurydice Network (eds) *Early Childhood Education and Care in Europe: tackling social and cultural inequalities*. Brussels: Education, Audiovisual and Culture Executive Agency, European Commission, 2009.

13 Belfield CR, Nores M, Barnett S, Schweinhart L. The High/Scope Perry Preschool Program: cost-benefit analysis using data from the age-40 follow-up. *Journal of Human Resources* 2006; 41(1): 162–190.

14 Halliday J, Asthana S. From evidence to practice: addressing health inequalities through Sure Start. *Evidence and Policy* 2007; 3(1): 31–45.

15 Waters E, Petticrew M, Priest N, Weightman A, Harden A, Doyle J. Evidence synthesis, upstream determinants and health inequalities: the role of a proposed new Cochrane Public Health Review Group. *European Journal of Public Health* 2008; 18(3): 221–223.

16 Petticrew M, Roberts H. Systematic reviews – do they 'work' in informing decision-making around health inequalities? *Health Economics, Policy and Law* 2008; 3(2): 197–211.

17 Shack L, Jordan C, Thomson CS, Mak V, Moller H. Variation in incidence of breast, lung and cervical cancer and malignant melanoma of skin by socioeconomic group in England. *BMC Cancer* 2008; 8(271).

18 Smith-Bindman R, Miglioretti DL, Lurie N, *et al*. Does utilization of screening mammography explain racial and ethnic differences in breast cancer? *Annals of Internal Medicine* 2006; 144(8): 541–543.

19 Sassi F, Luft HS, Guadagnoli E. Reducing racial/ethnic disparities in female breast cancer: screening rates and stage at diagnosis. *American Journal of Public Health* 2006; 96(12): 2165–2172.

20 Moser K, Patnick J, Beral V. Inequalities in reported use of breast and cervical screening in Great Britain: analysis of cross sectional survey data. *British Medical Journal* 2009; 338(b025): 1480–1484.

21 Currin LG, Jack RH, Linklater KM, Mak V, Moller H, Davies EA. Inequalities in the incidence of cervical cancer in South East England 2001–2005: an investigation of population risk factors. *BMC Public Health* 2009; 9(62).

22 Sabates R, Feinstein L. The role of education in the uptake of preventative health care: the case of cervical screening in Britain. *Social Science and Medicine* 2006; 62(12): 2998-3010.

23 Webb R, Richardson J, Esmail A, Pickles A. Uptake for cervical screening by ethnicity and place-of-birth: a population-based cross-sectional study. *Journal of Public Health* 2004; 26(3): 293–296.

24 Hagberg LA, Lindholm L. Is promotion of physical activity a wise use of societal resources? Issues of cost-effectiveness and equity in health. *Scandinavian Journal of Medicine and Science in Sports* 2005; 15(5): 304–312.

25 Panter J, Jones A, Hillsdon M. Equity of access to physical activity facilities in an English city. *Preventive Medicine* 2008; 46(4): 303–307.

26 Sassi F, Le Grand J, Archard L. Equity versus efficiency: a dilemma for the NHS. *British Medical Journal* 2001; 323(7316): 762–763.

27 Dolan P, Bekker H, Brennan A, *et al. The Relative Importance Attached to Access, Equity and Cost-Effectiveness by People and Organisations Providing Health Services*. London: NHS Service Delivery and Organisation, 2006.

28 Wagstaff A. QALYs and the equity–efficiency trade-off. *Journal of Health Economics* 1991; 10(1): 21–41.

29 Rawlins MD, Culyer AJ. National Institute for Clinical Excellence and its value judgments. *British Medical Journal* 2004; 329(7459): 224–227.

30 Murray CJL, Lopez AD. *The Global Burden of Disease*. Geneva: World Health Organization, Harvard School of Public Health, World Bank, 1996.

31 Cookson R, McCabe C, Tsuchiya A. Public health care resource allocation and the Rule of Rescue. *Journal of Medical Ethics* 2008; 34(7): 540–544.

32 Williams AH, Cookson RA. Equity–efficiency trade-offs in health technology assessment. *International Journal of Technology Assessment in Health care* 2006; 22(1): 1–9.

33 Nord E, Pinto J-L, Richardson J, Menzel P, Ubel P. Incorporating societal concerns for fairness in numerical valuations of health programmes. *Health Economics* 1999; 8(1): 25–39.

34 Lindholm L, Rosen M, Emmelin M. How many lives is equity worth? A proposal for equity adjusted years of life saved. *Journal of Epidemiology and Community Health* 1998; 52(12): 808–811.

35 Sassi F, Archard L, Le Grand J. Equity and the economic evaluation of health care. *Health Technology Assessment* 2001; 5(3): 1–138.

36 Culyer AJ. NICE's use of cost effectiveness as an exemplar of a deliberative process. *Health Economics, Policy and Law* 2006; 1(3): 299–318.

37 National Institute for Health and Clinical Excellence. *Social Value Judgements. Principles for the development of NICE guidance*, 2nd edn. London: National Institute for Health and Clinical Excellence, 2008.

38 Cookson R, Drummond M, Weatherley H. Explicit incorporation of equity considerations into economic evaluation of public health interventions. *Health Economics, Policy and Law* 2009; 4(3): 231–245.

39 National Institute for Health and Clinical Excellence. *Methods for the Development of NICE Public Health Guidance*, 2nd edn. London: National Institute for Health and Clinical Excellence, 2009.

40 National Institute for Health and Clinical Excellence. *Workplace Health Promotion: how to help employees to stop smoking*. London: National Institute for Health and Clinical Excellence, 2007.

41 Pearce D, Atkinson G, Mourato S. *Cost Benefit Analysis and The Environment: recent developments*. Paris: Organisation for Economic Co-operation and Development, 2006.

42 Shiell A. Still waiting for the great leap forward. *Health Economics, Policy and Law* 2009; 4(2): 255–260.

43 Shemilt I, Mugford M. Including economic perspectives and evidence in Campbell reviews to inform policy and practice: a critical review of current approaches. *Evidence and Policy* 2009; 5(3): 229–246.

44 Sefton TAJ, Byford S, McDaid D, Hills J, Knapp M. *Making the Most of It. Economic evaluation in the social welfare field*. York: Joseph Rowntree Foundation, 2002.

45 Levin HM. Waiting for Godot: costeffectiveness analysis in education. In: Light RJ (ed) *Evaluation Findings That Surprise: new directions for evaluation*. San Francisco: Jossey-Bass, 2001.

46 Marsh K, Chalfin A, Roman J. What does cost-benefit analysis add to decision making? Evidence from the criminal justice literature. *Journal of Experimental Criminology* 2008; 4(2): 117–135.

47 Swaray RB, Bowles R, Pradiptyo R. The application of economic analysis to criminal justice interventions: a review of the literature. *Criminal Justice and Policy Review* 2005; 16(2): 141–163.

48 Shemilt I, Mugford M, Byford S, *et al. Where does economics fit in? A review of economics in Cochrane reviews*. Oral paper presentation at the XV Cochrane Colloquium, Sao Paolo, Brazil, 23–27 October, 2007.

49 Dans AM, Dans L, Oxman AD, *et al.* Assessing equity in clinical practice guidelines. *Journal of Clinical Epidemiology* 2007; 60(6): 540–546.

50 Tugwell P, Maxwell L, Welch V, *et al.* Is health equity considered in systematic reviews of the Cochrane Musculoskeletal Group? *Arthritis and Rheumatism* 2008; 59(11): 1603–1610.

51 Main C, Thomas S, Ogilvie D, *et al.* Population tobacco control interventions and their effects on social inequalities in smoking: placing an equity lens on existing systematic reviews. *BMC Public Health* 2008; 8(178).

52 Tugwell P, Petticrew M, Robinson V, Kristjansson E, Maxwell L, for the Cochrane Equity Field Editorial Team. Cochrane and Campbell Collaborations, and health equity. *Lancet* 2006; 367(9517): 1128–1130.

53 Cochrane Health Equity Field-Campbell Equity Methods Group. *Cochrane Health Equity Field*. Oxford: Cochrane Collaboration, 2010. Available from: http://equity.cochrane.org/en/index.html.

54 Campbell and Cochrane Economics Methods Group and Cochrane Health Equity Field-Campbell Equity Methods Group. *Economics and equity in health care: current perspectives and evidence*. Special session at the XVI Cochrane Colloquium, Freiburg, Germany, 3–7 October, 2008.

55 Shemilt I, Mugford M, Byford S, *et al.* Incorporating economics evidence. In: Higgins JPT, Green S (eds) *Cochrane Handbook for Systematic Reviews of Interventions*. Version 5.0.1 (updated September 2008). Oxford: Cochrane Collaboration, 2008.

56 Shemilt I, Mugford M, Byford S, *et al. Campbell Collaboration Methods Policy Brief: economics methods.* Oslo: Campbell Collaboration, 2008.

57 Brazier J, Deverill M. A checklist for judging preference-based measures of health related quality of life: learning from psychometrics. *Health Economics* 1999; 8(1): 41–51.

58 Evans T, Brown H. Road traffic crashes: operationalizing equity in the context of health sector reform. *International Journal of Injury Control and Safety Promotion* 2003; 10(1–2): 11–12.

59 Ueffing E, Tugwell P, Welch V, Petticrew M, Kristjansson E, Cochrane Health Equity Field. *C1, C2 Equity Checklist for Systematic Review Authors*. Ottawa: Cochrane Health Equity Field, 2010. Available from: www.equity.cochrane.org/Files/equitychecklist.pdf.

60 Drummond MF, Jefferson TO, on behalf of the BMJ Economic Evaluation Working Party. Guidelines for authors and peer reviewers of economic submissions to the BMJ. *British Medical Journal* 1996; 313(7052): 275–283.

61 Evers S, Goossens M, de Vet H, van Tulder M, Ament A. Criteria list for assessment of methodological quality of economic evaluations: Consensus on Health Economic Criteria. *International Journal of Technology Assessment in Health care* 2005; 21(2): 240–245.

62 Heller RF, Verma A, Gemmell I, Harrison R, Hart J, Edwards R. Critical appraisal for public health: a new checklist. *Public Health* 2008; 122(1): 92–98.

CHAPTER 7

Searching for evidence for cost-effectiveness decisions

Julie Glanville[1], Suzy Paisley[2]

[1]York Health Economics Consortium, University of York, York, UK
[2]School of Health and Related Research, University of Sheffield, Sheffield, UK

Introduction

High-quality evidence is required to inform decision making. The information used to support the development of decision models also needs to be well sourced and reliable. Efficient and transparent searching is central to the tasks of both reviewing economic evaluations and creating new decision models. However, specifying information needs, preparing search strategies and selecting the resources to search differ depending on which of these two tasks is being undertaken.

This chapter describes current approaches to searching for (full) economic evaluations (cost-effectiveness analyses, cost-benefit analyses and cost-utility analyses) and for identifying evidence to support the development of new decision models. Approaches to identifying other forms of economic study, such as comparative effectiveness research presenting studies of resource or service use data, cost-of-illness studies and econometric studies, are not included. Studies of economic interventions (such as pricing and purchasing polices, financial incentives or reimbursement policies) are also excluded, but can be identified by using the search approaches used for other interventions in health care, social welfare, education or criminal justice.[1–3]

This chapter begins with a description of current approaches to searching for economic evaluations as

part of the research process of reviewing such studies and lists selected key resources and guidance. It then describes the different approaches required for identifying high-quality evidence to support the development of new decision models.

The examples and evidence used in this chapter mostly stem from health care information retrieval. In part, this reflects the relative dearth of economic evidence relating to social welfare, education and criminal justice.[4] It also reflects the developmental stage of methods for evidence identification to support economic evaluations in those areas. Organisations such as the Campbell Collaboration, the EPPI-Centre and the NICE Centre for Public Health Evidence in the UK are all involved in the development of search methods to support economic decisions.

We explore the published evidence base that informs search approaches to identifying economic evaluations and high-quality evidence to support the development of new decision models. Ongoing research is described and areas where further research would be helpful are highlighted. We argue for a systematic approach to the development of search strategies: capturing relevant search concepts, using relevant resources and combining search terms effectively. Finally, we recommend transparency in reporting search processes and sources of studies and data.

Reviews of economic evaluations

Identifying and assessing published and unpublished economic studies as part of a systematic review

Evidence-Based Decisions and Economics, 2nd edition. Edited by I. Shemilt, M. Mugford, L. Vale, K. Marsh and C. Donaldson. © 2010 Blackwell Publishing.

may be required if the review includes a primary or secondary focus on such studies. For example, if a systematic review of interventions specifies measures of resource use, costs and/or cost-effectiveness amongst target outcome measures, possibly alongside measures of beneficial and adverse effects, then a search for economic evaluations is required. The search approach used to identify evidence for systematic reviews tends to emphasise sensitivity, seeking to identify as many relevant published and unpublished studies as possible (specific to the question and within available resources) to minimise potential bias.[1-3]

The search process has two main elements: capturing the search question in a structured search strategy (a set of search terms) and applying the search strategy to a range of resources expected to yield economic evaluations. Obtaining the input of an experienced information professional or librarian to develop and conduct the search is recommended by systematic review methods guidance.[1-3]

Capturing the search question

Searches for economic evaluations to inform systematic reviews are likely to be conducted at one point in time, sometimes with an update search towards the end of the review process. Alternatively, it is possible to set up regular automatic alerts as new relevant records are added to databases.[2] The search terms used in the search strategy are likely to be those developed for the main topic of the review: the subject search. The subject search question is often structured into concepts using the PICO convention, which specifies the population(s), intervention(s), comparator(s) and outcome(s) of interest.[1,2,5] If the search is undertaken in a specialist economics resource, additional economic search terms may not be required. However, if the search is being undertaken in a general database, the subject search may be combined with search terms to capture economic concepts.[1,3,5,6] The size of the economics literature within a specific database may also influence the choice of concepts.

Box 7.1 presents an example of a (non-exhaustive) search strategy to find economic evaluations of traffic-calming measures to reduce road traffic accidents. Two PICO concepts are operationalised in the search: the concept of road traffic accidents (PICO outcome concept in sets 1–4) and the traffic-calming measures (PICO intervention concept in sets 6–7).

Box 7.1 Example search for economic evaluations of traffic-calming measures in Medline

1. Accidents, Traffic/
2. (traffic adj6 (accident$ or incident$)).ti,ab.
3. (road$ adj6 (accident$ or death$)).ti,ab.
4. exp Motor Vehicles/ and Accidents/
5. 1 or 2 or 3 or 4
6. (traffic adj3 calm$).ti,ab.
7. (speed adj3 (bump$ or limit$ or restrict$ or zone$)).ti,ab.
8. 6 or 7
9. economics/
10. exp "costs and cost analysis"/
11. exp "economics, hospital"/
12. economics, medical/
13. economics, nursing/
14. (economic$ or cost or costs or costly or costing or price or prices or pricing or pharmacoeconomic$).ti,ab.
15. (expenditure$ not energy).ti,ab.
16. (value adj1 money).ti,ab.
17. budget$.ti,ab.
18. or/9–17
19. 5 and 8 and 18

Key

Exp	Explode subject heading (identifies all more specific terms 'below' the heading)
/	Subject heading
Adj6	Terms must be within 6 words of each other
$	Truncation symbol to identify words with the same stem
.ti,ab.	Searches title and abstract
Or/1–3	Set combination: 1 or 2 or 3

The economic evaluation concept is captured in sets 9–17. The records which contain all three concepts are identified by combining the concept set numbers using the AND operator (see line 19 of Box 7.1). The choice of which PICO concepts feature in the search strategy is reached through iterative testing, using different combinations of concepts and assessing how many relevant records may be lost or gained in different combinations. Few search strategies use all the PICO concepts, because the use of four concepts in a search is very stringent given the amount of data available to be searched in database records.

Search terms need to be adapted to the different resources in which the strategy will be run, to reflect differences in database indexing, and database interface search commands and syntax. Focusing the search strategy onto economic evaluations can be achieved by using relevant available search filters. Search filters are collections of search terms developed to capture specific themes such as study design. Search filters can be developed using a range of research-based and other methods and there is currently no agreed standard approach.[7–9] For example, filters may be developed by analysing records from reference standards or by collecting search terms from experts. Filter performance in finding relevant records may be tested against reference standards in various ways. Finally, filter performance may be validated on further reference standards and compared to the performance of other filters.

The example search strategy in Box 7.1 incorporates an abbreviated version of the NHS Economic Evaluation Database (NHS EED) search filter for Medline.[10] Although many economic search filters are available, few have been extensively validated and there is currently little recent evidence on the comparative performance of the available filters to assist in choosing between them.[11–15]

Anecdotal reports from information professionals note that economic filters for biomedical databases tend to be as sensitive (i.e. retrieving a large proportion of the available relevant records) as some other study design filters, such as those for randomised controlled trials, but also imprecise (i.e. retrieving many irrelevant records). However, search filter imprecision may reflect imprecision about and within the target records. First, there is a lack of agreement about which specific study designs fall within the set 'economic evaluations' and also lack of agreement on the specific study design terms used to describe types of economic evaluation with specific sets of features, such as cost-benefit analysis and cost-effectiveness analysis. This lack of agreement means that search filter designers may have to overcompensate.[13,14] It also means that researchers and information professionals need to be clear about what they are seeking when preparing a search or using a filter. There is also the potential for mismatch between researchers' definitions and the indexing applied by database producers. For example, Medline indexes records containing all types of economic evaluations under a single term 'Cost-Benefit Analysis' despite the fact that many economists would consider that the term is assigned inaccurately. With all this uncertainty and the need to compensate in the search terms used, search results may be more numerous than desired. Second, some authors may not report their methods clearly, as noted in many abstracts in the NHS EED database.[15] Finally, the availability of indexing terms provided by database producers may not result in their consistent application by indexers. This means that search filters may not be able to benefit from sensitive but precise indexing and may, as a consequence, underperform in terms of precision.[11–14] As a result, a high proportion of irrelevant records may need to be processed to identify relevant records.

Guidance on assessing the value and reliability of search filters is available.[7–9] Search filters for economic evaluations are available for the major biomedical databases and they may be adaptable, with care, for non-biomedical databases.[2,10] However, any adaptations should take account of the differences in research reporting, and indexing between biomedicine and other fields such as the social sciences, including social welfare, education and criminal justice. Some commentators have noted that structured abstracts are less common in social science journals and that methods information is often less clearly reported.[2,16] This will carry over into the databases where research is recorded. As the assignment of methods indexing is also less widespread in social sciences databases, this makes retrieval more challenging than tends to be the case in biomedical databases.[16]

Which resources to search

A review of economic evaluations involves searching a range of information resources, and is similar to the process involved in finding effects evidence in systematic reviews.[1–3,5,6] The search is likely to include searches of bibliographic databases but may also include efforts to identify ongoing studies. It is also important to identify research which might have been published more informally (grey literature), perhaps as working papers or reports. The latter are noted to be particularly important in the social sciences where publication in non-journal formats is more frequent and key studies may appear in reports before they achieve journal publication.[2] REPEC offers access to economics grey literature (http://repec.org) and OAIster offers access to grey literature in all fields (http://www.oclc.org/oaister). Searching the websites of key relevant organisations may also increase retrieval of grey literature.

Checklists offer guidance on suitable resources to search and approaches to searching.[2,3,5,17–19] These tend to be pragmatic guides and their recommendations are often based on a combination of experience of searching the resources and research evidence. Most checklists recommend that the search should start with any specific resources which collect economic evaluations and then move to searches of large bibliographic databases. This approach is intended to maximise the efficiency of searching by looking in a focused resource first and supplementing with limited searches in larger general databases, where precision (i.e. proportion of relevant records) is likely to be comparatively low. To assist researchers and decision makers, a number of databases gather together economic evaluations from across a range of resources. Table 7.1 shows a selection of health economic evaluation databases. These include major international collections (NHS EED and the Health Economic Evaluations Database (HEED)), subject specific collections (Paediatric Economic Database Evaluation (PEDE)) and country-specific databases (COnnaissances et Décision en EConomie de la Santé (CODECS)).[15,20–22] Many are more than bibliographic databases, offering added value through critical appraisals (NHS EED, CODECS), extensive categorisations and enriched abstracts (HEED) or summaries (Cost-effectiveness Analysis Registry) (see also Chapter 8). The authors have not identified similar collections of economic evaluations in non-health care fields.

Economic evaluation databases overlap in terms of their coverage. Evidence on the scale of the overlaps, the currency of the resources, and their respective advantages is limited.[12,13,19,23] Sassi and colleagues compared the yield of search strategies in seven medical and social science databases, NHS EED and a published bibliography, for publications in the first quarter of 1997.[13] Their research suggested that Medline can be relied on as the key general database source for the identification of published economic evaluations in health care.[13] Royle & Waugh assessed

a sample of 19 English health technology assessments (retrieving 130 studies) to explore the yield of different databases in terms of the economic evaluations reviewed.[12] They found that Medline and Embase both identified 86.6% of the economic evaluations used in the reviews, with 86.7% of those studies common to both databases; 40.2% of studies were identifiable in NHS EED. Searching Medline, Embase and NHS EED reached a cumulative percentage of 94.8% of the included studies and they recommended searching these databases. The authors did not access and assess HEED. More recently, Alton and colleagues analysed the yield of searches of NHS EED, HEED, PubMed, Embase, Econlit and SciSearch.[23] They recommended that a search of NHS EED, supplemented by a search of a general database such as Medline, was effective.

The challenges for comparing studies which have assessed database yield include ensuring that the definitions of economic evaluation used in those studies are comparable and that the currency of the databases is comparable.

Inevitable identification, abstracting and publication lags may mean that tertiary databases such as those in Table 7.1 may not always be as current as secondary databases such as Medline. To compensate, it is advisable, when identifying economic evaluations of health care topics, to search major bibliographic databases and other resources for the last few years to identify further economic evaluations. These databases are likely to be the same as those recommended in checklists for systematic reviews.[1,3,6] For reviews of economic evaluations outside health care, searches of a range of resources are recommended.[2] The specific resources can be identified from search guidance and by consulting information professionals.[2,3]

A key element of systematic reviews is the importance of transparency and replicability which allow the reader to assess potential biases in the review. To assist with transparency, detailed recording of the search process is recommended and detailed descriptions of the search strategy should be included in the final report, made available on request and/or posted on a website.[1,2,5] The search report should include a list of the databases searched, which search terms were used and in which combinations. Examples of search reports are given in many guides to reviewing.[1,2,5]

Table 7.1 Selected databases of economic evaluations.

Database	Coverage	Availability	Value-added features
NHS Economic Evaluation Database (NHS EED)	Health care economic evaluations (worldwide), early 1990s to date	Free at: http://www.crd.york. ac.uk/crdweb/ Subscription service: http://eu.wiley. com/WileyCDA/ Brand/id-6.html	Detailed summaries plus critical appraisal
Health Economic Evaluations Database (HEED)	Economic evaluations (worldwide)	Subscription service: http://www3. interscience.wiley.com/cgi-bin/ mrwhome/114130635/HOME	Extensive categorisations; detailed abstracts
Cost-effectiveness Analysis (CEA) Registry	Health care cost-utility analyses	Free at: https://research.tufts-nemc. org/cear/default.aspx	Extracts cost-effectiveness ratios and utility weights
Health Technology Assessment (HTA) database	Health care technology assessments	Free at: http://www.crd.york. ac.uk/crdweb/ Subscription service: http://eu.wiley.com/WileyCDA/ Brand/id-6.html	Bibliographic details; links to technology assessments that often include integrated economic evaluations
Paediatric Economic Database Evaluation (PEDE)	Paediatric economic evaluations	Free at: http://pede.bioinfo.sickkids. on.ca/pede/index.jsp	Categorisations
European Network of Health Economic Evaluation Databases (EURONHEED)	European health care economic evaluations	Free at: http://infodoc.inserm.fr/ euronheed/publication.nsf	Summaries plus critical appraisal
COnnaissances et Décision en EConomie de la Santé (CODECS)	French health care economic evaluations	Free at: http://infodoc.inserm.fr codecs/codecs.nsf	Summaries plus critical appraisal

The research agenda

Development of reference sets of economic evaluations

Research would be assisted by the development of reference sets of economic evaluations that are judged to conform to specific definitions of the term 'economic evaluation'. Reference sets can be created by database searching, hand searching publications or by relative recall methods. NHS EED is an example of a reference set of records meeting a specific definition of 'economic evaluation' and built up through database searching and hand searching. Relative recall uses the included studies identified in published reviews of economic evaluations which have been compiled through extensive searching as a proxy for extensive hand searching (see Sampson and colleagues, 2006[24]). Reference sets could be used to develop search filters,

providing a source of search terms and a test set of data for testing search filter performance.

Search filters

The available search filters to identify economic evaluations need to be more extensively validated to better understand their performance. Research funded by the Canadian Agency for Drugs and Technologies in Health (CADTH) and undertaken by the York Health Economics Consortium (YHEC) explored the development and performance of health economic evaluation search filters for Embase and Medline. In fields beyond health care, the value of developing search filters for economic evaluations or adapting available health care filters remains to be determined. There is little published evidence on search filters for economic evaluations conducted in the applied fields of social welfare, education or criminal justice.

Which databases should be searched?

Within health care, evidence on the comparative unique yield of the large bibliographic databases and specialist economic evaluation databases is growing slowly, but in all fields a detailed analysis is elusive. More retrospective analyses of completed reviews where the identified studies are retraced to their original database could be undertaken to provide more information on the value of searching a range of databases. This type of analysis has been used for other study types.[25] Such record analyses are relatively easy to achieve at the end of a review and, to a limited extent, may be publishable. However, to build a performance picture more quickly, a group such as the Campbell and Cochrane Economic Methods Group (CCEMG) might wish to explore options to encourage such analysis and dissemination of the results, by providing, for example, guides to conducting such studies and a wiki to encourage researchers to record performance data on a website as a routine element of the search process.

Publication bias

Extensive searching (including unpublished literature) is advocated to inform systematic reviews to minimise the impact of potential biases, including publication bias. Reviews of publication bias in economic evaluations of health care interventions suggest that reporting or publication biases are present and describe approaches to further investigation.[6] A further research theme would be to investigate the extent of non-publication of economic evaluations and the implications for study identification. For example, analyses of the subsequent publication rates of health economic evaluations first presented at conferences, such as International Society for Pharmacoeconomics and Outcomes Research (ISPOR) and Health Technology Assessment International (HTAi) meetings, might indicate levels of publication bias and approaches to study identification if some studies are only published as grey literature.[26,27]

Identifying evidence to inform the development of decision models

Decision models are used increasingly to support policy decision making in the delivery of health care (see also, *inter alia*, Chapters 2 and 9).[28] Search methods for this type of evidence synthesis are not standardised and the reporting of the information-seeking processes that support decision models is not transparent.[29,30] This section explores the role of evidence in informing decision models for economic evaluations (see also, *inter alia*, Chapters 2 and 9). It draws comparisons between decision models and systematic reviews of published and unpublished economic evaluations in order to identify issues specific to modelling which should be considered in the development of search methods in this area.

Background

It is recognised that decision models need a broader range of evidence than costs and effects in order to derive estimates of clinical and cost-effectiveness.[29,31] This includes evidence on epidemiology, natural history and specific outcomes including adverse events and (in health care) health state utilities (see also Chapters 9 and 10). In order to satisfy this range of information need and to ensure that models reflect the context of the specific decision being made, it is necessary to draw on different types of evidence, in addition to randomised controlled trials (RCTs), including observational research and routine administrative data.[31,32]

The scope of the evidence base relevant to the development of decision models is therefore recognised as being broader and more diverse than that required to inform systematic reviews of existing economic evaluations. Conversely, there is a question as to how much evidence is required. It is suggested that a comprehensive approach to searching, characteristic of the procedures recommended by the Cochrane and Campbell Collaborations for systematic reviews, is not practical in terms of time and resources.[1,33] There is a further implication that this extensive approach is not necessarily required. Decision models do not seek to derive as precise an estimate as possible of cost-effectiveness but to support decision making in the absence of ideal evidence. What is required is *sufficient* evidence to understand the inevitable uncertainty associated with the outputs of the model and with the evidence available to inform the decision.[34,35] A formal definition or measure of sufficient evidence does not currently exist, although sensitivity analysis and value of information (VOI) analysis are potentially useful tools in deciding where more searching is required (see also Chapter 12). However, there are further considerations in determining what constitutes sufficient evidence to support a decision model and these will be discussed later in this chapter.

Despite these recognised differences, methodological guidelines in decision modelling and health technology assessment (HTA) give limited guidance on searching.[30,36] Where guidance does exist, it does not address the differences outlined above and, as a result, it is difficult to operationalise. Existing guidance is largely restricted to the process of identifying evidence to populate model parameters, in particular clinical effectiveness parameters, and refers, in the main, to an approach to searching such as that recommended by The Cochrane Collaboration.[1]

The absence of search methods to inform decision models is recognised as a gap in the methodological literature.[30] Golder and colleagues, assessing the feasibility of searching for evidence to populate model parameters, concluded that there was a need to develop search methods to meet the needs of decision models in health care.[33] Further research is currently exploring how factors associated with the model development process and with the use of evidence in models impact on the way searches should be undertaken.[34,37] Some of the ideas emerging from this research form the basis for the remainder of this chapter.

The Cochrane and Campbell approach to searching is intended to provide a systematic, transparent and replicable means of specifying and identifying the scope of evidence relevant to a systematic review. The procedures associated with this approach, in terms of focusing search questions and searching widely, have been shown to be difficult to apply in the context of decision models in health care. It is important to understand why this is so. In order to achieve a systematic, transparent and replicable approach to identifying evidence for decision models, search methods should be designed to fit the requirements of decision models. Factors associated with the development of decision models and with the use of evidence in supporting that development, together with a consideration of how they impact on the approach to searching, are discussed below.

Defining the scope of relevant evidence

The main question to be addressed by a systematic review or a decision model is typically structured according to the PICO convention (described earlier in this chapter).[5,28,38] In assessing effectiveness, systematic reviews tend to focus on evidence that seeks to address the same question as the review. The general methods of the *Cochrane Handbook for Systematic*

Reviews of Interventions describe eligibility criteria as being defined by the components of the PICO structured question.[38] Using this approach, studies that do not address the PICO question are considered to be outside the scope of relevant evidence. The PICO question therefore provides the analytical framework for the review and it is used to focus the conduct of the review.[38] Relevance is defined according to the PICO framework, which in turn directs the development of the search strategy (see Box 7.1), defines the inclusion and exclusion criteria, and so on.

In addressing the same question of effectiveness, a typical decision model draws widely on relevant sources of evidence that relate both directly and indirectly to the PICO question. The need to build a decision model is generated by the gaps between the PICO question, the available effectiveness evidence and the issues relevant to making a decision.[39,40] In the absence of evidence that addresses all these requirements, a decision model brings together, within a relevant analytical framework, indirect evidence from a range of sources.[39] As a consequence, the process of model development can generate a large number of information needs and many of these will not be stated explicitly in the PICO question. The PICO question therefore cannot focus the conduct of the search as it does in systematic reviews. It is not an adequate tool with which to translate all the information needs of a decision model into relevant search strategies. A description of information needs that typically arise as a result of addressing the gaps in the direct evidence is given below.

Randomised controlled trials control for differences between study participants. As a result, the study population might not reflect the characteristics of the population relevant to the context of a given decision and observational, epidemiological evidence is required to inform the baseline characteristics of the populations in the model.[31]

Randomised controlled trials might not assess comparisons that reflect current practice relevant to the context of a given decision either because placebo-controlled comparisons constitute the only available evidence or because head-to-head comparisons do not reflect current practice (see also Chapter 3). In this case an indirect comparison would be modelled, requiring one set of evidence relating to the intervention and additional sets of evidence relating to each of the relevant comparators.[39]

The available trial evidence might not provide adequate evidence of certain outcomes. Typical examples where indirect evidence is required include adverse events and health state utilities (see also Chapters 8 and 9). A further common problem is the length of follow-up in trials which provides only short-term evidence of overall survival or evidence of surrogate outcomes such as, for example, reductions in cholesterol rather than changes in the risk of cardiovascular events. Here modelling is used to extrapolate short-term and surrogate evidence to provide longer-term estimates of clinically relevant outcomes. Evidence might be required to inform the analytical approach to extrapolation and in addition, observational evidence of longer-term outcomes might be sought.

Due to the compound or complex nature of some information needs arising from the decision model, a breakdown of the need into multiple subquestions might be required. For example, the cost of a health care intervention might comprise multiple components including drug acquisition costs, drug delivery costs, monitoring and follow-up costs. The example in Figure 7.1 demonstrates a breakdown of the cost of delivering chemotherapy agents to treat colon cancer.[41] Whilst it is not suggested that a separate search would be required for each component, the example does demonstrate how a range of individual 'pieces' of information is required to inform one component of the model.

Decision models commonly include evidence relating to populations and interventions not specified in the PICO question. In assessing effectiveness, models may consider the long-term and broader impacts of the intervention. For example, a well-specified assessment of a screening or diagnostic test would not be limited to the immediate costs of the test nor to its effects in terms of its sensitivity and specificity. The test would also be assessed in terms of the impact on the consequent need for treatment and care, and the losses or gains in terms of overall survival and quality-adjusted life-years (QALYs) at later stages of the disease pathway. These are examples of key questions whose answers are likely to be of relevance to many decision makers in assessing the effectiveness and cost-effectiveness of a course of action.

The scope of this longer-term and broader impact is captured in the definition of the perspective and time horizon of the decision model. These will have an effect in determining the scope of evidence relevant to a decision model. For example, the perspective of the model can be defined in terms of the impact of the intervention on the management of the problem within the care setting (health and social care perspective) or on the individual and their carers (patient perspective) or from a societal perspective (for example, including loss of productivity). The time horizon determines the impact of an intervention on the development and management of a disease over time. For example, in Markov models this is handled through the definition and incorporation of relevant health states. A move from one state to another denotes a change in the characteristics of the population (for example, from early stage to advanced stage cancer) and in the management of that population (for example, from curative to palliative treatment). The assessment of the intervention takes into account the costs and effects associated with all included health states. As a result, the scope of relevant evidence, particularly with regard to epidemiology, treatment effects, costs and utilities, is not determined by the PICO question but by all the health states included in the model.

The final consideration in defining the scope of relevant evidence is its use in developing the analytical framework within which the decision problem is considered. Here the focus is on the use of evidence to gain a conceptual understanding of the decision problem and to translate it into a mathematical framework, as opposed to the use of evidence to populate the framework.

Whilst methods guidelines specify the elements that make up the analytical framework (in terms of the model structure, perspective, time horizon, modelling approach, data and data analysis), there is very little discussion in the HTA decision-modelling literature on the developmental process of establishing this framework.[30] The broader modelling literature, however, clearly identifies this process and describes it as having two levels: conceptualisation and specification.[42] Conceptualisation is the understanding of the decision problem and its context. In health care decision models, this can include the use of evidence on natural history and expert opinion to understand the condition of interest. Practice guidelines, prescribing rates and experts' advice might be consulted to understand what constitutes standard or current practice in the management of the condition in the setting.

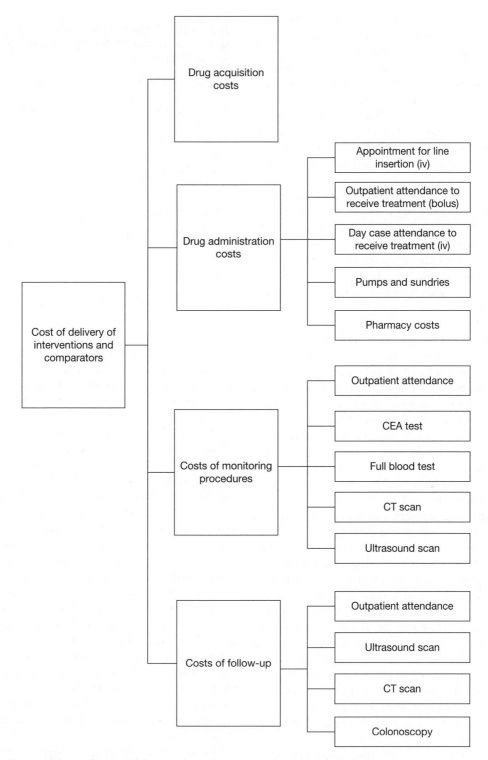

Figure 7.1 Breakdown of costs of delivering chemotherapy treatments for colon cancer.

It also includes understanding the direct evidence relating to the intervention(s) of interest in order to assess how to address the gaps in that evidence.

Specification is the translation of the conceptualisation of the problem into a mathematical framework which both reflects the conceptualisation of the decision problem (i.e. is relevant to and is an acceptable representation of the issues associated with the decision problem) and allows the analysis of those issues using relevant data and relevant analytical techniques.

In summary, the range of evidence relevant to a decision model is not clearly captured in the definition of the PICO focused questio n that the model is seeking to address. A broader range of evidence is needed to populate the model. In addition, evidence is required to inform the development of a relevant framework within which to analyse the decision problem.

Implications for the approach to searching

The scope of evidence relevant to a decision model and the process by which this scope is defined have implications for the conduct of searches. Ongoing research suggests that a diverse range of information is used to provide the data required to populate a decision model and to support other modelling activities, including the development of the analytical framework, sensitivity analysis and model validation.[37] The range of information used to support these activities is summarised in Box 7.2.

There are established standards for the retrieval of evidence of effects but little research has been undertaken to inform the efficient retrieval of other types of information.[1,5] Search filters for other types of information, most of which have not been validated, could be useful in supporting the retrieval of some of the information required to inform a decision model.[10] Research into the best approaches to identifying evidence on adverse events is ongoing and guidance on the identification of evidence on utilities is presented in Chapter 8 of this volume.[43] Standardised approaches to searching in response to other types of information, for example information on what constitutes established current practice, have not been developed.

The different types of evidence used to inform a decision model are drawn from diverse sources of

---

Box 7.2 Types of information used to support decision models in health care

- Adverse events
- Compliance
- Current practice (including treatment options and pathways)
- Epidemiology
- Modelling and analytical methods
- Natural history
- Prognosis
- Resource use
- Treatment effects
- Unit costs
- Utilities

---

information, including both research-based and non-research-based information sources (see Table 7.2). For example, in terms of research-based information, evidence derived from (a meta-analysis of) well-conducted RCTs remains the best source of evidence of effects (see also Chapter 9). Epidemiological information used to inform the baseline characteristics of the model population and the baseline risk of clinical events is more likely to come from observational studies.[31]

The 'real-world' context of decision making is reflected in the use of sources providing routinely collected rather than research-based information.[32] Examples in health care include national disease registers, claims databases, prescription rates and hospital activity statistics. They also include 'reference' sources or standard, authoritative sources that provide generic information common to many decision models. Examples of reference sources in health care might include drug formularies, classifications of disease and clinical practice guidelines. The relevance of reference sources and sources of routinely collected data will to some extent be specific to the context of the decision, for example geographically or to a specific decision-making authority (see also, *inter alia*, Chapters 3, 4, 5 and 10). The development of local knowledge of sources relevant to the context of the decision making is therefore required to make full use of such sources.

The use of information to support different decision-modelling activities is also reflected in

Table 7.2 Sources of information used to support decision models in health care.

Types of sources	Examples
Evidence syntheses	Systematic reviews of effectiveness, existing decision models
Expert judgement	Published opinion or personal advisers
Methodological sources	Methodological guidelines, empirical methodological evidence to justify modelling approach
Observational research	Epidemiological evidence, utilities evidence
RCTs	Effectiveness evidence
Reference sources	Drug formularies, disease classifications
Routine data	Disease registers, claims databases, activity data

the range of sources. Whilst expert opinion would not be considered a reliable source of evidence on treatment effects, the 'concurrence of experts' is a recognised form of model validation and strong anecdotal evidence suggests that expert advice is used in informing development of the scope and structure of decision models in health care.[31,34,44]

Bibliographic databases remain important sources for identifying research-based evidence. However, not all information relevant to a decision model can be identified using bibliographic databases. The remaining sources are scattered and diverse, and many are specific to the context of the decision. A better knowledge of non-research-based information is required, including techniques in locating and interrogating such sources, so that the evidence base of relevance to a decision model is fully exploited.

A further important consideration is the way in which the multiple information needs associated with a model are generated. In systematic reviews, information needs are defined *a priori* based on the PICO question and associated eligibility criteria. In decision models, the full range of information needs is not predefined but emerges as the analytical framework and the understanding of the decision problem and of the available evidence develops. Information needs are established through the processes of conceptualisation and specification. The use of evidence is

iterative and non-sequential and informs the process of model development.

As a result, searches cannot be conducted at one point in time as for systematic reviews. In order that searches can be conducted according to some form of systematic process, an iterative search process that facilitates the management of multiple information needs is required. This would involve matching the information found with the different requirements of the decision model, monitoring which information needs have been satisfied and auditing the links between the modelling process and the use of information in supporting that process. Most importantly, information needs are not expressed explicitly in the PICO question that the model is seeking to address; nor can they be known or fully defined before searching commences. There is a need, therefore, for the search process to capture emerging information needs so that the full scope of evidence identified as being relevant to the model is adequately explored. The usefulness of descriptive models of information-seeking behaviour, from the field of information science, in informing the development of such an approach is being investigated.[37]

The emergent process by which the scope of relevant evidence is defined has possible implications for how much information is required to inform a decision model. The decision-modelling literature focuses on two principal issues in discussing how much information is required. The first is that a less than comprehensive approach to searching may be required on pragmatic grounds, due to limited time and resources.[33] The second is that the decision to acquire further information rests on the value of further information to the decision-making process and should be guided by uncertainty analysis. Following this principle, further information should only be acquired where uncertainty might have an overall impact on model results or on the direction of the decision (see also Chapter 12).[34,35] Ideally, decisions on when to stop searching should not be guided by arbitrary factors such as time and resources. Further research is required to explore how the principles underlying value of information analysis can be used to inform and guide the search process.

There are two further considerations in determining what constitutes sufficient evidence that are not discussed in the literature in the context of searching. The first is the specific purposes for which evidence is used in a decision model. The second is the way in which the term 'all the relevant evidence' is interpreted. These are discussed briefly here.

Evidence is used to support different activities during the course of decision model development (see also, *inter alia*, Chapters 2 and 9) and the definition of 'sufficient evidence' will vary according to the nature of these activities. For example, the identification of evidence on effects to inform estimates of effectiveness will require a relatively sensitive approach to searching. A search for evidence on the natural history of a condition or pattern of behaviour, used to support the structure of the model, would need to identify sufficient evidence to establish an acceptable or credible description of, for example, disease or criminal pathways. It would not, however, be required to identify every occurrence of that description.

In the development of decision models, the term 'all the relevant evidence' acknowledges the consideration of evidence not directly related to the intervention and population specified in the PICO question. As such, it refers not to every occurrence of evidence that matches a set of focused, predefined criteria, as is the case in systematic reviews, but rather to the full breadth of evidence that informs (or could inform) an understanding of the decision problem. The scope of the full breadth of relevant evidence is not expressed explicitly in the PICO question. Moreover, and more importantly, the scope of relevant evidence is not predefined *and* it is open to interpretation. The completeness of the search process in terms of scope, and the extent to which it is able to recognise and conceptualise the full range of information needs relevant to a decision model, is clearly important in identifying 'all relevant evidence' in the context of decision modelling. The conceptualisation of a search question is recognised as an important measure of the quality of a search.[45] However, there is little procedural guidance on how to translate a research question or decision problem into a search strategy beyond using terms relating to the population and intervention of interest (see Box 7.1). In particular, there is a lack of search methods guidance for cases where the information need driving the search is not clearly understood or predefined. This is a key area where current search methods guidelines do not support a search process fit for the purpose of informing decision models.

The research agenda

Search methods for the identification of evidence to support decision models are not as well developed as search methods to support systematic reviews of existing economic evaluations. The iterative nature of decision model development and the wide-ranging use of evidence within the development process suggest that an approach to searching different from that commonly associated with systematic reviews is required. We suggest the following areas as priorities for further research.

- Development of systematic, non-sequential, iterative search procedures to support the iterative nature of model development.
- Development of methods to conceptualise and develop search queries that capture emerging concepts of relevance to a decision model systematically.
- Development of a definition and measures of sufficient evidence to inform search stopping rules.
- Development of search methods to identify the different types of evidence required to inform a decision model, in terms of both study design for research-based evidence and sources for non-research-based evidence, including routinely collected administrative data, reference sources and expert opinion.
- Definition of tasks undertaken as part of the model development process and their associated information-seeking processes.

Conclusion

Evidence on the best approaches to searching to inform systematic reviews of economic evaluations and decision models is currently limited. There is some evidence from health care of systematic approaches to searching which may assist with reviews, but their relevance to fields beyond health care has yet to be thoroughly investigated. There is also a wide range of resources available to assist with reviews of economic evaluations in health care, but information about the yield of resources beyond health care is, once again, limited.

We advocate that the systematic and transparent approach associated with systematic review search methods should inform the development of search methods specific to the development of decision models. However, systematic review search procedures have been developed for a specific purpose and cannot be transferred directly to the context of decision models. In order that search methods fit for the purpose of supporting decision models can be developed, it is important to understand the activities associated with the model development process and the role of evidence in supporting those activities.

To some degree, the search methods developed in health care will provide a model for the development of methods in other areas – for example, the identification and compilation of resource lists specific to social welfare, education and criminal justice, the development of specialist resources equivalent to NHS EED and the generation of search filters designed to incorporate study designs, index terms and vocabulary relevant to those fields.

On the other hand, the development of search methods in the fields of social welfare, education and criminal justice will also have to address issues of complexity that are only just beginning to be addressed in the field of health care. The synthesis of evidence relating to health care interventions relies heavily on a clearly focused question to direct the process of searching. Where this approach does not fit, as can be seen in the case of health care decision models, it is difficult to apply this retrieval model. Managing complexity is ubiquitous in the fields of social welfare, education and criminal justice and can be seen in the descriptions of interventions, in the definitions of outcome measures and in the theories of why and when interventions do or do not work. The development of search procedures that can handle these sorts of issues will progress information retrieval in all fields of evidence-based decision making.

Acknowledgements

Other contributors to this chapter: Karianne Thune Hammerstrøm, The Campbell Collaboration Social Welfare Group; Professor Mark Petticrew, London School of Hygiene and Tropical Medicine; Kath Wright, Centre for Reviews and Dissemination. Suzy Paisley's contribution is based on work undertaken for a Department of Health in England and Wales-funded personal fellowship.

How this chapter should be cited

Glanville J, Paisley S. Chapter 7: Searching for evidence for cost-effectiveness decisions. In: Shemilt I, Mugford M, Vale L, Marsh K, Donaldson C (editors). *Evidence-based decisions and economics: health care,*

social welfare, education and criminal justice. Oxford: Wiley-Blackwell, 2010.

References

1 Lefebvre C, Manheimer E, Glanville J. Searching for studies. In: Higgins JPT, Green S (eds) *Cochrane Handbook for Systematic Reviews of Interventions*. Version 5.0.2 (updated September 2009). Cochrane Collaboration, 2009.

2 Petticrew M, Roberts H. How to find the studies: the literature search. In: Petticrew M, Roberts H (eds) *Systematic Reviews in the Social Sciences: a practical guide*. Oxford: Blackwell Publishing, 2006.

3 Rothstein HR, Turner HM, Lavenberg JG. *The Campbell Collaboration Information Retrieval Policy Brief*. Oslo: Campbell Collaboration, 2004. Available from: http://camp.ostfold.net/ resources/methods_policy_briefs.shtml.

4 Swaray RB, Bowles R, Pradiptyo R. The application of economic analysis to criminal justice interventions: a review of the literature. *Criminal Justice Policy Review* 2005; 16(2): 141–163.

5 Centre for Reviews and Dissemination. *Systematic Reviews: CRD's guidance for undertaking reviews in health care*, 3rd edn. York: Centre for Reviews and Dissemination, 2009.

6 Shemilt I, Mugford M, Byford S, *et al.* Incorporating economics evidence. In: Higgins JPT, Green S (eds) *Cochrane Handbook for Systematic Reviews of Interventions*. Version 5.0.2 (updated September 2009). Cochrane Collaboration, 2009.

7 Bak G, Mierzwinski-Urban M, Fitzsimmons H, Morrison A, Maden-Jenkins M. A pragmatic critical appraisal instrument for search filters: introducing the CADTH CAI. *Health Information and Libraries Journal* 2009; 26(3): 211–219.

8 Glanville J, Bayliss S, Booth A, *et al.*, on behalf of the InterTASC Information Specialists' Sub-Group. So many filters, so little time: the development of a search filter appraisal checklist. *Journal of the Medical Library Association* 2008; 96(4): 356–361.

9 Jenkins M. Evaluation of methodological search filters – a review. *Health Information and Libraries Journal* 2004; 21(3): 148–163.

10 InterTASC Information Specialists Subgroup. *Search Filter Resource: economic evaluations*. InterTASC Information Specialists Subgroup, 2010. Available from: http://www.york.ac.uk/inst/ crd/intertasc/econ.htm.

11 McKinlay RJ, Wilczynski NL, Haynes RB. Optimal search strategies for detecting cost and economic studies in EMBASE. *BMC Health Services Research* 2006; 6: 67.

12 Royle P, Waugh N. Literature searching for clinical and cost-effectiveness studies used in health technology assessment reports carried out for the National Institute for Clinical Excellence appraisal system. *Health Technology Assessment* 2003; 7(34): 1–61.

13 Sassi F, Archard L, McDaid D. Searching literature databases for health care economic evaluations: how systematic can we afford to be? *Medical Care* 2002; 40(5): 387–394.

14 Wilczynski NL, Haynes RB, Lavis JN, Ramkissoonsingh R, Arnold-Oatley AE, HSR Hedges Team. Optimal search strategies for detecting health services research studies in

MEDLINE. *Canadian Medical Association Journal* 2004; 171(10): 1179–1185.

15 Centre for Reviews and Dissemination. *NHS Economic Evaluation Database.* York: Centre for Reviews and Dissemination, 2010. Available from: http://www.crd.york.ac.uk/crdweb.

16 Bradshaw JR. *Methodologies for socially useful systematic reviews in social policy (Economic and Social Research Council Research report).* Swindon: Economic and Social Research Council Research, 2005.

17 Canadian Agency for Drugs and Technologies in Health. *Grey Matters: a practical search tool for evidence-based medicine.* Ottawa: Canadian Agency for Drugs and Technologies in Health, 2008. Available from: http://cadth.ca/media/pdf/Grey-Matters_A-Practical-Search-Tool-for-Evidence-Based-Medicine.doc.

18 Kristensen FB, Sigmund H (eds). *Health Technology Assessment Handbook 2007.* Copenhagen: Danish Centre for Health Technology Assessment, 2008. Available from: http://www.sst.dk/publ/publ2008/mtv/metode/HTA_handbook_net_final.pdf.

19 Napper M. NHS economic evaluation database and the Health Economic Evaluation Database: a user perspective. In: Sassi F (ed) *Cochrane Collaboration Economics Methods Group Newsletter (Series 2, Number 2).* Norwich: Cochrane Collaboration Economics Methods Group, 2001. Available from: http://www.c-cemg.org.

20 Collège des Economistes de la Santé. *CODECS.* Paris: Collège des Economistes de la Santé, 2010. Available from: http://infodoc.inserm.frcodecs/codec.nsf

21 Hospital for Sick Children. *PEDE: Paediatric Economic Database Evaluation.* Toronto: Hospital for Sick Children, 2010. Available from: http://pede.bioinfo.sickkids.on.ca/ pede/index.jsp.

22 Wiley Interscience. *HEED: Health Economics Evaluation Database.* Chichester: Wiley Interscience, 2010. Available from: http://heed.wiley.com.

23 Alton V, Eckerlund I, Norlund A. Health economics evaluation: how to find them. *International Journal of Technology Assessment in Health care* 2006; 22: 512–571.

24 Sampson M, Zhang L, Morrison A, *et al.* An alternative to the hand searching gold standard: validating methodological search filters using relative recall. *BMC Medical Research Methodology* 2006; 6: 33.

25 Whiting P, Westwood M, Burke M, Sterne J, Glanville J. Systematic reviews of test accuracy should search a range of databases to identify primary studies. *Journal of Clinical Epidemiology* 2008; 61(4): 357–364.

26 Hopewell S, Clarke MJ, Stewart L, Tierney J. Time to publication for results of clinical trials. *Cochrane Database of Systematic Reviews* 2007, Issue 2. Art no. MR000011.

27 Hopewell S, Loudon K, Clarke MJ, Oxman AD, Dickersin K. Publication bias in clinical trials due to statistical significance or direction of trial results. *Cochrane Database of Systematic Reviews* 2009, Issue 1. Art no. MR000006.

28 National Institute for Health and Clinical Excellence. *Guide to the Methods of Technology Appraisal.* London: National Institute for Health and Clinical Excellence, 2008.

29 Cooper N, Coyle D, Abrams K, Mugford M, Sutton A. Use of evidence in decision models: an appraisal of health technology assessments in the UK to date. *Journal of Health Services Research and Policy* 2005; 10: 245–250.

30 Philips Z, Ginnelly L, Sculpher M, *et al.* Review of guidelines for good practice in decision-analytic modelling in health technology assessment. *Health Technology Assessment* 2004; 8(36): 1–172.

31 Coyle D, Lee K. Evidence-based economic evaluation: how the use of different data sources can impact results. In: Donaldson C, Mugford M, Vale L (eds) *Evidence-Based Health Economics: from effectiveness to efficiency in systematic review.* London: BMJ Books, 2002.

32 Garrison LP, Neumann PJ, Erickson P, Marshall D, Mullins CD. Using real-world data for coverage and payment decisions: the ISPOR Real-World Data Task Force report. *Value in Health* 2007; 10(5): 326–335.

33 Golder S, Glanville J, Ginnelly L. Populating decision-analytic models: the feasibility and efficiency of database searching for individual parameters. *International Journal of Technology Assessment in Health care* 2005; 21(3): 305–311.

34 Cooper NJ, Sutton AJ, Ades AE, Paisley S, Jones DR. Use of evidence in economic decision models: practical issues and methodological issues. *Health Economics* 2007; 16(12): 1277–1286.

35 Sculpher M, Claxton K. Establishing the cost-effectiveness of new pharmaceuticals under conditions of uncertainty – when is there sufficient evidence? *Value in Health* 2005; 8(4): 433–446.

36 International Society for Pharmacoeconomics Outcomes Research. *Pharmacoeconomics Guidelines Around the World.* Available from: http://www.ispor.org/peguidelines/index.asp.

37 Paisley S. *Identification of evidence for decision-analytic models.* PhD thesis, in preparation.

38 Higgins JPT, Green S (eds). *Cochrane Handbook for Systematic Reviews of Interventions.* Version 5.0 (updated September 2009). Cochrane Collaboration, 2009.

39 Buxton MJ, Drummond MF, van Hout BA, *et al.* Modelling in economic evaluation: an unavoidable fact of life. *Health Economics* 1997; 6(3): 217–227.

40 Brennan A, Akehurst R. Modelling in health economic evaluation: what is its place? What is its value? *Pharmacoeconomics* 2000; 17(5): 445–459.

41 Pandor A, Eggington S, Paisley S, Tappenden P, Sutcliffe P. The clinical and cost-effectiveness of oxaliplatin and capecitabine for the adjuvant treatment of colon cancer: systematic review and economic evaluation. *Health Technology Assessment* 2006; 10(41): 1–204.

42 Sargent R. Validation and verification of simulation models. In: Ingalls R, Rossetti M, Smith J, Peters B (eds) *Proceedings of the 2004 Winter Simulation Conference.* Washington, 2004.

43 Golder S, Loke YK. Search strategies to identify information on adverse effects: a systematic review. *J Med Libr Assoc* 2009; 97(2): 84–92.

44 Eddy D. Technology assessment: the role of mathematical modeling. In: Committee for Evaluating Medical Technologies in Clinical Use. *Assessing Medical Technology.* Washington DC: National Academy Press, 1985.

45 Sampson M, McGowan J, Lefebvre C, Moher D, Grimshaw J. *PRESS: peer review of electronic search strategies.* Ottawa: Canadian Agency for Drugs and Technologies in Health, 2008.

CHAPTER 8

Identifying and reviewing health state utility values for populating decision models

John Brazier[1], Diana Papaioannou[1], Anna Cantrell[1], Suzy Paisley[1], Kirsten Herrmann[2]

[1]School of Health and Related Research, University of Sheffield, Sheffield, UK
[2]ICF Research Branch of the World Health Organisation CC FIC, Germany

Introduction

A key component in economic evaluation is the way in which the benefits of interventions are valued. In health economics, a common way to value benefits has been in terms of the quality-adjusted life-year (QALY) in which the health benefits are summarised into a single measure combining length of life with health-related quality of life (HRQL).[1] This involves assigning a value to every health state on a scale where full health is equal to one and states regarded as being as bad as dead are given a value of zero. Thus, a chronic health state lasting 10 years with a value of 0.8 equates to eight QALYs. More complex multistate profiles are valued in a similar way by weighting each time period by the value of the health state experienced in that period. Thus health state values are crucial to the calculation of QALYs and it is important to ensure that the appropriate values are being used.

Health state values, or health state utility values (HSUVs) as they are often referred to in the literature, are key parameters in decision models that estimate the incremental cost per QALY of an intervention (see also, *inter alia*, Chapters 2, 7 and 9).[2] The use of decision models has seen a large increase in recent years, as reimbursement agencies such as the National Institute for Health and Clinical Excellence (NICE) in England now routinely assess the cost-effectiveness of new health care interventions. This has resulted in a corresponding increase in the demand for data on HSUVs, since decision models are typically built around a set of health states that patients are assumed to occupy over their lifetime. The role of systematic review in obtaining data used to populate decision models has tended to focus primarily on estimates of clinical efficacy built around clinical measures of outcome, such as mortality, fracture rates, heart attacks and so on. Such reviews have tended to adopt methods similar to those advocated by the Cochrane Collaboration to collect and synthesise clinical efficacy data in order to generate reliable estimates of the transition probabilities into different health states (see Chapters 7 and 9). However, relatively little attention has been focused on the role of systematic review methods in obtaining the utility values assigned to those health states.

The large and growing body of literature on methods for deriving HSUVs has been concerned mainly with techniques for valuing health states (e.g. time trade-off (TTO), standard gamble (SG) or visual analogue scales (VAS)) and determining from whom values should be obtained (e.g. patient or general public), and more recently there has been research into specific instruments (such as EQ-5D).[3,4] However, for many health states, such as hip fractures, vertebral fractures, cancer, stroke, osteo-arthritis, chronic obstructive pulmonary disease (COPD), cardiovascular disease,

Evidence-Based Decisions and Economics, 2nd edition. Edited by I. Shemilt, M. Mugford, L. Vale, K. Marsh and C. Donaldson. © 2010 Blackwell Publishing.

and HIV/AIDS, there are numerous utility values that could be used and these values have often been obtained from varied populations using different methods. For the analyst, this raises the question of how HSUVs should be selected from the literature.

In the past, decision models have often presented a single set of HSUVs with little justification as to why these have been selected over and above others.[5] Whilst a single set of HSUVs used may meet the broad methodological requirements of the agency for which a decision model is produced, any particular selection of values is prone to bias. Recent NICE methods guidelines for economic evaluation also recognise this problem: 'The use of utility estimates from published literature must be supported by evidence that demonstrates that they have been identified and selected systematically'.[6] However, no guidance is provided on how this might be achieved.

Where there are multiple values for a health state, it may be considered good practice to combine the evidence in order to provide more robust evidence. However, to date there has been little attempt to synthesise evidence on HSUVs. Additionally, it is clear from published reviews that decision models may require HSUVs for particular subgroups that may not be covered well by some or even all published studies. In these circumstances, published estimates of HSUVs require some manipulation in order to make them more relevant to the needs of a decision model.

This chapter starts to address the problem of how to identify and select HSUVs for use in decision models that aim to produce estimates of the incremental cost per QALY of health care interventions. The next section examines how to conduct a systematic search of the HSUVs literature. This is followed by a section on reviewing published studies in terms of quality and relevance to the decision model. We then consider how to synthesise data in order to yield combined estimates of HSUVs. The chapter finishes with suggestions for further research in this new and emerging area. Throughout the chapter, we refer to the case study of a systematic review of HSUVs undertaken to populate a decision model of interventions to prevent and treat osteoporosis.[7–10]

Although this chapter focuses exclusively on health care and HSUVs, we invite the reader to consider parallel issues that may be applicable to the identification and use of evidence on valuations of the outcomes of social welfare, education and criminal justice interventions (although primary data may be lacking as is discussed in Chapters 2, 4 and 7).

Searching the literature

This section covers various aspects of the process of searching the literature for studies that have measured and reported HSUVs data ('utility studies'), which is the first stage of research in a review of such data to populate a decision model: scoping the search; developing the search strategy; minimising the risk of missing relevant records; sensitivity and specificity; and key specialist resources.

Searching for HSUVs is challenging due to the lack of guidance and validated methods, as well as problems in deciding upon a focused or sensitive search approach. There is no specific guidance on searching for HSUVs from the Centre for Reviews and Dissemination and very little from the Cochrane Collaboration.[11,12] Furthermore, there are no validated methods or filters to ensure efficient retrieval and there are no directly relevant HSUVs terms within the MeSH (Medline) or EMTREE (Embase) thesauri. The sensitivity (i.e. the ability to retrieve relevant records) versus specificity (i.e. the ability to exclude irrelevant records) trade-off is particularly characteristic of searching in this area. Thesaurus terms are controlled terms or vocabulary applied to give an indication about the content of a database record, their main strength being that records are described by a consistent set of terms. Although there are broadly related thesaurus terms for HSUVs, there are no defined terms. Therefore, there is a need to decide between a more specific approach using HSUVs terms in a free-text search and a more sensitive approach using the best available thesaurus terms.

Scoping the search

The scoping process is used to provide a focus for development of a search strategy. It should aim to specify precisely the characteristics of the HSUVs data to be captured by the search. The standard approach to scoping a search conducted for a systematic review is to structure the strategy according to the PICO question (Patient, Intervention, Comparison, Outcome), focusing especially on keywords relating to the population(s), intervention(s) and study design(s) of interest.[13] This approach raises several issues in the context of searching for HSUVs, particularly in the context of populating a decision model (see Table 8.1). The discussion uses the example of a published systematic review and decision model of interventions for osteoporosis, described in Table 8.2 (see Kanis and colleagues for a full description[7]).

Using the osteoporosis review as an example, one question could be: 'Do bisphosphonates reduce the incidence of fractures in patients with osteoporosis?'. Breaking down this question using PICO gives:

- P – patients with osteoporosis
- I – bisphosphonates
- Comparator – no treatment
- Outcome – lower the number of fractures (including those of the hip, vertebra and wrist).

Conducting extensive searches for a review of evidence on clinical effects generally involves searching for studies of the target population(s) (osteoporosis) and intervention(s) (bisphosphonate) combined with a search filter developed to retrieve primary comparative effectiveness research (CER) studies, typically randomised controlled trials (RCTs), and/or previously published systematic reviews of such studies. These searches will typically retrieve studies in which HSUVs have been measured and reported as part of an RCT. However, the measurement of HSUVs is not restricted to RCTs; HSUVs data will

Table 8.1 Scoping issues.

Issues to consider	Possible solutions
Cost-effectiveness analysis requires HSUVs estimates relevant to the population, not just in combination with the treatment.	Search for population only, not the population and the treatment.
Cost-effectiveness analysis requires HSUVs relating to the relevant health states in the model.	Searches may need to be done for the condition being treated and additional health states that could occur.
Cost-effectiveness analysis requires HSUVs relating to specific subgroups of either the population or the relevant health state.	It may be necessary to search for specific ages, ethnicities relating to the condition.

Table 8.2 Decision model for osteoporosis.

Time Tx state	Event in time Tx +1	Health state at year 1 and subsequent years
	1. No event	• Population norm
	2. Hip fracture	• Non-fatal fracture • Fatal fracture
	3. Vertebral fracture	• Non-fatal fracture • Fatal fracture
Population in model (e.g. age/sex norm)	4. Proximal fracture	• Non-fatal proximal fracture • Fatal fracture
	5. Wrist fracture	• Non-fatal wrist fracture
⟶	6. Breast cancer	• Non-fatal breast cancer • Fatal breast cancer
	7. Coronary heart disease (CHD)	• Non-fatal CHD • Fatal CHD
	8. Death (excluding hip fracture, breast cancer and CHD)	• Fatality

Description: An individual starts in a 'normal' health state for their age and sex group, and then in year 1 (Tx + 1) are assumed to experience one of eight possible events listed in column 2. The probability of experiencing one of the events is Pn, where the sum of the probabilities of having one of these eight events is 1. Following each event, an individual may die or survive in one of seven health states that have associated costs and HSUVs. The model allowed for different values at year 1 and subsequent years. The purpose of the systematic review was to obtain estimates for mean HSUVs and their associated distributions. It was assumed that there will be a multiplier effect on the 'normal' for their age and sex group. In this paper, we only report on the review of evidence on fractures HSUVs. For more details about this decision model, see Kanis and colleagues[7] and Stevenson and colleagues.[8]

often be measured and reported within other forms of CER studies, such as health technology assessments and observational studies, as well as economic evaluations.

Simply replacing an RCT or systematic review filter with a search filter designed to retrieve studies containing HSUVs data would not be sufficient, as the search would only retrieve studies containing HSUVs relating to the target population/condition *and* the intervention. Many useful utility studies are not specific to a particular intervention and thus it would be more useful to search for the target population(s) or condition(s) combined with HSUVs terms, omitting terms relating to the intervention. The search would then retrieve available published HSUVs for outcomes associated with osteoporosis.

Health state utility values data might also be required for different age groups, ethnic groups and clinical subgroups that could be causing or have an impact on patients' osteoporosis. Relevant clinical subgroups could be patients within different age groups or with certain co-morbidities. Additionally, utilities terms need to cover the whole treatment pathway and disease progression. This is because decision models generally consider what happens to patients over a period of time – if they do or don't get the intervention, if it is effective or not, if the intervention causes adverse effects, and so on – and therefore a series of HSUVs, which may change as patients' health states change, are required over a period of time corresponding to the time horizon of the model.

Another key issue is to determine the exact health states required for the decision model. The HSUVs needed may extend beyond the health states specified in the 'P' of PICO. In our example review of interventions for the prevention and treatment of osteoporosis, the researchers also considered other relevant health states (see Table 8.2 for the full list). In particular, some of the interventions had implications (positive and negative) for breast cancer and cardiovascular disease. Once patients enter a different health state, they will have different characteristics, with the result that the 'P' in the main PICO developed for the review of clinical effects is no longer useful in the development of a search strategy for relevant HSUVs.

Developing the search strategy

Studies that include HSUVs data can be retrieved from electronic biomedical literature databases such as Medline and Embase. However, there are no defined or validated methods on how to search these resources for studies that include HSUVs and (as mentioned above) these data are not always provided in *evaluations* of health care interventions. We are aware of only one search filter for HSUVs that has not been validated.[14] In addition, the MeSH (Medline) and EMTREE (Embase) thesauri provide little coverage specific to this area. As a consequence, utility studies are difficult to retrieve using thesaurus terms. Managing the trade-off between the retrieval of large numbers of irrelevant records and the risk of missing relevant records is an important consideration when searching for studies containing HSUVs.

First, defined thesaurus terms for HSUVs (e.g. utilities, EQ-5D or SF-6D) do not exist. Instead, thesaurus terms that refer to the broader concept of quality of life are applied. Although a broader concept, the thesaurus term 'quality-adjusted life-years' is the most applicable to studies containing HSUVs data. A sample of 1000 records from Medline, retrieved using a set of HSUVs terms from an unvalidated quality of life search filter, were examined to determine the most frequently applied MeSH thesaurus terms, which are listed in Box 8.1.[15] Using thesaurus terms leads to a very sensitive search, reducing the likelihood of missing relevant records. However, this approach is low in precision (specificity) and can therefore result in large numbers of irrelevant records.

Second, relevant free-text terms fall into three categories: general terms (e.g. QALY, utility); instrument-specific terms (e.g. SF-6D, EQ-5D, etc.); and terms

---

Box 8.1 MeSH terms for HSUVs

- Quality of life
- Questionnaires
- Health status
- Health status indicators
- QALY
- Health surveys
- Psychometrics
- Severity of Illness Index

associated with methods of elicitation (e.g. standard gamble, time trade-off, etc.). Free-text searches are reliant on terms being present within the title, abstract or other fields of a database record. However, studies often report HSUVs data as a secondary outcome (this is particularly the case in clinical trials) and consequently related free-text terms may not be present within the abstract. Also, specific health utility instruments are referred to in different ways, including by their full names or their abbreviated names and using different spellings. Therefore, when searching for a specific instrument, it is important to list all the possible ways of naming an instrument, for example: 'euroqol or euro qol or eq-5d or eq5d or eq 5d' for the EQ-5D. Box 8.2 lists some free-text terms for use in searches for HSUVs.

> **Box 8.2 Free-text search terms adapted from a quality of life search filter**
>
> quality adjusted life
> (qaly$ or qald$ or qale$ or qtime$)
> disability adjusted life
> daly$
> (sf36 or sf 36 or short form 36 or shortform 36 or sf thirtysix or sf thirty six or shortform thirtysix or shortform thirty six or short form thirtysix or short form thirty six)
> (sf6 or sf 6 or short form 6 or shortform 6 or sf six or sfsix or shortform six or short form six)
> (sf12 or sf 12 or short form 12 or shortform 12 or sf twelve or sftwelve or shortform twelve or short form twelve)
> (sf6D or sf 6D or short form 6D or shortform 6D or sf six D or sfsixD or shortform six D or short form six D)
> (sf20 or sf 20 or short form 20 or shortform 20 or sf twenty or sftwenty or shortform twenty or short form twenty)
> (euroqol or euro qol or eq5d or eq 5d)
> (hql or hqol or h qol or hrqol or hr qol)
> (hye or hyes)
> health$ year$ equivalent$
> health utilit$
> utilit$
> (hui or hui1 or hui2 or hui3)
> disutili$

> rosser
> quality of wellbeing
> qwb
> standard gamble$
> SG
> time trade off
> time tradeoff
> tto
>
> Reproduced with permission from InterTASC Information Specialists' Sub-Group, 2010.[12]
> $, truncation symbol. In some databases, the truncation symbol is*.

Box 8.2 includes various free-text terms for studies using the instruments SF-36 and SF-12. Whilst these instruments are not utility measures in their own right, they can be used to generate HSUVs indirectly, either by generating the SF-6D or using functions available for mapping onto the EQ-5D.[16–18] This could be extended to other instruments, including those that are disease/condition specific, if appropriate mapping functions exist.[19] However, the use of mapping functions beyond the SF-36 is currently limited as most require individual-level data and in most cases reviewers will only have access to published aggregate data.

Minimising the risk of missing relevant records

Using supplementary search methods and looking within existing literature may assist in identifying records of additional, potentially relevant studies that a search may have failed to identify due to its high specificity or insufficient sensitivity.

Supplementary search methods

Once studies have been identified using the methods described above, highly relevant or 'reference standard' studies can be used to inform supplementary searches.

Citation searching

This involves taking the key relevant papers and identifying further papers which subsequently cite them. Electronic literature databases such as Web of Science, Medline, Embase and Cinahl offer a citation search facility. Google Scholar is also a useful resource in citation searching.

Author searching

Within search results, key author(s) may appear frequently. It is often worthwhile conducting supplementary searches using such author names, as it is likely they may have published other relevant studies.

Searching published literature

Supplementary searches for published cost-utility analyses are likely to return relevant results, since such studies will include references to studies containing HSUVs. Useful thesaurus terms on Medline (MeSH terms) are 'cost-benefit analysis' and 'cost and cost analysis' (free-text terms could include: cost-effectiveness analysis and cost-utility analysis). A good source of published economic evaluations, including cost-utility analyses, is the NHS Economic Evaluation Database (NHS EED). Additionally, reference lists from previously published systematic reviews and health technology assessments which include cost-utility analyses can be an effective way of locating studies containing HSUVs.

Sensitivity and specificity

There is a lack of empirical evidence on the optimal approach to searching for HSUVs data and no validated methodological search filters exist. As discussed, thesaurus terms that may be applied to records of studies containing HSUVs data are based on broader concepts and so are not directly relevant to HSUVs (i.e. low specificity). The absence of HSUVs terms within study abstracts means free-text searching will not necessarily find relevant records (i.e. low sensitivity). This makes a standard approach to locating HSUVs data difficult to formulate.

Depending on the disease and available research resources, searching using a sensitive approach, such as using thesaurus terms, may generate unmanageably large results sets. Alternatively, a more focused approach, which may involve limiting the numbers of search terms and searching in selected fields (e.g. title field), will reduce the number of records retrieved whilst potentially omitting relevant records.

Determining which health utility instruments are particularly important in the context of a specific review/decision model can inform the number and choice of terms. For example, in the NICE Technology Assessment process, the EQ-5D is the preferred measure of HRQL in adults.[6] Alternatively, if the aim is to ensure that all possible studies including HSUVs are retrieved and there are sufficient resources to sift through potentially large result sets, it may be more appropriate to undertake a sensitive literature search incorporating thesaurus terms as well as a number of free-text terms.

Key specialist resources

In addition to biomedical electronic literature databases such as Medline and Embase, the following specialist health economics electronic literature databases are selected key resources for identification of HSUVs:

Cost-Effectiveness Analysis Registry (formerly known as the Harvard CUA database)[20]

The CEA Registry is a free-access specialist register of health care cost-utility analyses maintained by the Center for the Evaluation of Value and Risk in Health at the Institute for Clinical Research and Health Policy Studies, Tufts Medical Center, USA. The registry is an electronic database containing over 1700 cost-utility analyses on a wide variety of diseases and treatments. The CEA registry can be searched for articles, ratios or utility weights using a basic or advanced search. In the basic search you can search for keywords within full records. Using the advanced search for one of the three types of information (articles, ratios or utility measures) allows the search to be restricted to a specific country, intervention type, disease, prevention type or utility weight range.

Centre for Reviews and Dissemination (CRD) NHS EED and HTA database[21,22]

The NHS EED contains 24,000 abstracts of health economics papers including over 7000 quality assessed economic evaluations. The HTA database brings together details of over 7000 completed and ongoing health technology assessments from around the world. It is maintained by the CRD in collaboration with the International Network of Agencies for Health Technology Assessment (INAHTA) secretariat, based in Sweden. Both databases are free access. Relevant health technology assessments and structured abstracts of full economic evaluations are likely to contain useful HSUVs data if a cost-utility analysis has been conducted. HSUVs data are abstracted into a specific field of NHS EED structured abstract records of cost-utility analyses.

Health Economics Evaluations database (HEED)[23]

This is an international, subscription access database containing in excess of 35,000 enriched abstract records and bibliographies of health economic studies obtained from biomedical databases such as Medline and Embase and over 5000 journals.

The EQ-5D website[24]

The EQ-5D website, developed by the EuroQol Group, provides a link to references related to the instrument. The list of references can be searched for specific diseases.

The MAPI Institute website[25]

The MAPI Institute is involved in translating health utility instruments into different languages and ensuring they are appropriate for cross-cultural use and interpretation. The Institute web pages also provide a link to a list of publications undertaken in the health utility instrument area.

There are also sources of unpublished HSUVs data available to researchers, such as the Health Outcomes Data Repository.[26]

Reviewing studies

This section covers other stages of research that may be undertaken as part of the process of reviewing utility studies to populate a decision model: screening and selecting studies; assessment of quality and relevance; data collection; presentation of results; synthesis and estimation of HSUVs for economic models, and (alternatively) adaptation of HSUVs. Again, the example of a systematic review and decision model of interventions for the prevention and treatment of osteoporosis is used to illustrate each stage of research.

Screening and selecting studies

For the osteoporosis review and decision model, electronic searching was undertaken using the search terms listed in Box 8.2 to identify studies containing empirical estimates of HSUVs for the following osteoporosis-related conditions: established osteoporosis, vertebral, hip, wrist and shoulder fractures.[10] This search identified 1000 unique papers. As with any review, a list of eligibility criteria was used as an aid to the process of selecting relevant studies. In our example, initial eligibility criteria were: adults (aged >17 years); men and postmenopausal women suffering primary or secondary osteoporosis; HSUVs empirically estimated using a recognised valuation technique (typically VAS, TTO or SG); English language or available translation. As discussed below, eligibility criteria could have been made tighter by stipulating specific health utility instruments (e.g. EQ-5D). One argument for excluding the latter stipulation at this stage is that it may be possible to adapt data obtained using other instruments or methods for the purposes of estimating HSUVs needed for a specific decision context (see our comment in the previous section of this chapter on indirect estimation through mapping outcomes to utility measures) or, alternatively, to combine HSUVs data using a meta-analysis (see below in this section).

Study selection uses standard systematic review processes of screening titles, abstracts and full texts.[11] At each stage, studies are rejected if they do not meet one or more eligibility criteria. In our osteoporosis example, this process identified 13 relevant studies amongst 1000 records retrieved for screening using electronic searches, which illustrates a potentially low specificity of electronic searches for HSUVs. Twelve additional studies were identified either through contacts with experts or from the reference lists of studies already retrieved, which (conversely) illustrates a potentially low sensitivity from electronic searches for HSUVs. The extent to which low levels of specificity and sensitivity of electronic searches for HSUVs are replicated in other areas of health care remains to be seen.

Assessment of quality and relevance

A conventional review of evidence on clinical effects involves an assessment of the quality of the evidence (usually in terms of potential risk of bias related to aspects of individual study design or conduct) in advance of evidence synthesis.[27] Experience with reviewing utility studies suggests that there is a need to assess the relevance of evidence alongside its quality.

In utility studies, quality can be hard to assess based on information provided in published reports. There are no accepted standards for reporting these types of studies, other than the overall standards for reporting research. At best, the report will contain information on recruitment procedures, inclusion and exclusion criteria and a description of the background characteristics of the sample population from whom values were obtained. As with any form of study involving repeated observations, it is also important to assess participants' response rates to invitations to participate in 'baseline' and follow-up data collection. However, these data are often not reported in utility studies.

As important in selecting data from utility studies is the relevance of the data to the decision model and to the agency to which the model will be submitted. The relevance of the data to the decision model depends on the precise population included in the utility study and how it compares to that being modelled. For this purpose, it is important to extract data on the characteristics of the patients recruited into the study such as age, gender, diagnosis and severity (see 'Data collection', below). Also, it will sometimes be necessary to adjust the values in the utility study in some way to make them more relevant for the decision model (see 'Adaptation of HSUVs for use in a decision model', below).

Some agencies have started to be more prescriptive about the type of HSUVs data they will accept in a submission. NICE have formulated a 'reference case' that prescribes a core set of methods that should be used in the main analysis of any submission.[6] NICE requirements for the reference case with respect to HSUVs include: the technique used to value health states (i.e. choice based such as TTO, SG or VAS), the population from whom values should be obtained (i.e. general population) and how the health states are described (i.e. generic preference-based instrument, preferably EQ-5D).[6] The rationale for developing a reference case is to enhance comparability across submissions and empirical studies have shown that different valuation techniques such as TTO, SG and VAS generate significantly different values for the same health state, whilst values from patients tend to be higher than those of the general public.[28,29] Also, numerous studies comparing the different health utility

instruments, such as EQ-5D, SF-6D and HUI3, have shown that these give different utility values from the same patients.[3,9,30,31]

One approach to reviewing utilities studies for decision models submitted to a specific agency might be to integrate reference case type criteria into eligibility criteria for the review. However, this is not advisable as it is important to collect data from studies using non-reference case methods as well, since (as in the example of the NICE reference case) the EQ-5D instrument is often not used on populations most relevant to the decision model and other utility data may provide evidence on important subgroups. A further consideration is that NICE allows non-reference case values where the EQ-5D can be shown to be inappropriate for the patient group, in which case HSUVs generated using other methods may be relevant.[6] Finally, there may be methods for synthesising values across studies using different methods that might improve the overall robustness and relevance of the values obtained (see 'Synthesis and estimation of HSUVs', below).

Data collection

The data that need to be collected from each utility study should include: study publication date; country of respondents; disease-related health state (e.g. established osteoporosis, hip, vertebral, wrist or shoulder fracture, along with the time period since any osteoporotic incident); health state description system (e.g. EQ-5D, HUI and QWB or vignettes); valuation technique (e.g. SG, TTO, VAS, including information on the version of the technique used, such as the definition of the best state (e.g. 'full health' or 'best for age')); and details of the participants who valued each health state (e.g. patients, general population; sample characteristics, such as age, sex, condition severity, co-morbidities and other sociodemographic or clinical variables). It is also necessary to enable assessments of the quality of primary data collection methods by collecting details of respondent selection and recruitment, inclusion and exclusion criteria and response rates from each study. Finally, descriptive statistics on the utility values need to be collected from each study, including sample size, means, medians, standard deviations and range, preferably by subgroup.

Presentation of results

As with a review of evidence on clinical effects, an important part of the review process is to tabulate detailed information on the characteristics of each study. Reporting only the HSUVs with little detail on the methods used to generate these data makes it impossible for users to understand why the values may differ across studies. Making such tables available to readers in some form (e.g. in a supporting electronic document) is important for this purpose, and also to allow users to fully assess the relevance of the HSUVs to their own context.

To provide an example of the range of results obtained in reviews of HSUVs, consider the values identified for hip fracture in the osteoporosis review undertaken by Peasgood and colleagues.[10] Across 12 studies containing HSUVs for hip fracture, values for the first year post fracture range from 0.05 to 0.73. A majority of studies were conducted on hip fracture patients at specific points in time post fracture and show a trend of recovery following hip fracture. The classification of hip fracture is clear in all studies and most studies exclude pathological fracture.

Six of the 12 studies report EQ-5D values using the UK tariff for patients following a hip fracture. These studies show a sharp decline in HSUVs immediately following the fracture, followed by rising utility (see Figure 8.1). EQ-VAS data, although broadly in line with other values at most time periods, is considerably higher compared with the EQ-5D at 2 weeks. The results from three Swedish studies give higher values both before and after hip fracture than those from the UK. The quality of one study was particularly poor in terms of response rates, with an initial rate of 18% for hip fracture patients at 2 weeks, falling to 9% at 12 months. Such low rates mean that the findings of this study should be viewed with caution.

A problem with this particular set of studies is that they either did not collect before-fracture data or else relied on retrospective recall of prefracture HSUVs that are prone to recall bias. None of the three studies with prefracture HSUVs suggest a return to full prefracture HRQL at final follow-up.

Health state utility values obtained using other generic preference-based utility measures follow a broadly similar pattern to those found using the EQ-5D. As expected, direct patient valuations tend to be higher than those obtained from the general population via EQ-5D and other generic preference-based measures. The three studies using vignettes representing a permanent hip fracture state find much lower utility values compared to those using patients' own health or one of the generic preference-based measures. For example, Salkeld and colleagues find a TTO-based (death/best imaginable for age) value of 0.05 for a bad hip fracture (involving a move to a nursing home, living away from friends, being unable to walk long distances, being unable to shower or dress without help from a nurse, being unable to pursue previous activities, feeling anxious and easily upset) and 0.31 for a good hip fracture (return to independent living, able to walk with a stick, unable to drive, unable to shop or manage the housework alone,

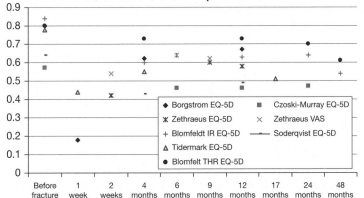

Figure 8.1 EQ-5D and EQ-VAS for hip fracture over time. Reproduced with permission from Peasgood *et al.*, 2009.[10]

periods of frustration and tearfulness, reduced previous activities), for an elderly sample of patients who had fallen at least twice in the past year.[32] This suggests that the vignette may have described a health state worse than that experienced on average by patients. Overall, the findings of the review indicate that the estimate of any HRQL loss from hip fracture depends crucially upon the choice of valuation method and whose values are used.

A weakness identified with the evidence found in these studies, and one likely to exist for other conditions, is that institutionalised adults and patients with co-morbidities, severe cognitive impairment and/or secondary osteoporosis are excluded to ensure that utility measures are purely identifying primary osteoporosis. However, the excluded groups might have different HRQL losses. Low response rates and high rates of losses to follow-up and drop-out may also influence average HSUVs obtained, if lost patients are non-representative of patients in the overall sample. For example, it is evident in the context of hip fracture that those patients providing full data have suffered, on average, a lesser impact on HRQL compared with patients in the overall sample. Such factors will inevitably influence the reliability of the results of a decision model that aims to predict HRQL for specific groups of patients, such as 'average' health service populations, who may not have been fully represented in the underlying utility studies.

Synthesis and estimation of HSUVs

Only a few reviews of HSUVs have attempted any kind of formal synthesis of results.[33,34] Most simply report what they find in a summary table and recommend one or two values for use in decision models.[35–38] Peasgood and colleagues use a simple pooling of values to estimate utility losses associated with the first and subsequent years following a hip fracture.[10] The reviewers estimate the QALY loss for the first year by taking EQ-5D results from five utility studies weighted by both the inverse of the variance and the sample size, assuming a linear progression in health change between time periods. This method produces estimated QALY losses of 0.228 in the first year following a hip fracture and 0.15 in year two.

More sophisticated approaches to synthesis have been attempted using techniques such as metaregression.[33,39] For example, in a systematic review of metastatic breast cancer, 118 HSUVs were identified from 19 included studies.[39] Included studies reported HSUVs for different states of disease progression (response, stable, progression, and terminal), treatment and side effects of the disease and used different valuation methods. Given the large number of values, it was decided to use metaregression based on pooled ordinary least squares (OLS) to estimate the impact on HSUVs of treatment and disease progression, co-morbidities and side effects, whilst controlling for 'moderator' variables related to the methods used to obtain values. Such methods of synthesis have not been widely used in utility studies but they show promise and will yield more reliable results (in terms of power and precision) as the number of published studies increases.

Adaptation of HSUVs

Health state utility values are often collected from patient groups with different characteristics from those required for decision models, in terms of sociodemographic (e.g. age and sex) and/or clinical variables (e.g. condition severity and the prevalence of co-morbidities). Furthermore, published HSUVs often come from cross-sectional studies, whilst decision models require estimates of how HSUVs change as a result of treatment and its associated impact on patients' health (such as reductions in event rates). In these circumstances, the analyst must adjust published utility values for these factors, and there are a number of methods for doing this.

In the osteoporosis model, it was necessary to know what HSUVs would have been without a fracture (i.e. the counterfactual). A common assumption is that the loss associated with the fracture is equivalent to 1.0 minus the value in the literature, but this may overestimate the value, since people prone to having fractures are likely to be less healthy. Some analysts have taken the age/sex norm of the general population to provide values for the control arm, but this only partially compensates for the problem of overestimation.[40] More accurate estimates of the impact of a condition require large-scale longitudinal studies of people experiencing such events. In the absence of such evidence, the minimum that should be done is to use age/sex norms, such as those that exist for the EQ-5D.

In our osteoporosis example, the values collected in the review did not cover all possible age groups.

Some studies were limited to one age group and others were based on small numbers of participants within age groups, so it was not possible to estimate reliable age-specific values. To extrapolate the findings from these studies to specific age groups used in decision model, one approach would be to assume a constant absolute reduction regardless of age. Another is to assume a constant proportional effect on HSUVs. A similar problem arises from co-morbidities, either in patients in the HSUV study or patients in the decision model who are experiencing multiple diseases or events. A more simple assumption is that co-morbidities are additive in their impact on HRQL and this can result in large negative values. Other potential assumptions are that the condition with the lower HSUV dominates or that each condition has a multiplicative effect. These different approaches can have a significant impact on decision model results. Evidence on the most appropriate method of adaptation is mixed, although a recent study suggests that a multiplicative formulation provides a better overall fit with the data.[17,18]

Discussion

Health state utility values play an important role in influencing the results of an economic evaluation, including decision models. It is therefore important for analysts to use the most appropriate mean HSUVs and quantify the uncertainty surrounding mean values based on all relevant evidence, rather than just the best known study. Selection bias is as important an issue in the choice of HSUVs for use in decision models as it is for any other parameter value, and so it is important to be systematic. The need to systematically review utility studies increases with the growth of the published literature on empirical HSUVs. This chapter has examined the process of systematically reviewing studies containing HSUVs, including methods of searching for, reviewing and synthesising studies of HSUVs.

Currently, research on searching for HSUVs is limited. One widely used but unvalidated quality of life filter has been adapted and presented in this chapter.[14] Paisley and colleagues present the most commonly used Medline (MeSH) and Embase (EMTREE) thesaurus terms for quality of life in a chapter looking at searching for general quality of life literature (i.e. not specifically for HSUVs data).[15] Clearly, an important area of future

research will be to develop these strategies and improve on their sensitivity and specificity in finding primary studies that report HSUVs.

The processes of screening and selecting studies and data collection are comparable in many ways to those used in other types of systematic review. However, in reviews of utility studies there is a need to assess the relevance of published HSUVs alongside study quality. This requires an assessment of the extent to which the population in the source study for the HSUVs matches the population used in the decision model. It also means assessing the extent to which they meet the 'reference case' criteria of the reimbursement agency, if applicable. The process of reviewing studies which include HSUVs can be frustrating since generating these data was not necessarily the main objective of the studies. With persistence, it has been possible for a number of authors to undertake such reviews. For a number of medical conditions, it has been shown that there are a number of relevant studies using the same measure, which improves the scope for attempting some kind of synthesis across studies.

The development of formal methods for synthesising HSUVs collected from multiple studies is at an early stage. Little is understood about the reliability of applying meta-analytic techniques to HSUVs data when there are so many sources of variability between studies. However, early attempts appear promising. With time, the amount of data available for such analyses will increase, making the use of such techniques more viable. It is important to persist with formal synthesis methods in order to make the most of the data available and to better understand the reasons for variations in values across studies.

The result of systematic reviews of HSUVs should be a public good made freely available to researchers around the world. Provided reviews are undertaken in a rigorous and systematic way, it should be possible to start to develop catalogues of values for different conditions and treatments. However, there will always be a concern that values will vary between countries owing to differences in the patient populations, accepted methods and patient valuations of the same states (e.g. there are now country-specific values set for the EQ-5D). Nonetheless, we believe there would be benefits from a wider sharing of these resources and for future reviews to build on past work.

How this chapter should be cited

Brazier JE, Papaioannou D, Cantrell A, Paisley S, Herrmann KH. Chapter 8: Identifying and reviewing health state utility values for populating decision models. In: Shemilt I, Mugford M, Vale L, Marsh K, Donaldson C (editors). *Evidence-based decisions and economics: health care, social welfare, education and criminal justice*. Oxford: Wiley-Blackwell, 2010.

References

1 Drummond MF, Sculpher MJ, Torrance GW, O'Brien BJ, Stoddart GL. *Methods for the Economic Evaluation of Healthcare Programmes*, 3rd edn. Oxford: Oxford University Press, 2005.

2 Torrance GW. Measurement of health state utilities for economic appraisal: a review. *Journal of Health Economics* 1986; 5(1): 1–30.

3 Brazier JE, Ratcliffe J, Tsuchiya A, Solomon J. *Measuring and Valuing Health for Economic Evaluations*. Oxford: Oxford University Press, 2007.

4 Tengs TO, Wallace A. One thousand health-related quality-of-life estimates. *Medical Care* 2000; 38(6): 583–637.

5 Tosh J, Longworth L. *Utility Values in NICE Technology Assessments (Health Economics and Decision Science Discussion Paper 06/09)*. Sheffield: University of Sheffield. Available from: www.shef.ac.uk/scharr/sections/heds/discussion.html.

6 National Institute for Health and Clinical Excellence. *Guide to the Methods of Technology Appraisal*. London: National Institute for Health and Clinical Excellence, 2008.

7 Kanis JA, Brazier JE, Stevenson M, Calvert NW, Lloyd-Jones M. Treatment of established osteoporosis: a systematic review and cost utility analysis. *Health Technology Assessment* 2002; 6(29): 1–146.

8 Stevenson MD, Brazier JE, Calvert NW, Lloyd-Jones M, Oakley J, Kanis JA. Description of an individual patient methodology for calculating the cost-effectiveness of treatments for osteoporosis in women. *Journal of the Operational Research Society* 2005; 56(2): 214–221.

9 Brazier JE, Green C, Kanis JA. A Systematic review of health state utility values for osteoporosis-related conditions. *Osteoporosis International* 2002; 13(10): 768–776.

10 Peasgood T, Herrmann K, Kanis JA, Brazier JE. An updated systematic review of health state utility values for osteoporosis related conditions. *Osteoporosis International* 2009; 20(6): 853–868.

11 Higgins JPT, Green S (eds). *Cochrane Handbook for Systematic Reviews of Interventions*. Version 5.0.1 (updated September 2008). Oxford: Cochrane Collaboration, 2008.

12 Centre for Reviews and Dissemination. *Systematic Reviews: CRD's guidance for undertaking reviews in healthcare*, 3rd edn. York: Centre for Reviews and Dissemination, 2009.

13 Lefebvre C, Manheimer E, Glanville J. Searching for studies. In: Higgins JPT, Green S (eds). *Cochrane Handbook for Systematic Reviews of Interventions*. Version 5.0.1 (updated September 2008). Oxford: Cochrane Collaboration, 2008.

14 InterTASC Information Specialists' Sub-Group. *Search Filter Resource: quality of life sample search filter*. InterTASC Information Specialists' Sub-Group, 2010. Available from: www.york.ac.uk/inst/crd/intertasc/qol1.htm.

15 Paisley S, Booth A, Mensinkai S. Health-related quality of life studies. In: *Etext on Health Technology Assessment (HTA) Information Resources*. Bethesda: US National Library of Medicine (NLM) National Information Center on Health Services Research and Healthcare Technology (NICHSR), 2005. Available from: www.nlm.nih.gov/ archive//2060905/nichsr/ehta/chapter12.html.

16 Brazier JE, Roberts J, Deverill M. The estimation of a preference based measure of health from the SF-36. *Journal of Health Economics* 2002; 21(2): 271–292.

17 Ara R, Brazier J. Deriving an algorithm to convert the 8 mean SF-36 dimension scores into a mean EQ-5D preference-based score from published studies (where patient level data are not available). *Value in Health* 2008; 11(7): 1131–1143.

18 Ara R, Brazier J. Predicting SF-6D preference-based utilities using the SF-36 health summary scores: approximating health related utilities when patient level data is not available. *Value in Health*, in press.

19 Brazier JE, Yang Y, Tsuchyia A, Rowen D. A review of mapping (or cross walking) from non-preference based measures of health to preference-based measures. *European Journal of Health Economics* 2009; 12(2): 346–353.

20 Centre for the Evaluation of Value and Risk in Health. *CEA Registry*. Boston: Tufts Medical Center, 2010. Available from: https://research.tufts-nemc.org/cear/Default.aspx.

21 Centre for Reviews and Dissemination. *HTA*. York: Centre for Reviews and Dissemination, 2010. Available from: www.crd.york.ac.uk/crdweb.

22 Centre for Reviews and Dissemination. *NHS Economic Evaluation Database*. York: Centre for Reviews and Dissemination, 2010. Available from: www.crd.york.ac.uk/crdweb.

23 Wiley Interscience. *HEED: health economics evaluation database*. Chichester: Wiley Interscience, 2010. Available from: http://heed.wiley.com.

24 EuroQol Group. *EQ-5D: a standardised instrument for use as a measure of health outcome*. Rotterdam: EuroQol Group. Available from: www.euroqol.org.

25 MAPI Research Institute. *MAPI Institute*. Lyon: MAPI Research Institute. Available from: www.mapi-institute.com/home.

26 Currie CJ, McEwan P, Peters JR, Patel TC, Dixon S. The routine collation of health outcomes data from hospital treated subjects in the Health Outcomes Data Repository (HODaR): descriptive analysis from the first 20,000 subjects. *Value in Health* 2005; 8(5): 581–590.

27 Deeks JJ, Higgins JPT, Altman DG. Analysing data and undertaking meta-analyses Higgins JPT, Green S (eds). *Cochrane Handbook for Systematic Reviews of Interventions*. Version 5.0.1 (updated September 2008). Oxford: Cochrane Collaboration, 2008.

28 Green C, Brazier J, Deverill M. A review of health state valuation techniques. *Pharmacoeconomics* 2000; 17(2): 151–165.

29 Ubel PA, Loewenstein G, Jepson C. Whose quality of life? A commentary exploring discrepancies between health state evaluations of patients and the general public. *Quality of Life Research* 2003; 12(6): 599–607.

30 Dolan P. Modelling valuations for EuroQol health states. *Medical Care* 1997; 35(11): 1095–1108.

31 Feeny D, Furlong W, Torrance GW, *et al*. Multiattribute and single-attribute utility functions for the Health Utilities Index Mark 3 System. *Medical Care* 2002; 40(2): 113–128.

32 Salkeld G, Cameron ID, Cumming RG, *et al*. Quality of life related to fear of falling and hip fracture in older women: a time trade-off study. *British Medical Journal* 2000; 320(7231): 241–246.

33 Tengs T O, Lin T H. A meta-analysis of utility estimates for HIV/AIDS. *Medical Decision Making* 2002; 22(6): 475–481.

34 Bremner KE, Chong CAKY, Tomlinson G, Alibhai SMH, Krahn MD. A review and meta-analysis of prostate cancer utilities. *Medical Decision Making* 2007; 27(3): 288–298.

35 Post PN, Stiggelbout AM, Wakker PP. The utility of health states after stroke: a systematic review of the literature. *Stroke* 2001; 32(6): 1425–1429.

36 Pickard AS, Wilke CT, Lin HW, Lloyd A. Health utilities using the EQ-5D in studies of cancer. *Pharmacoeconomics* 2007; 26(5): 365–384.

37 Muszbek N, Thompson MM, Soong CV, Hutton J, Brasseur P, van Sambeek MRHM. Systematic review of utilities in abdominal aortic aneurysm. *European Journal of Vascular and Endovascular Surgery* 2008; 36(3): 283–289.

38 Ruchlin HS, Insinga RP. A review of health-utility data for osteoporosis: implications for clinical trial-based evaluation. *Pharmacoeconomics* 2008; 26(11): 925–935.

39 Peasgood T, Brazier JE. *A Review of Utility Values in Breast Cancer (Health Economics and Decision Science Discussion Paper 07/09)*. Sheffield: University of Sheffield. Available from: www.shef.ac.uk/scharr/sections/heds/discussion.html.

40 Fryback DG, Dasbach EJ, Klein R, *et al*. The Beaver Dam Health Outcomes Study: initial catalog of health-state quality factors. *Medical Decision Making* 1993; 13(2): 89–102.

CHAPTER 9

Use of evidence in decision models

Doug Coyle[1], Karen M. Lee[2], Nicola J. Cooper[3]

[1]Department of Epidemiology and Community Medicine, University of Ottawa, Ottawa, Canada
[2]Canadian Agency for Drugs and Technology in Health, Ottawa, Canada
[3]Department of Health Sciences, University of Leicester, Leicester, UK

Introduction

The practice of conducting health economic evaluations through decision analysis based on secondary data sources has become wellestablished.[1,2] However, it has been argued that economic analysis conducted through decision analysis is open to bias.[3] This is evident from certain journals questioning the scientific rigour of decision analysis-based studies.[4] Concerns over bias have been particularly pertinent to analysis funded by industry.[5]

For any decision model, the results are only as reliable as the model's poorest data input. However, the extent to which this has a qualitative effect will depend on whether 'poor' evidence is used for parameters that strongly influence the model results (i.e. key driver(s) in the model). Thus, hierarchies which outline the quality of data elements within economic evaluation, including decision models, are desirable as a means of improving the 'evidence base' of inputs used in such analyses. The adoption of such a hierarchy should help to limit the potential for bias.

In a review of health economic evaluations conducted in the field of osteoporosis, all analyses were conducted using forms of decision modelling based on existing data. However, studies differed in their source of data inputs.[6] For example, a number of the studies identified obtained their estimates of

effectiveness from single clinical trials rather than from systematic reviews of all available trials.

This chapter addresses three specific objectives. First, a hierarchy developed in the health care context is presented. The hierarchy relates to five of the most common data elements within decision models for health economic evaluation: clinical effect size, baseline clinical data, costs, resource use and utilities.

Second, the chapter highlights results from a review of decision models developed as part of the NHS Research and Development Health Technology Assessment (HTA) programme between 1997 and 2003.[7] The review applies the hierarchy to determine the quality of the sources of evidence used to parameterise the decision models. Finally, we demonstrate the impact of using alternative data sources on the results of a decision model developed to evaluate the cost-effectiveness of alendronate compared to no therapy in the treatment of postmenopausal women with osteoporosis.

Different sources of data

Previous guidance

The hierarchy presented here was first developed by Coyle & Lee[7] and was later adapted by Cooper and colleagues.[8] The hierarchy relates to standards for the source of data inputs for health economic analysis and ranks sources on a scale from 1 (highest quality) to 6 (lowest quality). The focus is on five common data elements: clinical effect sizes, baseline clinical data, resource use, unit costs, and utilities (see Table 9.1). Although there are a number of quality assessment tools for health economic evaluation (see also, *inter alia*, Chapters 2 and 10), none of these provides

Evidence-Based Decisions and Economics, 2nd edition. Edited by I. Shemilt, M. Mugford, L. Vale, K. Marsh and C. Donaldson. © 2010 Blackwell Publishing.

Table 9.1 Hierarchies of data sources for health economic analyses.

Rank	Data Components
A	**Clinical effect sizes**
1+	Meta-analysis of RCTs with direct comparison between comparator therapies, measuring final outcomes
1	Single RCT with direct comparison between comparator therapies, measuring final outcomes
2+	Meta-analysis of RCTs with direct comparison between comparator therapies, measuring surrogate outcomes[a]
	Meta-analysis of placebo-controlled RCTs with similar trial populations, measuring final outcomes for each individual therapy
2	Single RCT with direct comparison between comparator therapies, measuring surrogate outcomes[a]
	Single placebo-controlled RCTs with similar trial populations, measuring final outcomes for each individual therapy
3+	Meta-analysis of placebo-controlled RCTs with similar trial populations, measuring surrogate outcomes[a]
3	Single placebo-controlled RCTs with similar trial populations, measuring surrogate outcomes[a] for each individual therapy
4	Case–control or cohort studies
5	Non-analytic studies, for example, case reports, case series
6	Expert opinion
B	**Baseline clinical data**
1	Case series or analysis of reliable administrative databases specifically conducted for the study covering patients solely from the jurisdiction of interest
2	Recent case series or analysis of reliable administrative databases covering patients solely from the jurisdiction of interest
3	Recent case series or analysis of reliable administrative databases covering patients solely from another jurisdiction
4	Old case series or analysis of reliable administrative databases. Estimates from RCTs
5	Estimates from previously published economic analyses: unsourced
6	Expert opinion
C	**Resource use**
1	Prospective data collection or analysis of reliable administrative data from same jurisdiction for specific study
2	Recently published results of prospective data collection or recent analysis of reliable administrative data – same jurisdiction
3	Unsourced data from previous economic evaluations – same jurisdiction
4	Recently published results of prospective data collection or recent analysis of reliable administrative data – different jurisdiction
5	Unsourced data from previous economic evaluation – different jurisdiction
6	Expert opinion
D	**Unit costs**
1	Cost calculations based on reliable databases or data sources conducted for specific study – same jurisdiction
2	Recently published cost calculations based on reliable databases or data sources – same jurisdiction
3	Unsourced data from previous economic evaluation – same jurisdiction
4	Recently published cost calculations based on reliable databases or data sources – different jurisdiction
5	Unsourced data from previous economic evaluation – different jurisdiction
6	Expert opinion

Continued on p.108

Table 9.1 *Continued.*

Rank	Data Components
E	**Utilities**

1	Direct utility assessment for the specific study from a sample:
	  a) of the general population
	  b) with knowledge of the disease(s) of interest
	  c) of patients with the disease(s) of interest
	Indirect utility assessment from specific study from patient sample with disease(s) of interest: using tool validated for the patient population

2	Indirect utility assessment from a patient sample with disease(s) of interest; using a tool not validated for the patient population

3	Direct utility assessment from a previous study from a sample:
	  a) of the general population
	  b) with knowledge of the disease(s) of interest
	  c) of patients with the disease(s) of interest
	Indirect utility assessment from previous study from patient sample with disease(s) of interest: using tool validated for the patient population

4	Unsourced utility data from previous study – method of elicitation unknown
5	Patient preference values obtained from a visual analogue scale
6	Delphi panels, expert opinion

Adapted from Coyle & Lee and Cooper and colleagues.[7,8]

[a] Surrogate outcomes = an endpoint measured in lieu of some other so-called true endpoint (including survival at end of clinical trial as predictor of lifetime survival).

explicit guidance on the relative merits of alternative sources for data inputs to decision models.

Clinical effect sizes

For health economic analysis, the source of clinical effect sizes of comparator treatments may be the most crucial data input. The hierarchy proposed for effect sizes follows previous hierarchies for clinical evidence, which demonstrate clear support for evidence synthesis over individual randomised controlled trials (RCTs) over observational studies and expert opinion, in assessing the relative quality of potential data sources for this data element.[9] However, the hierarchy also reflects that there can be many aspects of an RCT which may make it difficult to incorporate such data in economic analyses, such as the preponderance of placebo-controlled trials to evaluate drug therapies and the use of surrogate outcomes.

Baseline risks of clinical events

Characteristics of clinical trials, especially patient exclusion criteria, can lead to the incidence of clinical events being very different from what would be experienced in normal clinical practice. Clinical trial populations are often a select group of patients for which the incidence of events may be substantially lower or higher than the norm. In addition, the design of trial protocols often influences the detection of clinical events, leading to an overestimate of their baseline incidence.

Given these concerns with trial-based data, the hierarchy proposes that a preferred source for baseline risk data is likely to be the analysis of good-quality administrative or epidemiological databases. The question of what constitutes good-quality administrative data is less clear; but this is likely to involve considerations of risks of bias, accuracy and generalisability to broader populations.

Event rates can vary by geographical and political areas due to a number of factors, primarily because of the prevalence of risk factors (e.g. genetic predisposition, diet, exercise, weather, availability of health care). Given this, bias may be introduced into analyses based on databases from different locations and thus the hierarchy reflects the need for data to be applicable to the jurisdiction of interest.

Resource use

In the measurement of resource use, major potential data sources include prospective data collection within

RCTs and observational studies, retrospective analysis of RCTs and observational studies, and analysis of administrative databases. These sources can all be considered valid. However, of more importance is whether the data obtained are applicable to the jurisdiction of interest. Because of the substantial differences between jurisdictions in terms of clinical practice and health care financing, it is often considered preferable (if not essential) that data sources from the geographical or political area to which the study relates are employed in analysis (for further discussions on various aspects of this issue, see, *inter alia*, Chapters 2, 3, 5, 10 and 13). Some analysts utilise data from previous studies or expert opinion in decision models. The latter may be seen as the least preferred source, primarily due to concerns of accuracy and relevance. However, the former sources of data all have potential problems that need to be considered within each individual study.

Unit costs

In the measurement of unit costs, potential sources include prospective costing or analysis of administrative databases. Either of these approaches, conducted specifically for the study in question, is considered the most reliable source of unit cost data. However, the unthinking use of administrative databases must be discouraged. Administrative databases can provide good estimates of average costs associated with health care resource use. In situations where changes in practice are likely to significantly affect resource provision, analysts must consider how closely these costs mirror true opportunity costs (see also, *inter alia*, Chapters 2, 3 and 13).[10]

Unit cost data obtained for previous studies are the next preferred source, assuming they relate to the jurisdiction of interest, as the same contextual issues apply as for resource use (see also, *inter alia*, Chapters 2, 3, 5, 10 and 13). The use of data from previous studies which do not provide adequate reporting of the source of unit cost data is the least preferred option.

Utilities

There is a lack of consensus over the preferred source of utility values to be used in economic analysis (see also Chapter 8). Such lack of consensus relates to the preferred tools for utility elicitation and the preferred source for the estimation of utility values.[11,12] Some commentators argue that applying direct utility elicitation techniques to patients with a particular condition provides the most relevant and accurate representation of the quality of life associated with a particular health state. Others argue that, as decisions relating to health care provision are taken from the perspective of not knowing who will benefit from treatment, valuations should be obtained from the general public. The latter can be obtained through patient responses to indirect utility questionnaires or direct utility elicitation from the general public, based on preferences for health state scenarios (see Chapter 8).

Given this lack of consensus, the proposed hierarchy does not take a particular position within this debate. Rather, the hierarchy makes a distinction in terms of appropriateness between the use of utilities from studies specifically designed for the particular analysis, utility estimates derived from previously published sources and those based on expert opinion. Clearly, if consensus were reached on this issue, further revision of the hierarchy would be required.

Review of published decision models

Methods

All decision models developed as part of NHS Research and Development Health Technology Assessment programme reports published between 1997 and 2003 were reviewed by one of the authors.[7] The quality of evidence used to estimate model parameters was assessed using the hierarchy shown in Table 9.1. Within each of the data elements, there is the potential that data can be obtained from different sources of different quality. Here, results are presented only in terms of the highest source of data quality.

Results

Forty-two decision models, considering both costs and effects, were identified from a total of 180 HTA reports published between 1997 and 2003. For certain studies, some of the data elements were not relevant: clinical event sizes (two out of 42) and utilities (17 out of 42). For these elements, results are presented as a proportion of studies where they were relevant.

Table 9.2 presents the results of appraising these studies using the hierarchy shown in Table 9.1. It was difficult to ascertain the quality of sources used from many of the studies. The data source was described

Table 9.2 Quality of data sources used in decision models.

		Clinical effect size	Baseline clinical data	Resource use	Costs	Utilities
Hierarchies of evidence	1+	16 (40.0%)				
	1	7 (17.5%)	1 (2.4%)	5 (11.9%)	1 (2.4%)	2 (8.0%)
	2+	1 (2.5%)				
	2	3 (7.5%)	21 (50.0%)	8 (19.0%)	34 (81.0%)	1 (4.0%)
	3+	1 (2.5%)				
	3	0 (0.0%)	3 (7.1%)	0 (0.0%)	1 (2.4%)	9 (36.0%)
	4	4 (10.0%)	5 (11.9%)	3 (7.1%)	2 (4.8%)	6 (14.0%)
	5	1 (2.5%)	0 (0.0%)	6 (14.3%)	3 (7.1%)	1 (2.0%)
	6	2 (5.0%)	1 (2.4%)	2 (4.8%)	0 (0.0%)	2 (5.0%)
	Unclear	5 (12.5%)	11 (26.2%)	18 (42.9%)	1 (2.4%)	4 (10.0%)

clearly most often for unit costs (97.6%), clinical effect sizes (87.5%) and utilities (84.0%) parameters, but less often for baseline clinical data (73.8%) and resource use (57.1%) parameters.

The source of data was of higher quality (level 3 or better) for costs (85.7%) and clinical effect sizes (70.0%) parameters, compared to baseline clinical data (59.5%), resource use (31.0%) and utilities (48.0%) parameters.

Analysis of the impact of different sources of data

Methods

Analysis was conducted based on a previous decision model of the cost-effectiveness of alternative drug therapies for the treatment of osteoporosis.[13] Economic analysis was conducted using a Markov model based within an Excel spreadsheet. Results presented here relate to treatment with alendronate for women aged 65 years and over with a previous osteoporosis-related fracture.

In the base model, the clinical effectiveness of treatment was assessed by estimating the associated relative risk reductions for hip, wrist and vertebral fractures based on a meta-analysis of all published RCTs. The baseline population risk of fracture was estimated through an analysis of administrative databases for the Canadian province of Ontario. Cost data (combining resource use and unit costs) were obtained from a sample of patients treated in Canada. Health state utility values (HSUVs) were elicited from a group of osteoporotic women in Ottawa, Ontario, using a study conducted alongside the original economic analysis.[14]

First, to assess the potential impact of using individual trials rather than a meta-analysis, the analysis was repeated three times using effect sizes data collected from each of three RCTs which provided relative risks for hip, wrist and vertebral fractures for alendronate.[15–17] Second, to assess the impact of different sources of baseline risks of clinical events data on the results of analysis, analysis was repeated using event rates from non-Canadian cohort studies and from a UK economic study that used event rates from clinical trials.[16,18–21]

Third, to assess the impact of different sources of HSUVs data, analysis was repeated using utility values derived from a US study using direct methods and from a UK economic study which used hypothetical valuations based on indirect utility assessment.[21,22] Finally, to assess the impact of different sources of cost data, analysis was repeated using alternative estimates of costs from Canada and estimates from previous studies conducted in different jurisdictions, inflated and converted to 2000 Canadian dollars.[21,23–27]

Each of the above further analyses was conducted based on Monte Carlo simulation techniques using

Crystal Ball software, whereby 10,000 repeated estimates of incremental costs and quality-adjusted life-year (QALYs) associated with alendronate were obtained from random sampling of the probability distributions for clinical effect sizes.[28]

Results

Table 9.3 presents estimates of the cost per QALY gained for alendronate from both the base model and from revised analyses that utilise the alternative sources of data described above. Results presented here are the ratio of the mean incremental costs to the mean incremental QALYs. Although not shown here, the degree of uncertainty around the incremental cost-effectiveness of alendronate was also presented using cost-effectiveness acceptability curves.[29] Using the base model, the mean incremental cost per QALY gained was $47,800 CAN.

Estimates of the cost per QALY varied most when applying different data sources to estimate clinical effect sizes and baseline clinical events parameters. Based on the individual RCTs, the cost per QALY ranged from $23,700 to $78,700 CAN, compared to the mean estimate from the meta-analysis of $47,800 CAN.

Table 9.3 Cost per QALY based on different data sources.

	Cost per QALY
Base case (level 1+: clinical effects, level 1: utilities, level 2: costs, resource use and baseline clinical data)	$47,800
Clinical effect size	
Individual trial[16]: level 1	$23,700
Individual trial[17]: level 1	$37,200
Individual trial[18]: level 1	$78,700
Baseline clinical data	
Clinical trial[17,26]: level 4	$27,800
Non-Canadian data[21–24]: level 3	$154,600
Utility values	
Non-Canadian data[25]: level 2	$46,300
Expert opinion[26]: level 6	$54,700
Alternative sources of cost data	
Same jurisdiction[27]: level 2	$45,800
Other jurisdiction[26]: level 4	$51,800
Other jurisdiction[28]: level 4	$44,600
Other jurisdiction[29]: level 4	$51,500
Other jurisdiction[30]: level 4	$50,000
Other jurisdiction[31]: level 4	$48,300

Analysis based on baseline clinical event rates from the clinical trial led to a mean cost per QALY gained figure of $27,800 CAN. Analysis based on non-Canadian population databases estimated a mean cost per QALY of $154,600 CAN. Results were relatively insensitive to changes in the source for utility values (a range of $46,300 to $54,700 CAN) and for costs (a range of $44,600 to $51,800 CAN).

Discussion

The potential to bias results of economic evaluation through the use of different sources of data has long been recognised. In this chapter we present a hierarchy relating to the quality of data sources employed in decision models for health economic evaluation.

A review of existing decision models illustrates that parameter estimates for such models are obtained from diverse sources of evidence, ranging from RCTs to expert opinion. The review identified concerns relating to both the reporting of data sources within decision models and the quality of these data sources. The development of the hierarchy should help decision modellers to improve this practice. For future studies, all potential sources for model parameters should be identified, quality assessed and, where applicable, pooled using explicit criteria and reproducible methods. Furthermore, given the poor degree of transparency within existing decision models, it is imperative that methods used to determining data sources adopted within a model should be reported explicitly.

The review was based on a small sample of health technology assessments produced in the UK. It may be that the conclusions drawn are not generalisable to other countries or to the peer-reviewed literature as a whole. However, the review does provide useful insights to the quality of data sources within economic studies that have undergone a rigorous review process.

The findings relating to the adoption of higher quality data for clinical effects and costs are intuitive. For funding and licensing purposes, most health care technologies require reasonable standard clinical evidence prior to adoption. Similarly, over the last few years there has been an increase in the availability of good-quality cost data for use in economic evaluations. Conversely, the lack of data on resource use attributable to individual patients and HSUVs is a continued problem in the conduct of economic evaluation. Finally, the dearth of information and lack of grant funding opportunities to explore the epidemiology of disease to allow extrapolation beyond the time horizon of clinical trials are a major problem, not just for economic evaluation but for clinical research in general.

The example analysis relating to the decision model for osteoporosis highlights the potential concern over adoption of data from less reliable sources. The analysis suggests that uncertainty regarding the appropriate source of clinical data, be it effect sizes or baseline risks of clinical events, has most impact on the results of the analysis. Of particular concern is the high degree of impact on results of moving from a meta-analysis of RCTs (level 1+ evidence) to a single RCT (level 1 evidence). This suggests that concern over data quality may be greater for specific data elements, although which elements may vary by study.

Thus, although the hierarchy attempts to determine the quality of data within specific data elements, it may not be appropriate to assess the quality of data *across* data elements. The relative importance of good-quality data for specific parameters will be contingent on the importance of that parameter within the decision model. Thus, the quality of relatively unimportant parameters may not be a major issue. This will be true both within data elements (e.g. different utility parameters may have different degrees of importance) and across data elements (e.g. treatment effects will be more important than unit costs). The relative importance of such parameters determines the importance of the quality of data inputs and can be assessed through standard methods.[30]

In some instances, only data corresponding to sources lower in the hierarchy may be available. In these circumstances, analysts should be certain that there are not higher quality sources available. If not, then the results should be interpreted bearing the quality of data sources in mind and appropriate methods for handling the uncertainty around such elements should be considered.

Often, multiple sources of evidence from different levels of the hierarchy will be available for each model parameter. Combining this evidence together is nontrivial and there are concerns that the inclusion of poorer study designs will weaken the analysis through the introduction of biases. Equally difficult is pooling of estimates from studies which are from the same

level of evidence but which provide widely different estimates. However, generalised evidence synthesis methods, which adjust for potential biases (i.e. downweight less rigorous and less relevant studies rather than omitting them all together), have been proposed in the statistics literature.[31–34]

As economists become more concerned with the applicability of their analyses, any initiatives to reduce accusations of bias should be welcomed. Thus, the adoption of the hierarchy proposed in this chapter could in some way improve both the conduct of decision models for health economic evaluation and the review of such analyses, by promoting transparency and identifying the weakest aspects of the model for future work. Whilst decision models for health economic evaluation have been the exclusive focus of this chapter, the need for transparency and knowledge of limitations of analyses and data is not restricted to the health care context. Thus adaptation and further development of the proposed hierarchy for applications in other applied fields are to be encouraged.

How this chapter should be cited

Coyle D, Lee KM, Cooper NJ. Chapter 9: Use of evidence in decision models. In: Shemilt I, Mugford M, Vale L, Marsh K, Donaldson C (editors). *Evidence-based decisions and economics: health care, social welfare, education and criminal justice.* Oxford: Wiley-Blackwell, 2010.

References

1 Buxton MJ, Drummond MF, van Hout BA, *et al.* Modelling in economic evaluation: an unavoidable fact of life. *Health Economics* 1997; 6(3): 217–227.

2 Jefferson T, Mugford M, Gray A, Demicheli V. An exercise on the feasibility of carrying out secondary economic analyses. *Health Economics* 1996; 5(2): 155–165.

3 Freemantle N. Maynard A. Something rotten in the state of clinical and economic evaluations? *Health Economics* 1994; 3(2): 63–67.

4 Kassirer JP, Angell J. The Journal's policy on cost-effectiveness analyses. *New England Journal of Medicine* 1994; 331(10): 669–670.

5 Hillman AL, Eisenberg JM, Pauly MV, *et al.* Avoiding bias in the conduct and reporting of cost-effectiveness research sponsored by pharmaceutical companies. *New England Journal of Medicine* 1991; 324(19): 1362–1365.

6 Cranney A, Coyle D, Welch V, Lee KM, Tugwell P. A review of economic evaluations in osteoporosis. *Arthritis Care Research* 1999; 12(6): 425–434.

7 Coyle D, Lee KM. Improving the evidence base of economic evaluations. In: Donaldson C, Mugford M, Vale L (eds) *Evidence-Based Health Economics*. London: BMJ Books, 2002.

8 Cooper N, Coyle D, Abrams K, Mugford M, Sutton A. Use of evidence in decision models: an appraisal of health technology assessments in the UK since 1997. *Journal of Health Services Research and Policy* 2005; 10(4): 245–250.

9 Canadian Task Force on the Periodic Health Examination. The periodic health examination. *Canadian Medical Association Journal* 1979; 121(9): 1193–1254.

10 Mogyorosy Z, Smith PC. *The Main Methodological Issues in Costing Health care Services: a literature review (Centre for Health Economics Research Paper No.7)*. York: Centre for Health Economics, University of York, 2005.

11 Gold MR, Siegel JE, Russell LB, Weinstein MC (eds). *Cost-Effectiveness in Health and Medicine*. New York: Oxford University Press, 1996.

12 Coyle D, Maunsell E, Wells GA, *et al*. Differences in preference values between cultural groups: women's preferences over lifetime risks associated with postmenopausal osteoporosis therapy. *Annual Meeting of the International Society of Technology Assessment in Health care* 1999; 15: 81.

13 Coyle D, Cranney A, Lee KM, Welch V, Tugwell P. Cost-effectiveness of nasal calcitonin in postmenopausal women. Use of Cochrane Collaboration methods for meta analysis in economic evaluation. *Pharmacoeconomics* 2001; 19(5): 565–575.

14 Cranney A, Coyle D, Pham B, *et al*. The psychometric properties of patient preferences in osteoporosis. *Journal of Rheumatology* 2001; 28(1): 132–137.

15 Liberman UA, Weiss SR, Broll J, *et al.,* for the Alendronate Phase III Osteoporosis Treatment Study Group. Effect of oral alendronate on bone mineral density and the incidence of fractures in postmenopausal osteoporosis. *New England Journal of Medicine* 1995; 333(22): 1437–1443.

16 Black DM, Cummings SR, Karpf DB, *et al*. Randomised trial of effect of alendronate on risk of fracture in women with existing vertebral fractures. Fracture Intervention Trial Research Group. *Lancet* 1996; 348(9041): 1535–1541.

17 Cummings SR, Black DM, Thompson DE, *et al.,* for the Fracture Intervention Trial Research Group. Effect of alendronate on risk of fracture in women with low bone density but without vertebral fractures – results from the Fracture Intervention Trial. *Journal of the American Medical Association* 1998; 280(24): 2077–2082.

18 Kannus P, Parkkari J, Sievanen H, Heinonen A, Vuori I, Jarvinen M. Epidemiology of hip fractures. *Bone* 1996; 18(1): 57S–63S.

19 Karagas MR, Lu-Yao GL, Barrett JA, Beach ML, Baron JA. Heterogeneity of hip fracture: age, race, sex, and geographic patterns of femoral neck and trochanteric fractures among the US elderly. *American Journal of Epidemiology* 1996; 143(7): 677–682.

20 Donaldson LJ, Cook A, Thomson RG. Incidence of fractures in a geographically defined population. *Journal of Epidemiology and Community Health* 1990; 44(3): 241–245.

21 Best L, Milne R. *Bisphosphonates (Alendronate and Etidronate) in the Management of Osteoporosis (Development and Evaluation Committee Report No.79)*. Southampton: Wessex Institute for Health Research and Development, 1998.

22 Silverman SL, Simons R. Utility values for osteoporosis outcomes (Second Joint Meeting of the American Society for Bone and Mineral Research and the International Bone and Mineral Society, Abstract W443). *Bone* 1998; 23(5): S398.

23 Goeree R, O'Brien B, Pettitt D, Cuddy L, Ferraz M, Adachi J. An assessment of the burden of illness due to osteoporosis in Canada. *Journal of the Society of Obstetricians and Gynaecologists of Canada* 1996; 18(suppl); 15–22.

24 Kristiansen IS, Falch JA, Andersen L, Aursnes I. Bruk av alendronat ved osteoporose – er det kostnadseffektivt? *Tidsskrift for Den Norske Laegeforening* 1997; 117(18): 2619–2622.

25 Cheung AP, Wren BG. A cost-effectiveness analysis of hormone replacement therapy in the menopause. *Medical Journal of Australia* 1992; 156(5): 312–216.

26 Ankjaer-Jensen A, Johnell O. Prevention of osteoporosis: cost-effectiveness of different pharmaceutical treatments. *Osteoporosis International* 1996; 6(4): 265–275.

27 Tosteson ANA, Weinstein MC. Cost-effectiveness of hormone replacement therapy after the menopause. *Baillière's Clinical Obstetrics and Gynaecology* 1991; 5(4): 943–959.

28 Doubilet P, Begg CB, Weinstein MC, Braun P, McNeil BJ. Probabilistic sensitivity analysis using Monte Carlo simulation: a practical approach. *Medical Decision Making* 1985; 5(2): 157–177.

29 Briggs AH. Handling uncertainty in cost-effectiveness models. *Pharmacoeconomics* 2000; 17(5): 479–500.

30 Coyle D, Buxton MJ, O'Brien BJ. Measures of importance for economic analysis based on decision modeling. *Journal of Clinical Epidemiology* 2003; 56(10): 989–997.

31 Greenland S. Multiple-bias modelling for analysis of observational data. *Journal of the Royal Statistical Society: Series A* 2005; 168(2): 267–306.

32 Prevost TC, Abrams KR, Jones DR. Hierarchical models in generalised synthesis of evidence: an example based on studies of breast cancer screening. *Statistics in Medicine* 2000; 19(24): 3359–3376.

33 Spiegelhalter DJ, Best NG. Bayesian approaches to multiple sources of evidence and uncertainty in complex cost-effectiveness modelling. *Statistics in Medicine* 2003; 22(23): 3687–3709.

34 Trichtler D. Modelling study quality in meta-analysis. *Statistics in Medicine* 1999; 18(16): 2135–2145.

CHAPTER 10

Grading economic evidence

Massimo Brunetti[1], Francis Ruiz[2], Joanne Lord[3], Silvia Pregno[4], Andrew D. Oxman[5]

[1]Local Health Unit, Modena, Italy
[2]Centre for Clinical Practice, National Institute for Health and Clinical Excellence, London, UK
[3]Health Economics Research Group (HERG), Brunel University, Uxbridge, UK
[4]Public Health Physician, Modena, Italy
[5]Norwegian Knowledge Centre for the Health Services, Oslo, Norway

Introduction

In this chapter we describe the Grading of Recommendations Assessment, Development and Evaluation (GRADE) approach to rating the quality of evidence and how the standard GRADE profile can capture both clinical evidence and data on the impact of interventions on resource use. Where estimates of costs or cost-effectiveness are obtained using some form of decision model, we have described a separate summary table that may be used to report these types of evidence alongside a GRADE profile. This 'Economic Evidence Profile' has been recommended for use in National Institute for Health and Clinical Excellence (NICE) clinical guidelines in England. These approaches were developed to inform health care decisions, but they could plausibly be adapted for use in other areas of public policy, such as social welfare, education and criminal justice.

Economic evidence in clinical recommendations

Identifying the optimal allocation of available resources in order to maximise population health gains has been and continues to be a key challenge

Evidence-Based Decisions and Economics, 2nd edition. Edited by I. Shemilt, M. Mugford, L. Vale, K. Marsh and C. Donaldson. © 2010 Blackwell Publishing.

for health care systems. One of the main perceived drivers of rising health care expenditure has been the rapid pace of innovation in medical technologies.[1] Throughout the world, there is an increasing emphasis on instruments to determine value for money when adopting interventions and medical technologies.

Summarising the literature in order to produce recommendations for clinical practice is an important part of the process.[2] The health sciences community has reduced the bias and imprecision of traditional literature summaries and their associated recommendations through the development of criteria for both systematic reviews and practice guidelines.[3,4]

In 1979, the Canadian Task Force on the Periodic Health Examination made one of the first efforts to specify the strength of practice recommendations.[5] This group classified the quality of evidence of the benefit of interventions into one of four categories based on the quality of individual study designs. Their classification of the strength of their recommendations was based on the quality of the underlying evidence.[2]

Given the increased awareness of the importance of evaluating value for money in health care, there has been growth in the number of published economic evaluations in recent years.[6] However, the question of whether guideline developers should include resource use or costs as a criterion in their decision making has been controversial. In 1991, the Committee on

Clinical Practice Guidelines in the USA concluded that while guidelines should always include information on the costs as well as health effects of alternative interventions, recommendations need not always be based on formal judgements of cost-effectiveness.[7]

However, guideline developers around the world take different positions on the role of evidence on resource use, cost and cost-effectiveness in guideline decision making. Only a small proportion of published clinical guidelines have incorporated economic analysis and methodological approaches vary, some developing a new decision model, some presenting a synthesis of previous economic evaluations and some presenting budget impact evaluation.[8,9]

The new GRADE system

In 2004 the GRADE system was introduced to grade evidence and recommendations.[10] The World Health Organization (WHO), the American College of Physicians, the American Thoracic Society, UpToDate and the Cochrane Collaboration are amongst the more than 30 organisations that have adopted GRADE. The GRADE website is available from: www.gradeworkinggroup.org.

It is argued that GRADE has advantages over previous rating systems. For example, there is an explicit evaluation of the importance of outcomes resulting from alternative management strategies. In addition, there are explicit, comprehensive criteria for downgrading and upgrading the quality of evidence. The GRADE approach can be used when undertaking systematic reviews and health technology assessments, as well as developing guidelines.[11]

This new rating system focuses on grading the quality of evidence and the strength of recommendations derived from that evidence base. In the context of making recommendations, the quality of evidence is defined as the extent to which confidence in an estimate of effect is adequate to support recommendations. The strength of a recommendation indicates the extent to which one can be confident that adherence to the recommendation will do more good than harm.

As in a standard systematic review, the application of GRADE requires that initially a clinical question is defined in terms of the PICO framework (see, *inter alia*, Chapters 3 and 7). Outcomes are classified as either 'critical' or 'important but not critical': this judgement may be context specific (see also, *inter alia*, Chapters 3, 5 and 13). A systematic review is used as the basis for judgements about the quality of evidence and estimates of effect for each outcome.[11]

The first step in assessing the quality of evidence is to use explicit criteria to judge the risk of bias (study limitations) for each important outcome.[11] The next step is to use explicit criteria to rate the quality of evidence across studies for each outcome, as the quality may differ from one outcome to another both within and across studies. The final step is to use explicit criteria to assess the overall quality of evidence for a recommendation across all the outcomes that are considered critical for a decision.

To achieve transparency and simplicity, the GRADE system classifies the quality of evidence using one of four levels: high, moderate, low and very low.[12] Evidence based on randomised controlled trials (RCTs) begins as high-quality evidence, but the level of confidence in it may be decreased for several reasons, including study limitations (risk of bias), inconsistency of results, indirectness of evidence, imprecision and publication bias. The latter terms, developed for clinical evidence, can be applied, with some adaptation, to estimates of resource use and costs obtained from clinical studies, as discussed in the following section.

Although observational studies (e.g. cohort and case–control studies) start with a 'low-quality' rating, grading upwards may be warranted if the magnitude of the treatment effect is very large, if there is evidence of a dose–response relationship or if all plausible biases would decrease the magnitude of an apparent treatment effect.

After grading the quality of evidence, guideline developers consider the direction and strength of recommendation. The GRADE system offers two grades of recommendations: 'strong' and 'weak'.[13] When the desirable effects of an intervention clearly outweigh the undesirable effects, or clearly do not, guideline panels offer strong recommendations. On the other hand, when the trade-offs are less certain, either because of low-quality evidence or because evidence suggests that desirable and undesirable effects are closely balanced, weak recommendations are warranted. The implications of strong and weak recommendations are summarised in Table 10.1.

Table 10.1 Implications of recommendations. Adapted from Guyatt *et al.*, 2008.[13]

	The implications of a strong recommendation are:	The implications of a weak recommendation are:
For patients	Most people in your situation would want the recommended course of action and only a small proportion would not; request discussion if the intervention is not offered	Most people in your situation would want the recommended course of action, but many would not
For clinicians	Most patients should receive the recommended course of action	You should recognise that different choices will be appropriate for different patients and that you must help each patient to arrive at a management decision consistent with her or his values and preferences
For policy makers	The recommendation can be adopted as a policy in most situations	Policy making will require substantial debate and involvement of many stakeholders

In addition to the quality of the evidence, several other factors affect whether recommendations are strong or weak, including uncertainty about the balance between desirable and undesirable effects, uncertainty or variability in patients' values and preferences, and if the intervention represents a wise use of resources.[13]

The evidence table is a key tool for summarising a body of evidence, displaying the information about main outcomes for a given health care question in a tabular format. Different layouts of evidence tables are available, including the GRADE Evidence Profile and Summary of Findings tables. The former contains detailed information about the quality of evidence and the summary of findings for each of the included outcomes. The latter provides more focused information regarding the results of the available evidence for each important outcome in a quick and accessible format.[14]

The GRADE approach to economic evidence

GRADE recognises that balance sheets are one way of helping decision makers to explicitly consider resource use along with other outcomes when making recommendations.[15] The aim of a balance sheet is to help decision makers to develop an accurate understanding of the important consequences of the options being compared, including resource use.[16] Balance sheets present 'raw information' to which decision makers can apply their own judgements about the trade-offs between health benefits, harms and use of resources. Economic evaluations have some advantages over balance sheets; use of full economic evaluation, in particular decision models, should be considered when decisions involve multiple important outcomes and resource consequences over long periods of time, 'offering the analyst a flexible and timely framework for analysis, . . . aiming to forecast and/or predict events where little or no data exist'.[17]

GRADE recommends that Evidence Profiles (a specific form of balance sheet) should be constructed to inform recommendations whether or not a formal economic evaluation (including trial-based economic evaluations and decision models) is used, in order to ensure decision makers' understanding and appraisal of the quality of key estimates used in an economic evaluation.[16] GRADE also recommends that important differences in resource use and costs should be included in Evidence Profiles along with other important outcomes.[18] If a decision model is used in the recommendation process, it should be transparent and take into consideration the critical outcomes included in the Evidence Profile.[19] However, the GRADE approach excludes evidence derived from decision models (although in the UK, NICE has developed an approach to presenting modelled economic evidence alongside GRADE Evidence Profiles – see 'Grading clinical and economic evidence in NICE guidelines', below). The primary reasons for this exclusion are that decision models synthesise health and resource use information derived from primary sources that may already summarised in the Evidence Profile and because they synthesise evidence of varying quality and assumptions.

The key steps in considering resource use when making recommendations within the GRADE approach are:

- identification of types of resource use and costs that are potentially important and which may differ between alternative treatment options (these resources/costs are context specific)
- finding evidence of the differences in levels of identified types of resource use between the options compared
- appraising the quality of the evidence
- valuing the resources used in monetary terms for the specific setting for which recommendations are being made.

Judgements on which types of resource use are important are in part predicated on the viewpoint(s) or analytic perspective(s) being considered in the recommendations being made (see also, *inter alia*, Chapter 3). The analytic perspective(s) should be clearly stated and appropriate for the guideline developer. Some guideline developers may adopt the perspective of the payer, while others may wish to consider a broader range of resource impacts. In the economic Evidence Profile presented in Table 10.2, we adopted a societal perspective in a comparison of two opioid maintenance treatments. In this example, resource use associated with the impacts of criminal behaviour was considered to be an important economic outcome, even though the costs of these resources are incurred outside the health care system.

For each recommendation, only important resource use and costs should be included. We suggest doing this in two steps.

1. As for health outcomes, consider whether overall resource use is likely to be important for the recommendation.
2. If evidence on resource use is likely to be important for decision making, consider specific types of resource use and their relative impact on the cost difference between the interventions (i.e. decide on which should be included in a Summary of Findings table because they are critical to a decision). This judgement about main resource items that are likely to drive the cost difference can be difficult to make, but is an essential first step in any economic evaluation.

Within GRADE, as with health outcomes, resources should be classified as either critical or important but not critical to a decision.[11]

It is also necessary to decide in advance on the relevant time horizon for resource use outcomes. Decision makers may be concerned about longer-term resource use, although only short-term information may be available. Under these circumstances, short-term data may provide convincing (high- or moderate-quality) evidence for longer-term outcomes, even though it is indirect, or they may provide low- (or even very low-) quality evidence if there is substantial uncertainty about whether the long-term outcomes would be the same as short-term outcomes, or substantially different. For example, in chronic diseases we could have only short-term studies, providing indirect evidence of long-term outcomes. Alternatively, it is possible to indicate in an Evidence Profile that no evidence was found for longer-term outcomes.

Some outcomes, such as hospitalizations or days in hospital, can be considered as both patient-important in their own right and as an important component of resource use. For example, an RCT evaluating the effectiveness of a humanised respiratory syncytial virus monoclonal antibody on viral infections in high-risk infants used hospitalisation as a primary clinical outcome.[20] This outcome should also be considered in an Evidence Profile as a component of resource use.

Resource use and cost data can be found in systematic reviews, randomised trials and observational studies. They may be published in or separately from reports of clinical studies. The use of resources in a specific setting can be retrieved from national or local administrative databases, such as drug use from prescription databases or hospitalisations from hospital databases. Prospective data collection or analysis of reliable administrative databases for a specific study is posited as the most reliable source of data on resource use (see also Chapter 9).[21] Resource use should be presented in natural units, such as the number of clinician visits or hospitalisations. When only aggregated cost data are reported (i.e. the final results obtained from multiplying quantities of each item of resource use by its 'per-unit cost'), attempts should be made to collect further information regarding the data components underpinning aggregated cost data (i.e. quantities of resource use and their unit costs) from the investigators.

Table 10.2 Example of a resource use evidence profile.
Question: Should buprenorphine maintenance flexible doses vs methadone maintenance flexible doses be used for opioid maintenance treatment?
Patient or population: Opiate dependents
Setting: Outpatients in USA, Australia, Austria, Switzerland, UK
Viewpoint: Societal

Studies (follow-up)	Quality assessment					Summary of resources and costs			Overall quality
	Design	Limitations	Inconsistency	Indirectness	Imprecision	No. of patients	Resources Costs per patient (1999 AU $)		
							Methadone[h]	Buprenorphine[h]	
Drugs									
Harris 2005 (1 year)[a23]	RCT	Serious limitations[e]	No	Some uncertainty[g]	Small sample size	139	*Resources (mean daily)* 50 mg / *Costs (annual)* 1122 (85 SE)	14 mg / 1785 (204 SE)	Very low
Doran 2003 (6 months)[a24]	RCT	No	No	Some uncertainty[g]	–	405	*Resources (mean daily)* 57 mg / *Costs (6 months)* 37 (33 SD)	11 mg / 459 (461 SD)	Moderate
Other health care costs									
Harris 2005 (1 year)[b23]	RCT	Serious limitations[e]	No	Some uncertainty[g]	Small sample size	139	*Resources* NA / *Costs (annual)* 2500 (489 SE)	NA / 3316 (667 SE)	Very low

Doran 2003 (6 months)[c24]	RCT	No	No	Some uncertainty[g]	–	405	Resources NA NA	Moderate
Crime Costs							Costs (6 months) 1378 (NA) 1270 (NA)	
Harris 2005 (1 year)[d23]	RCT	Very serious limitations[f]	No	Some uncertainty[g]	Small sample size	139	Resources NA NA	Very low
							Costs (annual)[i] 13,223 NA (10,209 SE) 6265 (2,028 SE)	

In this example we decided not to pool resource data from different studies due to insufficient information provided.

NA, not available; SD, standard deviation; SE, standard error.

a Including dispensing fee

b Includes other prescription and OTC drugs, prescriber, inpatient, outpatient, emergency, ambulance, counseling, allied health and pathology services

c Include staff time (i.e. face-to-face contact and preparation time), diagnostic procedures and facility level (supplies, consumables, capital, equipment, ancillary support including administration, management, security, etc.)

d Health care costs from assault, loss of income by the victims of crime, depreciated value of property damaged, stolen or obtained fraudulently, detection, prosecution and imprisonment

e Some limitations because of incomplete outcome data

f Some limitations because of incomplete outcome data and crucial limitations for self-reported crime data

g All the studies were conducted within the Australian health system (while the recommendation was global)

h Doses for methadone and buprenorphine derived from Doran 2003 study, at the 10th week[24]

i The average cost of crime was substantial across the sample but these reported costs were associated with just a few participants. 90% of the sample randomized to methadone and 96% of that randomized on buprenorphine reported non-involvement in property crime. Indeed, the majority of patients reported no criminal activity during the trial (6/66 patients for methadone and 3/73 for buprenorphine)[23]

In our example (Table 10.2), information about health outcomes came from a systematic review.[22] In considering the relative importance of outcomes, overall resource use was considered to be important. In the next step, drugs, other health care costs and crime costs were identified as important specific resource use and costs. Travel costs were not considered important on the basis of the magnitude of their costs (i.e. they were unlikely to make a sizeable contribution to the overall cost difference between the interventions) and were therefore excluded from the Evidence Profile. Two studies provided evidence for the included outcomes.[23,24] Criminal behaviour was considered both as a clinically important outcome and as having an important overall impact on resource use and costs, as well as on specific types of resource use and costs (e.g. those associated with, *inter alia*, victimisation, policing, courts and incarceration).

Changes in the productivity of patients may be important. However, there is substantial controversy regarding the optimal methods to measure and value changes in productivity.[17] Along with others, we suggest that changes in productivity should be considered as a component of the value of changes in health status and therefore should only be included in Evidence Profiles as a health outcome, not as a component of resource use.[25]

When a recommendation is made in a specific context, attaching appropriate monetary values to resource use can help decision makers to value different items of resource use consistently and appropriately. In principle, the values should reflect opportunity costs, which are likely to be specific to the setting in which the option is implemented (see also, *inter alia*, Chapters 1 and 3).[26] Cost calculations based on reliable databases or data from a specific study in the same jurisdiction are posited as the most reliable source of data on costs (see also Chapter 9).[21]

Monetary valuation of resource use should therefore be made using data specific to the context of a recommendation (i.e. utilising locally applicable unit costs), which should be reported separately from aggregated cost data in the guideline. However, if locally applicable unit costs are not available, techniques based on purchasing power parity (PPP) exchange rates and/or inflation factors could be used to adjust unit cost data obtained from other localities with similar health systems.[27]

Discounting is used in economic evaluations to adjust for social or individual preferences over the timing of costs and health benefits. GRADE recommends that resource quantities and health outcomes should be reported in Evidence Profiles in their undiscounted form. If resources and costs are discounted, the data used to calculate discounted costs – including quantities of all types of resource use, unit costs and the discount rate – should be reported, if available. This will enable decision makers and guideline developers to adapt the cost estimates for their locality.

The quality of evidence on resource use should also be reported. There are more than 20 published checklists and instruments for assessing the quality of health economic analyses. However, none is specifically constructed to assess the quality of evidence as defined by GRADE. GRADE recommends that the quality of evidence should be appraised explicitly for each important resource use outcome using the same criteria as for health outcomes. Judgements about the quality of evidence should be based, as far as possible, on estimates of resource use rather than on estimates of the aggregated costs of those resources. As with health outcomes, only critical resource use outcomes should be taken into account in determining the overall quality of evidence across such outcomes.[16]

As with health outcomes, evidence on resource use collected from randomised trials starts at high quality and evidence collected from observational studies starts at low quality. Observational data can be upgraded using the same criteria as for health outcomes, and evidence from randomised trials can be downgraded based on the same five criteria: study limitations (risks of bias), inconsistency of results, indirectness of evidence, imprecision and reporting bias.[11]

Study limitations (risks of bias)

GRADE judges that study limitations (risks of bias) for resource use outcomes are similar to those for health outcomes (see Box 10.1), and they can be evaluated using a risk of bias tool.[28]

- Non-random allocation or inadequate allocation concealment can result in selection bias and important differences, for example, in disease severity, requiring more use of resources.[18]
- Effective blinding ensures that each treatment group receives a similar amount of attention,

Box 10.1 GRADE criteria to evaluate quality of economic evidence

1. Study limitations (risk of bias)
   - Non-random allocation
   - Inadequate allocation concealment
   - Inadequate blinding
   - Incomplete outcome data
   - Per protocol instead of an intention-to-treat analysis
   - Patient self-reported data with a long recall period
2. Inconsistency of results (estimates of resource use)
3. Indirectness of evidence
   - Different populations, including different providers or settings (e.g. teaching vs community hospitals)
   - Different interventions or comparisons, including older studies (e.g. changes in the use of technologies)
   - Indirect (surrogate) outcomes, including:
   - Inappropriate unit cost data
   - Inadequate follow-up period
   - Indirect comparisons (i.e. comparisons between studies)
4. Imprecision
5. Publication bias

ancillary treatment and diagnostic investigations. Risk of bias can be high for some outcomes and low for others, when there is a lack of blinding. Knowledge of treatment assignments may affect resource use.

- Incomplete outcome data can bias estimates of resource use. If resource use data are missing in both treatment groups, but reasons for missing data are both reported and balanced across groups, the risk of bias is likely to be low.
- As for health outcomes, adherence to the intention-to-treat principle is necessary to maintain prognostic balance.
- Ideally, there should be comparable resource data for an adequate follow-up period for the groups being compared. Sometimes, however, resource use is not measured for the entire follow-up period, but extrapolated from more time-limited measurements. As with sampling patients,

sampling time periods will introduce a risk of bias unless there is reason to believe that resource use will be stable over time (e.g. for long-term chronic diseases).

- Resource use data can be collected directly from patients, in which case there is a risk of errors and/or recall bias, especially if the recall period is relatively long and detailed information is requested.[29] Validation of self-reported data can reduce the risk of recall bias. For example, in a study of care for terminally ill patients, data regarding the use of health services were reported by patients and confirmed by providers.[30]

Inconsistency of results

As for clinical outcomes, consistency of results is likely to be important also for resource use and this should be measured using magnitude and direction of the difference in resource use and costs.[12] Variations can be expected if there are different patterns of resource use in the settings where studies were conducted or differences in populations or interventions (see also, *inter alia*, Chapters 3, 5 and 13). When variability exists but investigators fail to identify a plausible explanation, the quality of evidence decreases. Judgements about the consistency of estimates of resource use can be difficult due to poor reporting of study methods and results, including lack of discussion of study results in the context of the results of previous studies.

Indirectness of evidence

For clinical outcomes, guideline developers face two types of indirectness of evidence. The first occurs when we have no head-to-head comparisons of two different interventions. The second includes differences between the population(s), intervention(s), comparator(s) to the intervention, and/or outcome(s) of interest (PICO).[12] Generally, directness of evidence is likely to be important for resource consequences. As a consequence of variations in patterns of resource use across settings (see also, *inter alia*, Chapters 3, 5 and 13), guideline developers will frequently choose to focus on the evidence that is most direct, rather than on an average across different settings. Other indirectness criteria for resource use and costs may result from differences in providers. For example, teaching and research-based hospitals have higher costs relative to non-teaching hospitals.[31] Evidence from older studies may be indirect due to changes in the use of technologies and innovations in health care (e.g. decreasing prices for generic drugs could change prescribing patterns).

Imprecision

As for health outcomes, imprecision can lower the quality of evidence for resource use outcomes. Because of variability in health care resource use between patients (for example, some patients use exceptional amounts of costly services), larger sample sizes may be required to ensure that studies are adequately powered to detect differences in resource use between treatment groups, compared to health outcomes.[32]

Publication bias

As with clinical studies, there is a risk of publication bias (and/or other forms of reporting bias) with respect to economic studies.[33]

Key points in considering resource implications when applying the GRADE approach are summarised in Box 10.2.

Box 10.2   Key points in considering resource implications using the GRADE approach[16]

- Only important resource use should be included in an evidence profile.
- Evidence must be found providing an estimate of the difference in resource use resulting from the implementation of the intervention between the intervention and the comparison group.
- Resource use should be presented in natural units.
- The quality of evidence should be appraised explicitly for each important resource consequence using the same criteria as for health outcomes (with focus on resources and costs).
- Evidence profiles should be constructed to inform recommendations whether or not an economic model is used.
- If an economic model is used in making the recommendation, it should be transparent, comprehensive and take into consideration the same outcomes included in the evidence profile.

Table 10.3 is a Summary of Findings table for the comparison of buprenorphine and methadone for opioid maintenance treatment. Estimates of effect and the quality of evidence are summarised for each critical outcome. Resource use and cost outcomes for which there is very low-quality evidence, such as crime costs, were not included in this table, but were included in the Evidence Profile (see Table 10.2). In our example there is little or no difference in health outcomes between buprenorphine and methadone, and buprenorphine costs more. A GRADE Summary of Findings table, such as Table 10.3, facilitates transparent decision-making processes that take account of important health outcomes and resource consequences, and the quality of evidence for these.

Grading clinical and economic evidence in NICE clinical guidelines

The NICE clinical guideline programme

Cost-effectiveness is a core element of decision making in NICE clinical guidelines, alongside evidence of effectiveness and other key social values.[34,35] The methods and processes employed by NICE and its National Collaborating Centres (NCCs) are described in detail in the *Guidelines Manual*.[36] To summarise these briefly, once a topic is referred to NICE, an NCC is commissioned to develop the guideline. A guideline development group (GDG) is convened, comprising health care professionals, patient and carer representatives and a technical team, which includes a health economist. The economist assists the GDG by reviewing relevant published economic evidence and developing decision models for selected topics. In effect, NICE guidelines use a combination of published literature, balance sheets and decision models to assess the cost-effectiveness of their recommendations.

NICE and the GRADE approach

The GRADE system for rating the quality of clinical evidence and for presenting it in the form of an Evidence Profile is being introduced into the NICE guidelines programme. Although NICE is not adopting the GRADE approach for classifying the 'strength' of recommendations, it is using an alternative method of wording guideline recommendations to reflect its own general principles of decision making.[37]

Table 10.3 Example of Summary of Findings table.

Question: Should buprenorphine maintenance flexible doses versus methadone maintenance flexible doses be used for opioid maintenance treatment?

Patient or population: Opiate dependants

Setting: Outpatients in USA, Australia, Austria, Switzerland, UK

Intervention : Maintenance flexible doses buprenorphine

Comparison: Maintenance flexible doses methadone

Outcomes	Illustrative comparative risks (95% CI)		Relative effect (95% CI)	No. of participants (studies)	Quality of the evidence	Comments
	Assumed risk	Corresponding risk				
	methadone	buprenorphine				
Clinical outcomes (12)						
Retention in treatment	63 per 100[1]	52 per 100 (45–60)	RR 0.82 (0.72–0.94)	976 (7)	High	Length of follow-up: 6–48 weeks
Use of opiate during the treatment[2]		The average difference in standard deviations for the mean number of morphine-positive urinalyses in the intervention group was 0.12 lower (−0.26 to + 0.02)		837 (6)	High	Data based on morphine urinalysis; only SMD is provided Interpretation: little or no difference
Use of cocaine during the treatment[2]		The average difference in standard deviations for the mean number of cocaine-positive urinalyses in the intervention group was 0.11 lower (−0.03 to + 0.25)	–	779 (5)	High	Data based on urinalysis; SMD is provided Interpretation: little or no difference
Use of benzodiazepine during the treatment[2]		The average difference in standard deviations for the mean number of benzodiazepine-positive urinalyses in the intervention group was 0.11 lower (−0.04 to + 0.26)	–	669 (4)	High	Data based on urinalysis; SMD is provided Interpretation: little or no difference
Criminal behaviour[2,3]		The average difference in standard deviations of the mean criminal activity score in the intervention group was 0.14 lower (−0.41 to + 0.14)	–	212 (1)	Moderate	Criminal activity as measured by self-report Interpretation: little or no difference
Resource use[4]						
Drugs[5]	57 mg daily 37 AU $ every 6 months	11 mg daily 422 AU $ more per patient every 6 months		405 (1)	Moderate	Drug and dispensing fee
Other health care costs[5]	1378 AU $ every 6 months	108 AU $ less per patient every 6 months		405 (1)	Moderate	Staff time, diagnostic and facilities costs

[1] Mean control group values.

[2] A standardized mean difference was calculated for continuous outcomes (urine results, self-reported heroin use and criminal activity). The urine data are presented as a continuous outcome measure but are based on data requested directly from authors. This was necessary as urine results in the literature are routinely reported as the percentage of urine samples collected per treatment group that were positive or negative for a given drug (e.g. heroin) across the study period. This "count data" is not compatible with the analyzable data fields in RevMan (i.e. continuous, dichotomous, individual patient data). Based on advice provided by Cochrane statisticians, we asked authors to calculate the number of positive urines for each patient in each treatment group and derive a mean number of positive urines with a standard deviation, allowing for analysis of urine results as continuous data.

[3] Criminal activity measured on a scale (Opiate Treatment Index) from 0, no criminal activity, to 16, daily criminal activity in all items.[22]

[4] Crime costs were not presented because of very low quality.

[5] Costs expressed in AU S (1999).

As stated earlier in this chapter, the GRADE approach excludes evidence derived from results of decision models from Evidence Profiles and Summary of Findings tables, but such estimates are a routine input to decision making in NICE guidelines. Indeed, decision modelling is ubiquitous if it is an aim to assess long-term costs and health outcomes from, inevitably limited, trial and epidemiological data.[38] Therefore, economists working in the NICE guideline programme have developed an approach for presenting modelled economic evidence alongside GRADE profiles of clinical evidence. This is intended to assist GDGs in weighing up the broad balance of benefits, harms and costs, and to provide a clearer depiction of the clinical and economic rationale underlying their recommendations.

The following sections describe the format for the NICE Economic Evidence Profile and its underpinning logic. A case study is presented from a NICE guideline to illustrate the use of such profiles. This is followed by a discussion of some of the practical and conceptual challenges that remain.

Format of the Economic Evidence Profile

One key difference between clinical and economic evidence is that there are currently no agreed-upon methods for pooling the results of decision models (and/or other economic evaluations) using meta-analysis or other quantitative evidence synthesis methods.[33] Economic evidence may be obtained from published sources or from a new analysis (often a decision model) developed specifically for the guideline.

A new analysis, reflecting the best available clinical and economic evidence and the specific guideline context, will generally supersede published studies, in which case the corresponding Economic Evidence Profile need only contain one row, to summarise the quality and findings of this new decision model. Similarly, when a single published analysis is used to inform the GDG decision (for example, when a recent Health Technology Assessment (HTA) report is available, which includes a decision model or other economic evaluation covering the population of interest), this is also presented in one row of the Economic Evidence Profile. However, sometimes a guideline panel may wish to compare the results of more than one published decision model or of

different versions of their own decision model, for example to evaluate the impact on results of different model structures or scenarios. In these circumstances, each study is presented in a separate row of the Economic Evidence Profile (see example in Table 10.4).

Quality assessment

As with clinical evidence, it is important to appraise the quality of economic evaluations (including decision models) before they are used to inform guideline decisions. As described earlier in this chapter, the GRADE Evidence Profile contains five main quality criteria. Some of these are redundant or inappropriate for modelled estimates. For example, there is no clear hierarchy of study design for economic evaluations: an analysis conducted alongside a single randomised trial is not necessarily superior or inferior to a decision model utilising data collected from various sources (see, *inter alia*, chapters 3, 7 and 9). Also, in the NICE approach to constructing an Economic Evidence Profile, there is no need to include 'consistency' as a separate criterion as in the GRADE approach, since if two or more economic evaluations are included, they will be reported separately.

The quality of economic evaluations can therefore be simplified into two main dimensions: *applicability* to the decision context (part of the directness criterion in GRADE) and the *methodological quality* of the evaluation performed (part of the study limitations criterion in GRADE). This approach is broadly consistent with earlier advice on the evaluation of economic evidence in Australian clinical guidelines, and recommendations made in methods guidance produced by the Campbell & Cochrane Economic Methods Group.[33,39]

There is currently no clear basis for merging these dimensions to provide an overall quality rating. Instead, the NICE guideline panel is asked to consider both the applicability and methodological quality (study limitations; risks of bias) of studies included in the Economic Evidence Profile. Each of these two dimensions is described below. Any additional information considered important to help inform the panel's deliberations can be provided in an 'other comments' column of the profile.

Applicability

The relevance of an economic evaluation to a guideline decision depends on:

- whether it directly addresses the same clinical question (defined by the population, intervention and comparator of interest)
- whether the results can be reliably transferred to, or generalised within, the health care system of interest (the UK National Health Service (NHS) in the case of NICE)
- whether the analysis reflects the correct decision-making framework (for NICE guidelines, this is specified in the NICE 'reference case' and Social Value Judgements criteria).[40,41]

NICE has developed a checklist to help NCC health economists to assess the applicability of economic evidence (see Figure 10.1). In Appendix H of the NICE *Guidelines Manual*, this checklist is accompanied by extensive notes giving guidance on each criterion.[36]

An overall judgement on applicability is summarised in the Economic Evidence Profile using one of three classifications.

1. *Directly applicable* – the study meets all applicability criteria, or fails to meet one or more criteria but this is unlikely to change the conclusions about cost-effectiveness.

Study identification		
Including author, title, reference, year of publication		
Guideline topic:		**Question no:**
Checklist completed by:		
Section 1: Applicability (relevance to specific guideline review question(s) and the NICE reference case[a]) *This checklist should be used first to filter out irrelevant studies.*	**Yes/Partly/No/ Unclear /NA**	**Comments**
1.1 Is the study population appropriate for the guideline?		
1.2 Are the interventions appropriate for the guideline?		
1.3 Is the health care system in which the study was conducted sufficiently similar to the current UK NHS context?		
1.4 Are costs measured from the NHS and personal social services (PSS) perspective?		
1.5 Are all direct health effects on individuals included?		
1.6 Are both costs and health effects discounted at an annual rate of 3.5%?		
1.7 Is the value of health effects expressed in terms of quality-adjusted life-years (QALYs)?		
1.8 Are changes in health-related quality of life (HRQL) reported directly from patients and/or carers?		
1.9 Is the valuation of changes in HRQL (utilities) obtained from a representative sample of the general public?		
10.10 **Overall judgement:** Directly applicable/Partially applicable/Not applicable There is no need to use section 2 of the checklist if the study is considered 'not applicable'.		
Other comments:		

[a]As detailed in the NICE *Guide to the Methods of Technology Appraisal*, Box 5.1 (page 30).[37] Section 5.2.3 of the guide states: 'There may be important barriers to applying reference-case methods. In these cases, the reasons for a failure to meet the reference case should be clearly specified and justified, and the likely implications should, as far as possible, be quantified.'

Figure 10.1 NICE applicability checklist: economic evaluations. See Appendix H of the NICE *Guidelines Manual*.[36]

Table 10.4 Omega 3 acid ethyl ester supplements versus control in people within 3 months of an acute myocardial infarction (MI). GRADE evidence profile.

Quality assessment

Outcome	Design (No. studies)	Study limitations	Inconsistency	Indirectness	Imprecision	Summary of findings		
						Supplements	Control	Relative risks	Quality
All-cause mortality	RCT (3)	Serious limitations[a]	No	Some indirectness[b]	No	581/6830 (8.5%)	755/6830 (11.1%)	0.83 (0.75 to 0.93)	Low
Combined CV events	RCT (3)	Serious limitations[a]	No	Some indirectness[b]	No	755/6830 (11.1%)	839/6826 (12.3%)	0.90 (0.82 to 0.99)	Low
Cancers	RCT (3)	Serious limitations[a]	No	Some indirectness[b]	No	150/6830 (2.2%)	138/6826 (2.0%)	1.09 (0.86 to 1.36)	Low

Economic evidence

Quality assessment				Summary of findings			
Study	Applicability	Limitations	Other comments	Incremental cost[c]	Incremental effect	ICER	Uncertainty
Franzosi 2001[71]	Partially applicable[d]	Potentially serious limitations[e]	Based on measured resource use and survival in 3.5 years follow-up in GISSI-P trial	£871	0.0332 LY	£26,243 per LY	£16,769 to £56,025 per LY gained (best /worst case SA)
Lamotte 2006[72]	Partially applicable[f]	Very serious limitations[g]	Based on measured resource use and survival over 3.5 years in GISSI-P, plus longer term survival benefits attributed to non-fatal events using Canadian database. Belgian results presented	£1090	0.282 LY	£3860 per LY	>98% probability ICER less than 120,000 per QALY gained (PSA)

| NCC analysis[73] | Directly applicable[h] | Minor limitations[i] | Based on morbidity and mortality estimated from Markov model using pooled effectiveness data fr.... GISSI-P and DART. Results sensitive to the size of treatment effects and over their assumed duration | £1073 | 0.09 QALY | £12,480 per QALY | £3912 to £130,705 per QALY gained (range in one-way SA) |

LY, life-years; QALY, quality-adjusted life-years; ICER, incremental cost-effectiveness ratio; SA, sensitivity analysis; PSA, probabilistic sensitivity analysis.

[a] Increase in statin use over follow-up in GISSI-P trial differed between the groups (from 4.4% to 46.0% in the omega-3 group and from 5.1% to 44.4% in the control group)

[b] High baseline rate of fish consumption in GISSI-P (more than 70%) – may not reflect usual diet in UK

[c] Costs estimated in 2006 UK pounds – converted using PPP exchange rates (www.oecd.org/std/ppp) and UK HCHS inflation index (www.pssru.ac.uk/pdf/uc/uc2006/uc2006.pdf)

[d] Uses Italian estimates of resource use and unit costs. Some uncertainty over the applicability of Italian effectiveness data to UK

[e] This study is relatively conservative, as it does not impute any quality of life or longer-term survival benefit to supplements. Conversely, it omits GI side effects

[f] Uses Belgian estimates of resource use and unit costs. 5% discount rate for costs and effects. Some uncertainty over the applicability of Italian effectiveness data to UK

[g] Methods and data used to estimate life expectancy are questionable, and were not subjected to sensitivity analysis. This is likely to have biased the results

[h] Costs estimated following the NICE reference case, using UK resource use and unit cost estimates. Some uncertainty over applicability of Italian effectiveness estimates in UK population

[i] Analysis is based on best available effectiveness estimates and follows NICE methodological guidance. Minor limitations in reporting (e.g. for inputs taken from NICE statins appraisal)

2. *Partially applicable* – the study fails to meet one or more applicability criteria, and this could change the conclusions about cost-effectiveness.

3. *Not applicable* – the study fails to meet one or more of the applicability criteria and this is likely to change the conclusions about cost-effectiveness. Such studies would be excluded from further consideration and there is no need to continue with the quality assessment.

It should be noted that this overall judgement is not straightforward, in part because there is currently no objective 'measure' to inform the specific judgement as to whether failure to meet one or more criteria is likely (or unlikely) to change conclusions about cost-effectiveness. In practice, the checklist and guidance notes are used to help guide judgements on each applicability criterion and health economists are encouraged to include justifications of their overall judgement within summaries of each individual study, presented in the main text of the guideline.

Study limitations

As noted earlier in this chapter, there are many published checklists and scales for assessing the quality of reporting and conduct of published economic evaluations.[41–62] Whilst there are differences between published checklists in the dimensions of quality and reporting covered, arguably all essentially build on a set of principles first proposed by Drummond and colleagues to underpin 'Guidelines for authors and peer reviewers of economic submissions to the British Medical Journal' (BMJ checklist).[45] Additional criteria and instruments have been proposed for assessment of decision models.[19,63-66] Most of these instruments were developed with little or no validation. However, two recent initiatives have taken a more formal approach to development and testing: the *Consensus on Health Economic Criteria* (CHEC) and *Quality of Health Economic Studies* (QHES) projects.[41,44,46,67,68] The Campbell & Cochrane Economic Methods Group currently recommends use of either the CHEC or BMJ checklists (or both) to inform critical appraisal of economic evaluations conducted alongside single effectiveness studies, and *Quality Assessment in Decision-Analytic Models: a suggested checklist* (Philips checklist) to inform critical appraisal of decision models.[19,33,41,45]

Following an unpublished review of available instruments and discussion amongst NICE and NCC economists, it was decided to adapt items from CHEC and the Philips checklist to create a tool suitable for NICE clinical guidelines (see Figure 10.2). Questions concerned with the quality of reporting were excluded, as were items already included in the NICE applicability checklist. Each criterion is accompanied by detailed notes in Appendix H of the *Guidelines Manual.*[36]

The overall methodological quality of economic evaluations is summarised as follows.

- *Minor limitations* – the study meets all quality criteria, or the study fails to meet one or more quality criteria but this is unlikely to change the conclusions about cost-effectiveness.
- *Potentially serious limitations* – the study fails to meet one or more quality criteria, and this could change the conclusions about cost-effectiveness.
- *Very serious limitations* – the study fails to meet one or more quality criteria and this is highly likely to change the conclusions about cost-effectiveness. Studies with very serious limitations should usually be excluded from the Economic Profile table.

The robustness of the study results to methodological limitations may sometimes have been demonstrated through sensitivity analysis. In the absence of relevant sensitivity analyses, however, judgement will be required to assess whether a limitation is likely to change the results.

Summary of findings

The results of economic evaluations may be summarised in a variety of ways. The base case results may be presented as an incremental cost-effectiveness ratio (ICER) or net benefit (NB) statistic. Uncertainty around this finding may be shown as a range of ICER or NB estimates from a deterministic sensitivity analysis, and/or as the probability of cost-effectiveness (for a given cost-effectiveness threshold, say £20,000 per QALY).

Case study: omega 3 supplements for secondary prevention of myocardial infarction

An example of a GRADE Evidence Profile (clinical evidence) and parallel NICE Economic Evidence Profile is presented in Table 10.4. Both were compiled

Section 2: Study limitations (the level of methodological quality) *This checklist should be used once it has been decided that the study is sufficiently applicable to the context of the clinical guideline.*[a]	Yes/Partly/ No/ Unclear/ NA	Comments
2.1 Does the model structure adequately reflect the nature of the health condition under evaluation?		
2.2 Is the time horizon sufficiently long to reflect all important differences in costs and outcomes?		
2.3 Are all important and relevant health outcomes included?		
2.4 Are the estimates of baseline health outcomes from the best available source?		
2.5 Are the estimates of relative treatment effects from the best available source?		
2.6 Are all important and relevant costs included?		
2.7 Are the estimates of resource use from the best available source?		
2.8 Are the unit costs of resources from the best available source?		
2.9 Is an appropriate incremental analysis presented or can it be calculated from the data?		
2.10 Are all important parameters whose values are uncertain subjected to appropriate sensitivity analysis?		
2.11 Is there no potential conflict of interest?		
2.12 **Overall assessment**: Minor limitations/Potentially serious limitations/Very serious limitations		
Other comments:		

[a]Items and notes in this checklist have been developed from guidance in the NICE *Guide to the Methods of Technology Appraisal*, CHEC and the Philips checklist.[19,37,46]

Figure 10.2 NICE study limitations checklist: economic evaluations· See Appendix H of the NICE *Guidelines Manual.*[36]

to address a question about the use of omega 3 supplements in a NICE guideline on secondary prevention of myocardial infarction.[69]

Further issues

It is important to emphasise that the Economic Evidence Profile cannot substitute for an in-depth description of the methods and results of decision models developed for guidelines, nor for a detailed appraisal of published economic evaluations used to inform guideline decisions. Rather, it provides a complementary, top-level summary to assist GDGs in their deliberations.

There are various practical challenges to summarising often very complicated clinical and economic evidence in a clear but compact way. There is not always a simple relationship between research questions, a body of clinical evidence, an economic evaluation (or a set of economic evaluations) and a set of recommendations. For example, a cost-effectiveness analysis might combine information from several treatment

comparisons and thus a single economic analysis might relate to several GRADE profiles, one for each comparison. In such cases, it will not always be appropriate to present an ICER for all comparisons, since in an incremental analysis each option should only be compared with the next most expensive, non-dominated option. Conversely, when an economic evaluation is based on an indirect or mixed treatment comparison, there may be comparative economic results in the absence of direct clinical comparisons.[70] Thus summary tables might contain blank cells to show where clinical or economic evidence is missing.

Another presentational challenge arises when clinical and/or economic results vary between patient groups. If the clinical results for different patient groups are presented in separate GRADE profile tables, each of these may be accompanied by an Economic Evidence Profile. However, if the relative treatment effects are constant across subgroups but the economic results differ (for example, if cost-effectiveness varies with baseline risk), it might be better to present a single GRADE profile and an associated Economic Evidence Profile with separate rows for each patient group. Or, if economic results vary across a continuum of risk, it may be simpler to present a threshold at which treatment becomes cost-effective.

The availability and choice of outcome measures can introduce a further layer of complexity. Early experience with GRADE in the NICE guidelines programme has highlighted the extreme difficulty that some GDGs have in selecting outcome measures. It is important that they do so to avoid information overload and bias from *post hoc* focusing on outcomes that give desired results. In fact, one real advantage of the GRADE approach is that this issue is forced at an earlier stage, since it is not practical to produce or use profiles with many outcomes. This may also be seen as an advantage of decision models, which force an explicit judgement about the (sometimes complex) trade-offs between multiple outcomes. In contrast, the balance sheet approach may compound difficulties when there are multiple outcomes by adding yet more cost or resource estimates.

Another common problem faced by guideline groups is the lack or scarcity of data on important outcomes. When this happens, a blank row in the GRADE profile may be used to indicate the missing data. By analogy, a blank row could be inserted in an Economic Evidence Profile when economic outcomes are missing. This problem arises in NICE guidelines when there are no published economic evaluations of adequate quality and relevance, and the topic is not prioritised for modelling. In such cases, the guideline economist could insert a simple estimate of cost or resource use (for example, drug prices or length of inpatient stay) in the Economic Evidence Profile, which alongside the GRADE profile would provide a balance sheet for the consideration of the GDG. If this is not possible or if the cost implications of the question are thought to be negligible, this should be stated explicitly.

Conclusions

We believe that the approaches to grading economic evidence described in this chapter can help to give health care decision makers, clinical guideline panels, patients and the wider stakeholder community a better appreciation of the overall health benefits, harms and costs of alternative interventions, and assist them in interpreting this evidence and communicating it to their readers.

In addition, we consider that these techniques can be usefully adapted for application in other fields of public policy such as social welfare, education and criminal justice. However, as outlined in other chapters of this volume, there are important differences between the health care and non-health care sectors that will need to be taken into account when designing economic evaluations. For example, there is a need to develop quality assessment methods that can be used when assessing economic information collected alongside non-experimental study designs, as for observational design, such as might routinely be the case when informing choices of interventions in criminal justice. In addition, certain areas of public policy, such as social care, are characterised by multiple and diverse outcomes. There may be particular difficulties therefore in applying GRADE-like approaches with respect to identifying the main outcomes to include in a profile. Finally, there will also be challenging issues to overcome when attempting to use a NICE-derived Economic Evidence Profile in the absence of general measures of outcome (such as the QALY), which is likely to be the case in many non-health areas at present. Under these circumstances, economic profiles may be difficult to construct and not easy to interpret.

How this chapter should be cited

Brunetti M, Ruiz F, Lord J, Pregno S, Oxman AD. Chapter 10: Grading economic evidence. In: Shemilt I, Mugford M, Vale L, Marsh K, Donaldson C (editors). *Evidence-based decisions and economics: health care, social welfare, education and criminal justice.* Oxford: Wiley-Blackwell, 2010.

References

1 Fuchs V, Sox H. Physicians' views of the relative importance of thirty medical innovations. *Health Affairs* 2001; 20(5): 30–42.

2 Guyatt GH, Sackett DL, Sinclair JC, Hayward R, Cook DJ, Cook RJ. Users' guides to the medical literature IX. A method for grading health care recommendations. *Journal of the American Medical Association* 1995; 274(22): 1800–1804.

3 Oxman AD, Schünemann HJ, Fretheim A. Improving the use of research evidence in guideline development: 8. synthesis and presentation of evidence. *Health Research Policy and Systems* 2006; 4: 20.

4 Oxman AD, Fretheim A, Schünemann HJ. Improving the use of research evidence in guideline development: 16. evaluation. *Health Research Policy and Systems* 2006; 4: 28.

5 Antman EM, Lau J, Kupelnick B, Mosteller F, Chalmers TC. A comparison of results of meta-analyses of randomized controlled trials and recommendations of clinical experts: treatments for myocardial infarction. *Journal of the American Medical Association* 1992; 268(2): 240–248.

6 Elixhauser A, Halpern M, Schmier J, Luce BR. Health care CBA and CEA from 1991 to 1996: an updated bibliography. *Medical Care* 1998; 36(5 suppl): MS1-9, MS18–147.

7 Field MJ, Lohr KN (eds). *Guidelines for Clinical Practice: from development to use.* Washington: National Academy Press, 1992.

8 Tan-Torres Edejer T. Improving the use of research evidence in guideline development: 11. Incorporating considerations of cost-effectiveness, affordability and resource implications. *Health Research Policy and Systems* 2006; 4: 23.

9 Eccles M, Mason J. How to develop cost-conscious guidelines. *Health Technology Assessment* 2001; 5(16): 1–69.

10 GRADE Working Group. Grading quality of evidence and strength of recommendations. *British Medical Journal* 2004; 328(7454): 1490–1499.

11 Guyatt GH, Oxman AD, Vist GE, *et al.*, for the GRADE Working Group. GRADE: an emerging consensus on rating quality of evidence and strength of recommendations. *British Medical Journal* 2008; 336(7650): 924–926.

12 Guyatt GH, Oxman AD, Kunz R, *et al.*, for the GRADE Working Group. GRADE: what is 'quality of evidence' and why is it important to clinicians? *British Medical Journal* 2008; 336(7651): 995–998.

13 Guyatt GH, Oxman AD, Kunz R, *et al.*, for the GRADE Working Group. GRADE: going from evidence to recommendations. *British Medical Journal* 2008; 336(7652): 1049–1051.

14 Grade Working Group. *GRADEpro Help 'About evidence tables'.* Available from: www.gradeworkinggroup.org.

15 Guyatt GH, Oxman AD, Kunz R, *et al.*, for the GRADE Working Group. GRADE: incorporating considerations of resources use into grading recommendations. *British Medical Journal* 2008; 336(7654): 1170–1173.

16 Eddy DM. Comparing benefit and harms: the balance sheet. *Journal of the American Medical Association* 1990; 263(18): 2493–2498, 2501.

17 Drummond MF, Sculpher MJ, Torrance GW, O'Brien BJ, Stoddart GL. *Methods for the Economic Evaluation of Health care Programmes,* 3rd edn. Oxford: Oxford University Press, 2005.

18 Brunetti M, Oxman AD, Pregno S, *et al.* GRADE guidelines: 10. Special challenges – resource use. *Journal of Clinical Epidemiology,* in press.

19 Philips Z, Ginnelly L, Sculpher M, *et al.* Review of guidelines for good practice in decision-analytic modelling in health technology assessment. *Health Technology Assessment* 2004; 8(36): 1–172.

20 Impact-RSV Study Group. Palivizumab, a humanized respiratory syncitial virus monoclonal antibody, reduces hospitalization from respiratory syncytial virus infection in high risk infants. *Pediatrics* 1998; 102: 531–537.

21 Cooper N, Coyle D, Abrams K, Mugford M, Sutton A. Use of evidence in decision models: an appraisal of health technology assessments in the UK since 1997. *Journal of Health Services Research and Policy* 2005; 10(4): 245–250.

22 Mattick RP, Kimber J, Breen C, Davoli M. Buprenorphine maintenance versus placebo or methadone maintenance for opioid dependence. *Cochrane Database of Systematic Reviews* 2008, Issue 2.

23 Harris A, Gospodarevskaya E, Ritter A. A randomised trial of the cost effectiveness of buprenorphine as an alternative to methadone maintenance treatment for heroin dependence in a primary care setting. *Pharmacoeconomics* 2005; 23 (1): 77–91.

24 Doran CM, Shanahan M, Mattick RP, Ali R, White J, Bell J. Buprenorphine versus methadone maintenance: a cost-effectiveness analysis. *Drug and Alcohol Dependence* 2003; 71(3): 295–302.

25 Luce BR, Manning WG, Siegel JE, Weinstein MC. Estimating costs in cost-effectiveness analysis. In: Gold MR, Siegel JE, Russell LB, Weinstein MC (eds) *Cost-Effectiveness in Health and Medicine.* New York: Oxford University Press, 1996.

26 Palmer S, Raftery J. Economic notes: opportunity cost. *British Medical Journal* 1999; 318(7197): 1551–1552.

27 Shemilt I, Thomas J, Morciano M. A new web-based tool for adjusting costs to a common currency and price year. *Evidence and Policy,* in press.

28 Higgins JPT, Altman DG (eds) Assessing risk of bias in included studies. In: Higgins JPT, Green S (eds) *Cochrane Handbook for Systematic Reviews of Interventions.* Version 5.0.1 (updated September 2008). Oxford: Cochrane Collaboration, 2008.

29 Petrou S, Murray L, Cooper P, Davidson LL. The accuracy of self-reported health care resource utilization in health economic studies. *International Journal of Technology Assessment in Health care* 2002; 18(3): 705–710.

30 Hughes SL, Cummings J, Weaver F, Manheim L, Braun B, Conrad KA. A randomized trial of the cost effectiveness of VA hospital-based home care for the terminally ill. *Health Service Research* 1992; 26(6): 801–817.

31 Baltussen RMPM, Ament AJHA, Leidl RM. Making cost assessment based on RCTs more useful to decision makers. *Health Policy* 1996; 37(3): 163–183.

32 Briggs A. Economic evaluation and clinical trials: size matters. *British Medical Journal* 2000; 321 (7273): 132–133.

33 Shemilt I, Mugford M, Byford S, *et al.* Incorporating economics evidence. In: Higgins JPT, Green S (eds) *Cochrane Handbook for Systematic Reviews of Interventions.* Version 5.0.1 (updated September 2008). Oxford: Cochrane Collaboration, 2008.

34 National Institute for Health and Clinical Excellence. *Social Value Judgements. Principles for the development of NICE guidance,* 2nd edn. London: National Institute for Health and Clinical Excellence, 2008.

35 Culyer AJ. NICE's use of cost effectiveness as an exemplar of a deliberative process. *Health Economics Policy and Law* 2006; 1(3): 299–318.

36 National Institute for Health and Clinical Excellence. *The Guidelines Manual*. London: National Institute for Health and Clinical Excellence, 2009.

37 National Institute for Health and Clinical Excellence. *Guide to the Methods of Technology Appraisal*. London: National Institute for Health and Clinical Excellence, 2008.

38 Buxton MJ, Drummond MF, van Hout BA, *et al*. Modelling in economic evaluation: an unavoidable fact of life. *Health Economics* 1997; 6(3): 217–227.

39 National Health and Medical Research Council. *How to Compare the Costs and Benefits: evaluation of the economic evidence*. Canberra: Commonwealth of Australia, 2001.

40 Adams ME, McCall NT, Gray DT, Orza MJ, Chalmers TC. Economic analysis in randomized control trials. *Medical Care* 1992; 30(3): 231–243.

41 Ament A, Evers S, Goossens M. Criteria list for conducting systematic reviews based on economic evaluation studies – the CHEC project. In: Donaldson C, Mugford M, Vale L (eds) *Evidence-Based Health Economics*. London: BMJ Books, 2002.

42 Blackmore CC, Magid DJ. Methodologic evaluation of the radiology cost-effectiveness literature. *Radiology* 1997; 203(1): 87–91.

43 Bradley CA, Iskedjian M, Lanetot KL, *et al*. Quality assessment of economic evaluations in selected pharmacy, medical and health economics journals. *Annals of Pharmacotherapy* 1995; 29(7): 681–689.

44 Chiou C-F, Hay JW, Wallace JF, *et al*. Development and validation of a grading system for the quality of cost-effectiveness studies. *Medical Care* 2003; 41(1): 32–44.

45 Drummond MF, Jefferson TO, on behalf of the BMJ Economic Evaluation Working Party. Guidelines for authors and peer reviewers of economic submissions to the BMJ. *British Medical Journal* 1996; 313(7052): 275–283.

46 Evers S, Goossens M, de Vet H, van Tulder M, Ament A. Criteria list for assessment of methodological quality of economic evaluations: Consensus on Health Economic Criteria. *International Journal of Technology Assessment in Health care* 2005; 21(2): 240–245.

47 Ganiats TG, Wong AF. Evaluation of cost-effectiveness research. A survey of recent publications. *Family Medicine* 1991; 23(6): 457–462.

48 Gerard K. Cost-utility in practice: a policy maker's guide to the state of the art. *Health Policy* 1992; 21(3): 249–279.

49 Gerard K, Seymour J, Smoker I. A tool to improve quality of reporting published economic analyses. *International Journal of Technology Assessment in Health care* 2000; 16(1): 100–110.

50 Gonzalez-Perez JG. Developing a scoring system to quality assess economic evaluations. *European Journal of Health Economics* 2002; 3(2): 131–136.

51 Heyland DK, Kernerman P, Gafni A, Cook DJ. Economic evaluations in the critical care literature: do they help us improve the efficiency of our unit? *Critical Care Medicine* 1996; 24(9): 1591–1598.

52 Holloway RG, Benesch CG, Rahilly CR, Courtright CE. Systematic review of cost-effectiveness research of stroke evaluation and treatment. *Stroke* 1999; 30(9): 1340–1349.

53 Sacristán JA, Soto J, Galende I. Evaluation of pharmacoeconomic studies: utilization of a checklist. *Annals of Pharmacotherapy* 1993; 27(9): 1126–1133.

54 Sanchez LA. Evaluating the quality of published pharmacoeconomic evaluations. *Hospital Pharmacy* 1995; 30(2): 146–152.

55 Severens JL, van der Wilt GJ. Economic evaluation of diagnostic tests. A review of published studies. *International Journal of Technology Assessment in Health care* 1999; 15(3): 480–496.

56 Udvarhelyi IS, Colditz GA, Rai A, Epstein AM. Cost-effectiveness and cost-benefit analyses in the medical literature. Are the methods being used correctly? *Annals of Internal Medicine* 1992; 116(3): 238–244.

57 Weinstein MC, Siegel JE, Gold MR, Kamlet MS, Russell LB. Recommendations of the panel on cost-effectiveness in health and medicine. *Journal of the American Medical Association* 1996; 276(15): 1253–1258.

58 Huijsman R. Economic evaluation of care for the chronically ill: a literature review. *European Journal of Public Health* 1995; 5(1): 8–19.

59 Iskedjian M, Trakas K, Bradley CA, *et al*. Quality assessment of economic evaluations published in Pharmacoeconomics. The first four years (1992 to 1995). *Pharmacoeconomics* 1997; 12(6): 685–694.

60 Maetzel A, Ferraz MB, Bombardier C. A review of cost-effectiveness analyses in rheumatology and related disciplines. *Current Opinion in Rheumatology* 1998; 10(2): 136–140.

61 Neumann PJ, Greenberg D, Olchanski NV, Stone PW, Rosen AB. Growth and quality of the cost-utility literature, 1976–2001. *Value in Health* 2005; 8(1): 3–9.

62 Siegel JE, Weinstein MC, Russell LB, Gold MR. Recommendations for reporting cost-effectiveness analyses. *Journal of the American Medical Association* 1996; 276(16): 1339–1341.

63 McCabe C, Dixon S. Testing the validity of cost-effectiveness models. *Pharmacoeconomics* 2000; 17(5): 501–513.

64 Sculpher MJ, Fenwick E, Claxton K. Assessing quality in decision analytic cost-effectiveness models: a suggested framework and example of application. *Pharmacoeconomics* 2000; 17(5): 461–477.

65 Soto J. Health economic evaluations using decision analytic modelling. Principles and practices – utilization of a checklist to their development and appraisal. *International Journal of Technology Assessment in Health care* 2002; 18(1): 94–111.

66 Weinstein MC, O'Brien BJ, Hornberger J, *et al*. Principles of good practice for decision analytic modeling in healthcare evaluation: report of the ISPOR Task Force on Good Research Practices – Modeling Studies. *Value in Health* 2003; 6(1): 9–17.

67 Ofman JJ, Sullivan SD, Neumann PJ, *et al*. Examining the value and quality of health economic analyses: implications of utilizing the QHES. *Journal of Managed Care Pharmacy* 2003; 9(1): 53–61.

68 Spiegel BM, Targownik LE, Kanwal F, *et al*. The quality of published health economic analyses in digestive diseases: a systematic review and quantitative appraisal. *Gastroenterology* 2004; 127(2): 403–411.

69 Cooper A, Skinner J, Nherera L, *et al. Clinical Guidelines and Evidence Review for Post Myocardial Infarction: secondary prevention in primary and secondary care for patients following a myocardial infarction*. London: National Collaborating Centre for Primary Care and Royal College of General Practitioners, 2007.

70 Caldwell DM, Ades AE, Higgins JPT. Simultaneous comparison of multiple treatments: combining direct and indirect evidence. *British Medical Journal* 2005; 331(7521); 897–900.

71 Franzosi MG, Brunetti M, Marchioli R, Marfisi RM, Tognoni G, Valagussa F. Cost-effectiveness analysis of n-3 polyunsaturated fatty acids (PUFA) after myocardial infarction. Results from the Gruppo Italiano per lo Studio della Sopravvivenza nell'Infarto (GISSI)-Prevenzione Trial. *Pharmacoeconomics* 2001; 19(4): 411–420.

72 Lamotte M, Annemans L, Kawelec P, Zoellner Y. A multicountry health economic evaluation of highly concentrated N-3 polyunsaturated fatty acids in secondary prevention after myocardial infarction. *Pharmacoeconomics* 2006; 24(8): 783–795.

73 Hooper L, Harrison RA, Summerbell CD, *et al*. Omega 3 fatty acids for prevention and treatment of cardiovascular disease. *Cochrane Database of Systematic Reviews* 2004, Issue 4.

CHAPTER 11

Meta-regression models of economics and medical research

T. D. Stanley

Department of Economics, Hendrix College, Conway, AR, USA

Introduction

In an era characterised by rapid expansion of research publications and a flood of empirical findings on nearly any given topic, knowledge and sensible policy discussions are being drowned. Without some balanced way to integrate this sea of research, ideology and self-serving deceit will dominate the public discussion of research and social policy. Meta-regression analysis (MRA) provides an objective, yet critical, method to integrate and evaluate diverse research findings. MRA methods developed to understand economics research can enrich medical research and vice versa. Such methods are routinely used in health care, medical, and social research and have been accepted as valid methods for use in both Cochrane and Campbell systematic reviews.[1,2] Furthermore MRA can identify publication bias and filter its effects from the research base.

This chapter describes the use of meta-analysis in economics with a focus on the statistical analysis of collected systematic data that minimises potential biases. It presents rigorous statistical methods to identify and correct for publication biases, which are often present in the research base, and to control for systematic heterogeneity, which has the potential to contaminate any summary of a policy's effect when ignored. Differences in research designs and

Evidence-Based Decisions and Economics, 2nd edition. Edited by I. Shemilt, M. Mugford, L. Vale, K. Marsh and C. Donaldson. © 2010 Blackwell Publishing.

perspectives between economics and medical research are discussed and illustrated by examples from both.

The meta-regression analysis of economics research

Two decades ago, MRA was developed for applied econometrics (i.e. empirical economics that employs regression on observational data).[3] Unlike medical and psychological research, MRA was designed to integrate and correct estimated regression coefficients, or transformations of regression coefficients, such as elasticities. Since then there have been literally hundreds of applications of MRA to different areas of economics research. Nelson & Kennedy list 114 meta-analyses of environmental economics alone.[4] Environmental economics has been a leading subfield employing meta-analysis, largely in an effort to estimate environmental values of unstudied sites.[5–7] Labour economists have also been quick to exploit the potential of meta-analysis to investigate union wage differentials, minimum wage and employment, labour demand, gender wage discrimination, union membership and productivity, and the wage curve.[8–13] More recently, health economists have employed MRA methods and models to test key hypotheses and reduce publication bias.[14,15] Dozens of MRA applications in economics are produced each year. As a consequence of this growing interest, an international network of scholars, the Meta-Analysis of Economics Research Network (MAER-Net), has coalesced and holds annual colloquia (www.hendrix. edu/maer-network).

A difference by design

Econometrics has several connotations and denotations. At one level, it is the statistical theory and methods found especially useful when dealing with economic data, which are largely observational. At another, it is the application of these methods to actual economic problems and data. Nearly all empirical research in economics is applied econometrics. MRAs integrate and explain the many empirical results that are routinely reported about important economic phenomena or questions. Empirical economics is very often forced to resort to observational data, usually collected by governmental or other potentially interested agencies. As a result, it is argued that reported econometric estimates are full of biases due to model mis-specification (for example, using the wrong type of mathematical model, linear versus logarithmic, or omitting an important explanatory variable), inappropriate estimators or data errors and limitations. In economics, summary and integration was never thought to be sufficient. The point was always to model explicitly these mis-specification and data biases and thereby to correct or at least reduce them.[3]

In contrast, medical researchers are often content to combine available estimates to achieve greater clarity and to ensure the statistical significance of the treatment in question. In medical research, the systematic review community relies more on the quality of the individual estimates themselves, often demanding that each comes from a randomised controlled trial (RCT). RCTs are widely regarded as the 'gold standard' by the systematic review community because they are thought to maximise internal validity. Studies using observational data are therefore frequently excluded from systematic reviews altogether.[16] However, due to potential risks of bias in RCTs (e.g. selective outcome reporting, subject attrition, early stopping, unexplained heterogeneity, inconsistency of results) and the strengths of well-designed or well-modelled observational studies, medical researchers have begun to accept observational studies.[17,18] As Kristiansen & Gosden have argued, 'In recent years . . . in the light of new evidence, the arguments for ignoring observational study designs have weakened'.[16]

The observational nature of applied econometrics and resulting mis-specification biases makes any simple summary of economics research results problematic.

Typically, to overcome the well-known weakness of applied econometrics, many studies are published, each containing multiple estimates, on the same topic. For any important economic question, there is a smorgasbord of empirical estimates, generated from different datasets, countries and sets of control variables, using different estimation techniques and econometric models. What economics research lacks in quality is compensated for by sheer quantity. This chaos may be a blessing in disguise. Such a rich, multifaceted research enterprise lends itself naturally to multivariate statistical analysis. Thus, MRAs of economics research are much the same as the original econometric applications; that is, both are complex multivariate statistical analyses of observational data.

Medical systematic research appears to ignore the fact that its data are, by their nature, observational. A given log odds ratio derived from a particular RCT is not a double-blind experiment when compared to another estimated log odds ratio calculated from a different RCT. Reported treatment effects may depend, in part, on differences in research protocols (e.g. the dosage, follow-up or other treatment dimension) as well as pre-existing differences in the populations from which both control and treatment groups were selected. Since systematic reviews of medical research are inescapably observational research, such reviews could be improved if they were to use more rigorous and comprehensive statistical methods that were designed for the task at hand. This is precisely what econometrics does. Thus, systematic reviews of medical research may be improved through the adoption of econometric methods in general, and MRA in particular. These are not new recommendations, as methods handbooks for systematic reviews already recognise that differences in methods, interventions and populations should be accounted for.[1,2]

For example, consider the cases of publication bias and other forms of reporting bias. It is widely acknowledged that not all outcomes of even the best designed RCTs get reported. The Paxil and Vioxx scandals have focused medical research on publication bias.[19] What is especially pernicious about these examples is that life-threatening side effects were well known from clinical trials, but the reporting of these side effects was suppressed by the sponsors of the trials. As a consequence, the more prestigious medical journals now require prior registration of clinical trials before the subsequent findings from these clinical trials can be published.[19]

When research findings are in conflict with conventional wisdom or with the financial interests of the funders, they may go unreported or under-reported. Or, when a treatment effect is measured in several different ways, the measure that is statistically significant is more likely to be reported. When publication bias and/or other forms of reporting bias are present in an area of medical research, conventional systematic reviews can give the wrong impression, and any summary of the treatment effect may exaggerate its efficacy or effectiveness. For example, as shown later in this chapter, the effectiveness of nicotine replacement therapy may be exaggerated fourfold. The design of the experiment, itself, is powerless to control how experimental results are reported and interpreted. Only observational methods (preferably MRA) can minimise these common types of research bias.

The conventional meta-regression model

The standard MRA model used in the vast majority of economic applications is:

$$e_j = \beta + \Sigma \alpha_k Z_{jk} + \varepsilon_j \, (j = 1, 2, ...L) \qquad (1)$$

where e_j is the empirical effect in question, and Z_{jk} are the moderator variables used to explain the large study-to-study heterogeneity (or biases) routinely found in economics research.[3] Moderator variables might include:

- dummy variables which reflect whether potentially relevant independent variables have been omitted from (or included in) the primary study
- specification variables that account for differences in functional forms, types of regression, and data definitions or sources, etc; and
- sample size.

As discussed later in this chapter, one of these moderator variables should be the standard error of the estimate of empirical effect, if we are to identify and control for publication bias.

As an illustration of an MRA application, take the popular and controversial topic of the effect of the minimum wage.[9,20] Here, we use the minimum wage *elasticity* of employment, an estimated regression coefficient, as the comparable measure of

effect, e_j, and confine our meta-analysis to studies of the US only.[21] We find 1474 separate estimates of this one economic effect. Each empirical minimum wage effect is estimated from observational data by a regression coefficient (or calculated from a regression coefficient). This plethora of estimates allows us to estimate and statistically control for many factors that might affect or threaten the validity of a given estimate. From about two dozen such factors, significant moderator variables include: the average year of the data used (the adverse employment effect is declining over time), whether a study measures minimum wage by using the Kaitz Index, whether a study uses a log-log model of employment, and whether it uses panel data (see Table 11.3). We also identify a large amount of publication bias that overwhelms any genuine adverse employment effect that raising the minimum wage might have (see also the next section of this chapter).

As another illustration, consider the research on gender wage discrimination. Stanley & Jarrell found that how wages were measured (hourly, annually or weekly) had a practically large effect on the magnitude of the gender wage gap.[11] Several moderator variables that reflect the omission of potentially important explanatory variables and therefore represent mis-specification bias were also found to have important effects on estimates of the wage gap. Even the gender of the researcher was identified to affect what he or she finds. In total, a dozen moderator variables were found to be statistically significant, explaining 87% of the variation among the reported estimates of gender wage discrimination.[11]

A word about quality

Although there are differences in research quality in economics, it is necessary to aim to include all available research results in an MRA, published or not. First, questions about a study's methodological quality often serve as a smoke screen to discount or ignore results contradictory to the reviewer's favoured theory or ideology. Too often, reviews are conducted 'in a subjective and selective manner for the purpose of disqualifying findings which run contrary to the beliefs of the author'.[22] Given the observational nature of economic data, the reviewer can always pick and choose their methodological preferences in order to skew the selected research. Like medical practice, the first rule of systematic reviewing should be: 'Do no harm'.

Second, objective criteria of research quality in economics are problematic. The most widely used measure of quality is journal impact factor or some similar index of citations. At best, such criteria are circular. It is like using TV ratings to measure the quality of the news. In economics, there is empirical evidence that journal impact factor is not correlated with an objective statistical measure of quality such as precision (i.e. the inverse of an estimate's standard error, $1/SE_i$). As discussed in the next section, precision is the most obvious measure of research quality but has yet to be widely accepted for this purpose.

Third, there are statistical reasons to include all estimates, regardless of their presumed quality. Even the worst estimates contain important information about the effect of making various methodological errors. Because all econometric studies contain some threat to their validity or potential methodological error, the resulting biases cannot be eliminated through further selection. Rather, it is a central objective of MRA to estimate the effects of these potential errors and biases. All credible MRAs in economics use multivariate MRA to explain the typically large systematic variation among reported effects and to estimate the size of potential biases. With enough data, we can sensibly estimate the effects that various methodological choices have upon the magnitude of the reported empirical results. Then, everyone can judge for themselves whether or how much the effect in question is affected by a given methodological choice. A rigorous and objective sensitivity analysis is not possible without MRA estimates of disputed methodological choices and specifications. If we were to omit many empirical estimates for quality reasons, using MRA to estimate methodological errors and biases would become either impossible or much inferior.

Against this recommendation to include all research results, others have argued that only the highest quality research, usually RCTs, should be incorporated into a systematic review.[23,24] When many well-designed RCTs are available, then rigorous selection on design quality may be warranted. If strict selection for high-quality designs (such as true and quasi-experiments) were imposed on systematic reviews of general economics (applied micro-, macro-, labour, international, etc.), most specific research areas would have no studies to review (the exception to this rule is the area of experimental research – although an important and growing area, its findings represent a small percentage of empirical economics). For economic, health and social interventions, it would be better to include all studies and code any observable difference in quality. Then, these differences in research quality can be incorporated explicitly into, and estimated by, MRA.

It is the duty of the systematic reviewer not to worsen existing biases. Quality is not somehow ignored as the result. Quite the contrary – only when various dimensions of quality are explicitly incorporated into the MRA model and their effects estimated by the full range of research results can we have any objective basis upon which to assess the importance of research 'quality' on the phenomenon in question.

Publication bias and its discontents

'Publication bias, the phenomenon in which studies with positive results are more likely to be published than studies with negative results, is a serious problem in the interpretation of scientific research.'

(Begg & Berlin 1988)[25]

Publication bias and other reporting biases have long been regarded by both economists and medical researchers as a severe threat to scientific inference.[9,25–33] If the majority of reported findings are selected in part for their statistical significance, empirical phenomena can be manufactured, mere artefacts of the publication selection process. For example, the efficacy of some new pharmacological treatment or the adverse employment effect of raising the minimum wage may be seen by many researchers as established fact, yet these effects may be nothing more than publication bias.[19,21] Two-thirds of areas of economics research contain substantial or severe publication bias.[34] As mentioned previously, many leading medical journals now require the prior registration of clinical trials to mitigate publication bias and other reporting biases. Nonetheless, a recent systematic review of publication bias of clinical medical trials found that 'trials with positive findings had nearly four times the odds of being published compared to findings that were not statistically significant'.[33] So what can be done to identify and minimise this pernicious problem?

Funnel graphs

'The simplest and most commonly used method to detect publication bias is an informal examination of a funnel plot.'

(Sutton *et al.*, 2000)[32]

Funnel graphs have been widely used in medical research and the social sciences to identify publication bias. A funnel graph is a scatter diagram of a reported empirical estimate (e_i) and its precision ($1/SE_i$). Funnel plots should resemble an inverted funnel (see Figure 11.1). As the estimates become more precise (i.e. moving from the bottom to the top of the diagram), the reported estimates become less spread out and tend to converge to the 'true' value. In the absence of publication bias, the plot will be symmetrical (see Figure 11.1).

Publication bias for a specific directional effect (whether positive or negative) will skew the reported results and make the funnel graph asymmetrical. Asymmetry is the hallmark of publication bias, and it is routinely observed in most areas of economics research.[34] Figure 11.2 appears to be more heavily weighted on the left, especially for moderate values

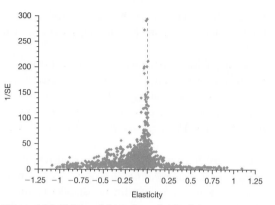

Figure 11.2 Trimmed funnel graph of minimum wage employment effects (n = 1424). Note: In order to see the shape of the vast majority of these estimates of the minimum wage effect, we had to trim a few (50, or 3.4%) of the most extreme estimates. Data from Doucouliagos & Stanley, 2009.[21]

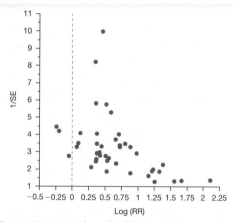

Figure 11.3 Funnel graph of the log risk ratio of nicotine replacement therapy: patch. Data from Stead *et al.*, 2008.[36]

of precision. Is this evidence of publication bias for an adverse employment effect from minimum wage? Similarly, Figure 11.3 appears asymmetrical, skewed to the right and favouring the use of the patch as a nicotine replacement therapy (NRT) for smoking cessation. But how can we be sure that these causal observations are not imagined, not the result of mere random variation? Any visual inspection of a funnel graph is inherently subjective and often ambiguous. Fortunately, we have a more objective, statistical test for the presence of publication bias.

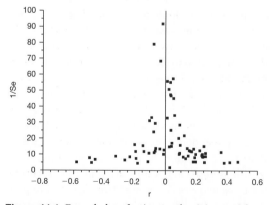

Figure 11.1 Funnel plot of union productivity partial correlations. Data from Doucouliagos & Laroche, 2003.[12]

Funnel asymmetry and precision effect tests (FAT-PET-MRA)

'Several of the regression based methods consistently outperformed the Trim and Fill estimators.'

(Moreno *et al.*, 2009)[37]

The conventional model of publication bias in both economics and medical research is a simple MRA between a study's estimated effect and its standard error.[9,30,38,39]

$$e_i = \beta_1 + \beta_0 SE_i + \varepsilon_i \qquad (2)$$

When there is no publication bias, estimated effects will vary randomly around the 'true' effect, β_1. $\beta_0 SE_i$ represents systematic selection for statistical significance. Studies with smaller samples and hence larger standard errors (SE_i) will need to run and re-run their models more intensely to achieve a statistically significant result. More precise studies (i.e. those with a larger $1/SE_i$) will require less searching and less selection to obtain the desired significant result. Egger and colleagues use the test of H_0: $\beta_0 = 0$ as a test for the presence of publication bias, which has been termed a funnel asymmetry test (FAT).[30,38,39] Simulations show that a FAT provides a valid, but low-power, test for publication bias.[39] MRA model (2) can be used to explain systematic bias and heterogeneity by adding back the moderator variables from equation (1).

An obvious statistical problem for these MRA models is that estimated effects in equation (2) will have different variances (i.e. heteroscedasticity). Weighted least squares (WLS) is the conventional correction for heteroscedasticity. The WLS version of (2) may be obtained by weighting the squared errors by the inverse of the estimates' individual variances (i.e., $1/SE_i^2$) or by dividing the entire equation (2) through by SE_i. Doing so gives:

$$t_i = e_i/SE_i = \beta_0 + \beta_1 (1/SE_i) + \nu_i \qquad (3)$$

where $\nu_i = \varepsilon_i/SE_i$.

Note that the dependent variable becomes the estimate's reported t-value, and the independent variable is its precision, $1/SE_i$. As SE_i approaches zero in equation (2), the expected effect will approach β_1, regardless of publication bias. For this reason, medical researchers have suggested use of the estimate of β_1 in equation (2) or (3) as the corrected empirical effect.[32,37] Unfortunately, this estimate is known to be biased downward when there is a genuine non-zero effect.[39] To reduce this bias, Stanley & Doucouliagos[35] offer an alternative MRA estimator (see also Moreno *et al.*, 2009[37]). It should also be noted that rather than dividing all the observations of each variable by SE_i, many meta-analysts choose to use a canned statistical routine for WLS using $1/SE_i^2$ as the weights. Estimating equation (3) using ordinary least squares (OLS) gives the same results as standard statistical routines for WLS on equation (2). A recent 'comprehensive simulation study' by a team of medical researchers found that variations of these MRA models consistently outperformed other methods in reducing publication bias.[37]

Both the funnel graph and this MRA model of publication bias reveal the central importance of precision in evaluating research. Testing precision's coefficient (H_0:$\beta_1 = 0$) serves as a powerful statistical test – precision effect test (PET) – for a genuine empirical effect beyond publication selection.[39] The PET's validity has been confirmed in simulations and in several economic applications.[21,38–40]

Table 11.1 estimates the FAT-PET-MRA for the three funnels graphs presented above. As our visual inspection suggested, there is strong evidence of publication bias in the minimum wage literature (FAT t = –16.6; p < 0.01) and in NRT studies using the patch (t = 3.01; p < 0.01). Consistent with the funnel graph, there is little evidence of publication selection of union productivity estimates (t = 1.72; p > 0.05).

After accommodating publication bias, identifying genuine empirical effects is more complicated. The PET (H_0:$\beta_1 = 0$) finds no evidence of union productivity effects (PET t = –1.06; p > 0.05), borderline evidence of the patch's effectiveness in smoking cessation (t = 2.00; p ≈ 0.05), and clearer evidence of minimum wage's adverse employment effect (t = –3.55; p < 0.01). Because the question of the patch's efficacy in smoking cessation is clearly a directional hypothesis, its PET can be honestly interpreted as providing some evidence in favour of its effectiveness (t = 2.00; one-tail p < 0.05).

The case for a genuine adverse employment effect from the minimum wage is more problematic, but instructive. Systematic reviewers should always make a clear distinction between statistical significance and practical significance. Failure to make this important distinction is a source of the 'significance controversy' in the social sciences. Although there is evidence of

Table 11.1 Simple meta-regression tests.

Variables	Union productivity	Minimum wage	Nicotine replacement therapy: patch
Intercept: β_0 (FAT)	0.65 (1.72)*	−1.60 (−16.6)*	1.10 (3.01)*
$1/SE_i$: β_1 (PET)	−0.0179 (−1.06)	−0.009 (−3.55)	0.197 (2.00)
n	73	1474	42

Dependent variable = t-value. *t-values are reported in parenthesis.

a statistically significant minimum wage effect, the magnitude of this effect has no practical import. This effect implies that a 10% increase in minimum wage reduces teenage employment by 0.09% or, in other words, a doubling of the minimum wage would cause a reduction in teenage employment of less than 1%. Such a small effect has no practical relevance or policy consequence. Also, simulations show that the PET can have inflated type I errors (i.e. finding a genuine empirical effect that is not there) when there is excess unexplained variation in the FAT-PET-MRA.[39] Because there is evidence of such excess variation (see the next section of this chapter), we cannot rule out the possibility that this practically small but nonetheless statistically significant effect is a type I error. If this small employment effect were taken at face value, it implies that publication bias inflates the adverse employment effect 20-fold because the average minimum wage elasticity is −0.19.

Correcting for publication bias also makes a large practical difference to the size of the patch's effect on smoking cessation. The average unadjusted relative risk ratio is 1.93, implying a 93% increase in smoking cessation attributable to NRT, but precision's estimated coefficient implies only a 22% increase ($e^{0.197} = 1.22$). Correcting for likely publication bias greatly reduces the patch's estimated effectiveness.

Conducting a meta-regression analysis: a brief sketch

In this section, we use the minimum wage employment effect as an illustration of an economic MRA (see Doucouliagos & Stanley 2009 for an extended discussion of this example[21]).

Identifying studies

The most challenging part of any meta-analysis is finding and coding the relevant research. To identify potentially relevant studies, several search engines such as, *inter alia*, Econlit, Google and Google Scholar should be searched using broadly defined keywords. References to seminal papers as well as those contained in identified empirical papers should also be added to the lists produced by the search engines. For minimum wage effects, this strategy identified 65 studies reporting US minimum wage effects and containing approximately 1500 estimated elasticities.[21]

Coding studies

The next step is to read carefully the seminal papers in the relevant area of research along with several of the better empirical studies, noting what the research literature considers to be the important theoretical, methodological, econometric and data issues. Along with past MRAs, these considerations should define the moderator variables to be coded. Although some may regard this approach as circular, it is an important stage of research. Past MRAs strongly suggest many specific and generic moderator variables that account for: potential omitted-variable bias, time, differences in econometric techniques, differences in outcome measure, data sources, and other potential sources of bias.

The most critical coding issue facing the meta-analyst is how to measure the empirical effect in question. The chosen measure of effect is the focus of MRA and needs to be comparable widely across studies. When possible, a 'unitless' measure should be used, such as elasticity, representing the percentage increase in the target phenomenon (say, teenage employment) caused by a 1% increase in the stimulus or treatment (say, minimum wage). Economists often use elasticity to measure empirical effect, and it is routinely considered to be stable. Partial correlations are another good choice. These are also pure numbers without units and can be calculated from almost any reported regression coefficient.[12] Alternatively, the gender wage gap can be measured using the difference in log wages between men and women. This log difference is quite similar to measures used in medical research (log odds ratio or log relative risk) and is easily converted to the 'unitless' percentage difference. In our example MRA, to represent the effect of minimum wage on employment, we used the employment elasticity of minimum wage, because it is, by far, the most commonly employed measure of effect in this particular research literature.

Descriptive statistics

The meta-analyst is obligated to report descriptive statistics (e.g. means, standard deviations, funnel graphs) for their chosen area of research. For minimum wage, the average elasticity is –0.19 (implying that a 10% increase in minimum wage leads to a 2% decline in teenage employment) with a standard deviation of 1.10. We find that showing a funnel graph is always helpful and sometimes enlightening. It is surprising just how often coding errors can be identified simply by looking at a funnel graph.

Economists are not fond of fixed effects and random effects estimators, because they are unlikely to be valid and are often misleading. The terms 'fixed effects' and 'random effects' estimators, as used by medical researchers, are mere weighted averages. These same terms have entirely different meanings when used by econometricians. The econometric use of 'fixed effects' and 'random effects' refers to complex multivariate and multilevel models (for example, see the random effects multilevel (REML) model in Table 11.3). When there is excess heterogeneity, as there *always* is in economics research, any simple or fixed effects weighted average will not be strictly valid. The Q-statistic is the conventional test for heterogeneity. It is distributed as a chi-square and can be calculated from the sum of the square errors of the simple FAT-PET-MRA, equation (3).[41] For minimum wages, there is clearly excess heterogeneity ($Q_{(1472)}$ = 12,232; p < 0.01), implying that there is no common minimum wage effect across these studies. With excess heterogeneity, the simple average and the fixed effect weighted average are inappropriate. Instead, the random effects weighted average would seem to be the proper choice.

The random effects estimator has two serious limitations for economic applications. First, when there is publication bias, the typical case in economics, it will contain considerably more bias than the fixed effects

estimator.[35] Second, there is always systematic variation that can be explained. The random effects weighted average assumes that all the excess heterogeneity is random, which is almost never true in economics research. Thus, economists often skip over the reporting fixed and random effects weighted averages to spend more time developing and reporting multivariate MRAs that explain both systematic and strictly random variation among reported empirical estimates. In a multivariate MRA context, we do not have to choose between random and fixed effects. Instead we have mixed effects, in which multivariate MRA incorporates both approaches – 'fixed effects' to model the systematic variation and 'random effects' to allow for any remaining excess random heterogeneity (see the REML reported in Table 11.3, which includes both types of effects in a multi-level and multivariate context).

Accounting for publication selection: FAT-PET-MRA

Publication bias has already been discussed above. There is strong evidence of publication bias in the minimum wage literature (recall Table 11.1). Researchers tend to select for evidence of adverse employment effects that are consistent with conventional economics theory (t = –16.6; p < 0.01). When evidence of publication bias is found, the standard error becomes an additional moderator variable, as in equation (2).

Multivariate MRA

Much of the variation in economics research can be explained by obvious moderator variables. MRA models (2) and (3) can be expanded to include moderator variables, Z_k, that explain variation in genuine effect and other factors, K_j, that are correlated with the publication selection process itself.

$$e_i = \beta_1 + \Sigma\alpha_k Z_{ik} + \beta_0 SE_i + \Sigma\gamma_j K_{ij} SE_i + \varepsilon_i \quad \text{(OLS)} \quad (4)$$

$$t_i = \beta_0 + \Sigma\gamma_j K_{ij} + \beta_1 (1/SE_i) + \Sigma\alpha_k Z_{ik}/SE_i + v_i \quad \text{(WLS)} \quad (5)$$

Table 11.2 lists the potential Z-K variables which were coded by this minimum wage MRA. This choice of MRA control variables was driven by debates in the literature and past experience. Many of these variables represent potential mis-specification error; hence they also reflect the 'quality' of the associated

Table 11.2 Potential explanatory variables for meta-regression analysis.

Z- & K-variables	Definition
1/Se	is the elasticity's precision
AveYear	is the average year of the data used; 2000 is the base year
Panel	=1, if estimate relates to panel data
Cross	=1, if estimate relates to cross-sectional data
Adults	=1, if estimate relates to young adults (20–24)
Male	=1, if estimate relates to male employees
Non-white	=1, if estimate relates to non-white employees
Region	=1, if estimate relates to region-specific data
Lag	=1, if estimate relates to a lagged minimum wage effect
Hours	=1, if the dependent variable is hours worked
Double	=1, if estimate comes from a double log specification
Agriculture	=1, if estimates are for the agriculture industry
Retail	=1, if estimates are for the retail industry
Food	=1, if estimates are for the food industry
Time	=1, if time trend is included
Yeareffect	=1, if year-specific fixed effects are used
Regioneffect	=1, if region/state fixed effects are used
Un	=1, if a model includes unemployment
School	=1, if model includes a schooling variable
Kaitz	=1, if the Kaitz measure of the minimum wage is used
Dummy	=1, if a dummy variable measure of the minimum wage is used
Published	=1, if the estimate comes from a published study

estimate. Table 11.3 presents the MRA results of general-to-specific modelling.[42] That is, all *Z* and *K* variables listed in Table 11.2 were included in a general meta-regression model, and then the statistically insignificant ones were removed, one at a time. Although there is no guarantee, general-to-specific modelling is much less likely to settle on a spurious

MRA model than adding moderator variables one at a time (e.g. stepwise). The art of regression model building is beyond the scope of this chapter. However, as Charemza & Deadman have observed, 'The strength of general-to-specific modelling is that model construction proceeds from a very general model in a more structured, ordered (and statistically valid) fashion, and in this way avoids the worst of data mining'.[42] It should be considered that the issue of selecting the proper multivariate MRA model would disappear if systematic reviewers were required to register their proposed MRA model specifications before collecting their research data.

The first column of Table 11.3 reports the MRA results using clustered data analysis which is one way to account for potential dependence among estimates within the same study. An alternative approach to

Table 11.3 Multivariate meta-regression analysis model (general to specific).

Moderator variables	Cluster robust	REML
Genuine empirical effects (Z-variables)		
1/SE	0.120 (4.39)*	0.107 (7.00)
Panel/SE	−0.182 (−4.72)	−0.155 (−12.31)
Double/SE	0.064 (3.20)	0.044 (5.96)
Region/SE	0.040 (0.92)	0.087 (6.37)
Adult/SE	0.024 (2.68)	0.021 (3.76)
Lag/SE	0.026 (1.60)	0.012 (2.05)
AveYear/SE	0.004 (4.34)	0.003 (7.40)
Un/SE	−0.042 (−3.04)	−0.041 (−6.14)
Kaitz/SE	0.052 (3.06)	0.033 (4.48)
Yeareffect/SE	0.069 (1.98)	0.068 (7.83)
Published/SE	−0.041 (−2.69)	−0.039 (−5.60)
Time/SE	−0.022 (−2.08)	−0.020 (−3.07)
Publication bias (K-variables)		
Intercept (β_0)	−0.359 (−0.11)	−1.222 (−3.82)
Double	−1.482 (−3.23)	−1.091 (−4.31)
Un	−0.840 (−1.87)	0.852 (2.64)
n	1474	1474
k	64	64

*Dependent variable = t-value.

modelling the intra-study dependence is reported in the second column – a random effects multilevel (REML). Here, the term 'REML' refers to a multilevel model that accounts for potential dependence of estimates within studies and allows for both fixed and random effects (whereas the data analysis and statistical software Stata uses the term 'REML' to refer to restricted maximum likelihood). For technical discussion of how to make modelling choices for MRA, see Stanley & Doucouliagos and Feld & Heckemeyer.[35,43]

The intercept of equation (5), by itself, is no longer a measure of the magnitude of the average publication bias. Rather, it is the combination of the intercept and all the K-variables (*Un* and *Double*), and clear evidence of publication bias remains in this multivariate MRA ($F_{(3,1459)} = 84.2$; $p < 0.01$). Likewise, genuine effect corrected for publication bias is no longer a single MRA coefficient but rather the combination of all Z-variables and *1/SE*. The Wald test is again easily passed ($F_{(11,1459)} = 50.8$; $p < 0.01$), providing evidence of a genuine, if heterogeneous, minimum wage effect. Thus, the central findings from our simple FAT-PET-MRA are confirmed by more sophisticated multivariate MRAs. Also, to economists, the magnitudes of many of the individual MRA coefficients are of interest in themselves.[21]

Because no single MRA coefficient represents the overall employment effect of minimum wage, some judgement about what constitutes 'best practice' must be used. Once such a professional judgement is made, the implied values of the moderator variables can be substituted into the MRA model to make a 'prediction' of the value of genuine empirical effect after controlling for publication bias and other potential biases. In our example, we substituted a range of values into the MRA based upon what researchers in the field regard as best practice to ensure that our conclusions about minimum wage effects are robust. Regardless of how 'best practice' is defined, no practically significant adverse employment effect remains.[21] The implicit flexibility of MRA is another great advantage. If any researcher disagrees with the range of values that is used to define some interpretation of 'best practice', the estimated MRA coefficients can generate another estimate for some other judgement of 'best practice'. In this way, robustness and consensus can be achieved even in controversial areas of research like the employment effects of minimum wage.

Conclusions

Meta-analysis was originally developed by psychologists and medical researchers and then imported into economics. Economists have refined these methods to suit the demands of sophisticated econometric research. Economics research always contains excess heterogeneity that needs to be explained if a given area of research is to be understood. MRA is the result.

Meta-regression analysis has been found to be especially helpful in identifying and correcting publication bias, a problem that also plagues medical research.[30,32,37,39] Funnel graphs and the FAT-PET-MRA go a long way towards identifying and correcting publication bias. Furthermore, the observational nature of medical systematic reviews makes them fertile ground for MRA. For example, wouldn't it be helpful to know how the dosage, type of drug and delivery system influence the outcomes of nicotine replacement therapy (NRT)? Perhaps other variables, such as the subjects' age, educational level and years of smoking, might help to explain the observed difference in NRT effectiveness.

However, using MRA in medical research does have serious pitfalls.[44] When there are few clinical trials but many potential moderator variables, MRA is not feasible. In such cases, there are actually 'negative' degrees of freedom available for statistical analysis. This is where economics research has the advantage, because many areas of economics research contain many dozens and often several hundred estimates. In medical research, the meta-analyst is forced to choose one or a few additional research dimensions to be investigated before conducting the meta-analysis, if the risk of finding a spurious relation is to be minimised. In economics, where there is no scarcity of degrees of freedom, data mining is nonetheless a real threat, but one that can be made manageable through general-to-specific modelling or prior registration of all MRA models to be investigated.

How this chapter should be cited

Stanley TD. Chapter 11: Meta-regression models of economics and medical research. In: Shemilt I, Mugford M, Vale L, Marsh K, Donaldson C (editors). *Evidence-based decisions and economics: health care, social welfare, education and criminal justice.* Oxford: Wiley-Blackwell, 2010.

References

1 Deeks JJ, Higgins JPT, Altman DG. Analysing data and undertaking meta-analyses. In: Higgins JPT, Green S (eds) *Cochrane Handbook for Systematic Reviews of Interventions*. Version 5.0.1 (updated September 2008). Oxford: Cochrane Collaboration, 2008.

2 Becker BJ, Hedges LV, Pigott TD. *Campbell Collaboration Statistical Analysis Policy Brief*. Oslo: Campbell Collaboration, 2004.

3 Stanley TD, Jarrell SB. Meta-regression analysis: a quantitative method of literature surveys. *Journal of Economic Surveys* 1989; 3(2): 161–170.

4 Nelson JP, Kennedy PE. The use (and abuse) of meta-analysis in environmental and natural resource economics: an assessment. *Environmental Resource Economics* 2009; 42(3): 345–377.

5 Rosenberger RS, Loomis JB. Benefit transfer. In: Champ PA, Boyle KJ, Brown TC (eds) *A Primer on Nonmarket Valuation*. Dordrecht: Kluwer Academic Publishers, 2003.

6 Rosenberger RS, Loomis JB. Panel stratification in meta-analysis of economic studies: an investigation of its effects in the recreation valuation literature. *Journal of Agricultural and Applied Economics* 2000; 32(3): 459–470.

7 Smith VK, Pattanayak SK. Is meta-analysis a Noah's Ark for non-market valuation? *Environmental Resource Economics* 2002; 22(1–2): 271–296.

8 Jarrell SB, Stanley TD. A meta-analysis of the union–nonunion wage gap. *Industrial and Labor Relations Review* 1990; 44(1): 54–67.

9 Card D, Krueger AB. Time-series minimum-wage studies: a meta-analysis. *American Economic Review* 1995; 85(2): 238–243.

10 Doucouliagos C. The aggregate demand for labour in Australia: a meta-analysis. *Australian Economics Papers* 1997; 36(69): 224–242.

11 Stanley TD, Jarrell SB. Gender wage discrimination bias? A meta-regression analysis. *Journal of Human Resources* 1998; 33(4): 947–973.

12 Doucouliagos C, Laroche P. What do unions do to productivity: a meta-analysis. *Industrial Relations* 2003; 42(4): 650–691.

13 Nijkamp P, Poot J. The last word on the wage curve? *Journal of Economic Surveys* 2005; 19(3): 421–450.

14 Gemmill MC, Costa-Font J, McGuire A. In search of a corrected prescription drug elasticity estimate: a meta-regression approach. *Health Economics* 2007; 16(6): 627–643.

15 Costa-Font J, Gemmill M, Rubert G. *Re-Visiting the Health care Luxury Good Hypothesis: aggregation, precision and publication bias (Documents de Treball No. E08/197)*. Barcelona: Universitat de Barcelona, 2008.

16 Kristiansen IS, Gosden T. Evaluating economic interventions: a role for non-randomised designs. In: Donaldson C, Mugford M, Vale L (eds) *Evidence-based Health Economics: from effectiveness to efficiency in systematic review*. London: BMJ Books, 2002.

17 Higgins JPT, Altman DG. Assessing risk of bias in included studies. In: Higgins JPT, Green S (eds) *Cochrane Handbook for Systematic Reviews of Interventions*. Version 5.0.1 (updated September 2008). Oxford: Cochrane Collaboration, 2008.

18 Reeves BC, Deeks JJ, Higgins JPT, Wells GA. Including non-randomized studies. In: Higgins JPT, Green S (eds) *Cochrane Handbook for Systematic Reviews of Interventions*. Version 5.0.1 (updated September 2008). Oxford: Cochrane Collaboration, 2008.

19 Krakovsky M. Register or perish. *Scientific American* 2004; 291(12): 18–20.

20 The Economist. *Economics Focus: debating the minimum wage (Finance and economics)*. London: Economist Group, 2001, February 3rd.

21 Doucouliagos C, Stanley TD. Publication selection bias in minimum-wage research? A meta-regression analysis. *British Journal of Industrial Relations* 2009; 47(2): 406–428.

22 Stanley TD. Wheat from chaff: meta-analysis as quantitative literature review. *Journal of Economic Perspectives* 2001; 15(3): 131–150.

23 Kunz R, Oxman AD. The unpredictability paradox: review of empirical comparisons of randomised and non-randomised clinical trials. *British Medical Journal* 1998; 317(7167): 1185–1190.

24 Deeks JJ, Dinnes J, d'Amico R, Sowden AJ, Sakarovitch C, Song F. Evaluating non-randomised intervention studies. *Health Technology Assessment* 2004; 7(27): 1–173.

25 Begg CB, Berlin JA. Publication bias: a problem in interpreting medical data. *Journal of the Royal Statistical Society: Series A* 1988; 151(3): 419–445.

26 Sterling TD. Publication decisions and their possible effects on inferences drawn from tests of significance – or vice versa. *Journal of the American Statistical Association* 1959; 54: 30–34.

27 Tullock G. Publication decisions and tests of significance – a comment. *Journal of the American Statistical Association* 1959: 54(287); 593.

28 Rosenthal R. The 'file drawer problem' and tolerance for null results. *Psychological Bulletin* 1979; 86(3): 638–641.

29 Cooper HM, Hedges LV (eds). *Handbook of Research Synthesis*. New York: Russell Sage, 1994.

30 Egger M, Davey Smith G, Scheider M, Minder C. Bias in meta-analysis detected by a simple, graphical test. *British Medical Journal* 1997; 315(7109): 629–634.

31 Copas J. What works? Selectivity models and meta-analysis. *Journal of the Royal Statistical Society: Series A* 1999; 161: 95–105.

32 Sutton AJ, Abrams KR, Jones DR, Sheldon TA, Song F. *Methods for Meta-analysis in Medical Research*. Chichester: John Wiley, 2000.

33 Hopewell S, Loudon K, Clarke MJ, Oxman AD, Dickersin K. Publication bias in clinical trials due to statistical significance or direction of trial results. *Cochrane Database of Systematic Reviews* 2009, Issue 1.

34 Doucouliagos C, Stanley TD. *Theory Competition and Selectivity (Deakin Working Paper, Economics Series 2008–06)*. Melbourne: Deakin University, 2008.

35 Stanley TD, Doucouliagos C. *Identifying and Correcting Publication Selection Bias in the Efficiency-Wage Literature: Heckman meta-regression (Deakin Working Paper, Economics Series 2007–11)*. Melbourne: Deakin University, 2007.

36 Stead LF, Perera R, Bullen C, Mant D, Lancaster T. Nicotine replacement therapy for smoking cessation. *Cochrane Database of Systematic Reviews* 2008, Issue 1.

37 Moreno SG, Sutton AJ, Ades A, *et al.* Assessment of regression-based methods to adjust for publication bias through a comprehensive simulation study. *BMC Medical Research Methodology* 2009; 9(2).

38 Stanley TD. Beyond publication selection. *Journal of Economic Surveys* 2005; 19(3): 309–345.

39 Stanley TD. Meta-regression methods for detecting and estimating empirical effect in the presence of publication bias. *Oxford Bulletin of Economics and Statistics* 2008; 70:103–127.

40 Roberts CJ, Stanley TD (eds). *Meta-Regression Analysis: issues of publication bias in economics*. Oxford: Blackwell, 2005.

41 Higgins JPT, Thompson SG. Quantifying hetergeneity in meta-analysis. *Statistics in Medicine* 2002; 21(11): 1539–1558.

42 Charemza W, Deadman D. *New Directions in Econometric Practice*, 2nd edn. Cheltenham: Russell Edward Elgar, 1997.

43 Feld LP, Heckemeyer JH. *FDI and Taxation - a meta-study (Zentrum für Europäische Wirtschaftsforschung GmbH Discussion Paper No. 08–128)*. Mannheim: Zentrum für Europäische Wirtschaftsforschung. Available from: ftp://ftp.zew.de/pub/zew-docs/dp/dp08128.pdf.

44 Thompson SG, Higgins JPT. How should meta-regression analyses be undertaken and interpreted? *Statistics in Medicine* 2002; 21(11): 1559–1573.

CHAPTER 12

From evidence-based economics to economics-based evidence: using systematic review to inform the design of future research

Ed Wilson[1], Keith Abrams[2]

[1]Health Economics Group, University of East Anglia, Norwich, UK
[2]Department of Health Sciences, University of Leicester, Leicester, UK

Introduction

The purpose of much health services research is to assist in decisions about whether or not to adopt a given technology (e.g. a drug, device, programme or technique). Economic evaluations using decision models are a means of assessing the relative value for money (cost-effectiveness) of technologies (see also, *inter alia*, Chapters 2 and 9). This is usually expressed as the incremental cost-effectiveness ratio (ICER), defined as the difference in mean cost between a technology and its comparator, divided by the difference in mean outcome. If the ICER is below some threshold, then the technology is considered good value for money and should be adopted in place of its comparator (see the Appendix to this chapter, equation A1). A common outcome metric is the quality-adjusted life-year (QALY) and an 'acceptable' threshold in the UK is in the region of £20,000–30,000 per QALY gained.[1]

It is convenient to rearrange the ICER into the incremental net benefit (INB), so that the decision rule becomes 'adopt the technology if the expected INB is greater than zero'. This generalises to 'choose the technology with the maximum expected net benefit (NB)', which is a mathematically convenient decision rule when comparing more than two options (see Appendix, equations A2–A4).

Decision uncertainty can be summarised in the cost-effectiveness acceptability curve (CEAC) (or preferably the cost-effectiveness acceptability frontier), which shows the probability a decision will be 'correct' as a function of willingness to pay for a unit of outcome.[2]

In order to maximise expected NB, decisions should be based solely on the expected net benefit, irrespective of the degree of uncertainty. Uncertainty should instead be used to inform the decision as to whether to pursue future research.[3] This contrasts with the classic frequentist statistical paradigm, which focuses on hypothesis testing and statistical significance, and where the decision rule would be to 'choose the option with the highest net benefit only if this is statistically significantly higher' (in this classic frequentist view, if there is no such option then there is too much uncertainty to make a recommendation).

There are therefore two separate decisions to be made: whether to adopt an intervention, and whether to collect further evidence to inform reassessment of the decision in the future (although these decisions are not truly independent of one another – see 'Discussion', below).

In this chapter, we first summarise the iterative approach to the evidence-gathering cycle of systematic

Evidence-Based Decisions and Economics, 2nd edition. Edited by I. Shemilt, M. Mugford, L. Vale, K. Marsh and C. Donaldson. © 2010 Blackwell Publishing.

review and meta-analysis, decision making and primary research, which could be referred to as 'economics-based medicine'. We then consider a number of ways in which research may be prioritised, classifying these different approaches as either 'economic' or 'non-economic'. We argue that economics-based approaches are the only ones consistent with health gain maximisation for the population as a whole, as they are the only ones that take into account the opportunity cost of research. After this, we focus on value of information (VoI) analysis as an economics-based approach to prioritising research.[4–7] We conclude the chapter with a discussion of the strengths and weaknesses of the VoI approach.

An iterative approach to evidence gathering and decision making

It has been argued that evidence gathering to answer a specific decision question should be an iterative process (see also Chapter 7).[8–11] This can be summarised in a number of steps, as follows (see also Figure 12.1).

1. Define the decision problem
2. Systematic review and decision model based on current evidence
3. Adoption decision
4. Research decision
5. Primary research

The process begins with the definition of a specific decision question. This must be specified fully; for example, 'Is Intervention X cost-effective compared with Intervention Y from the perspective of Health care organisation Z?'. Following on from this, a systematic review of the existing literature should be carried out to assemble evidence needed to address the specific decision question (including evidence on effects and costs), and this evidence synthesised in a decision model (see also, *inter alia*, Chapters 2, 3, 7, 8 and 9).

It is critical to specify appropriate decision model input parameters, carefully estimate their mean values and characterise the uncertainty (probability distribution) at this stage. Where no data exist for a particular parameter, expert judgement is required to define a likely range of values (and suitably uninformative distribution, such as a uniform distribution or Normal with a 'large' variance). Parameter uncertainty within the model should ideally be analysed using probabilistic sensitivity analysis (PSA).[12,13]

The next stage is the adoption decision: based on current evidence, will society be better off with or without adoption of the new technology? This is a straightforward case of selecting the option with the highest expected INB, irrespective of whether there is a statistically significant difference between options.

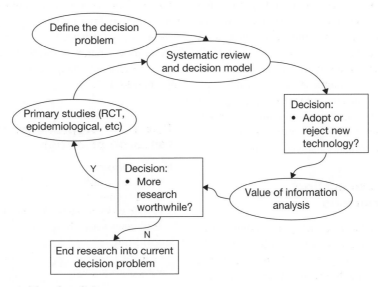

Figure 12.1 'Economics'-based medicine.

Following the adoption decision is the research decision. We propose VoI methodology as an appropriate tool for informing this (other approaches are considered in the next section of this chapter). The uncertainty within model parameters should be used in the VoI analysis to determine whether new information has a probability of changing the adoption decision. If not, then no further research into the current decision problem should be carried out, and the decision made on the basis of current evidence alone. However, if so, there may be a case for conducting additional primary research. This may be a randomised controlled trial (RCT), with or without piggybacked economic evaluation, but equally could be an epidemiological study or utility elicitation exercise (see also Chapter 8), the choice depending on which uncertain parameters have the greatest impact on decision uncertainty. Finally, the new data generated by the primary research should be fed back into an updated systematic review, and the cycle repeated.

A consequence of this approach is that decision models and RCTs or other primary studies are not mutually exclusive but complementary. Fully informed decision making should be based on all available evidence on both the costs and benefits associated with all possible alternative interventions over an appropriate time horizon (typically lifetime in health economic evaluation), in all relevant patient groups.[11] Furthermore, the evidence needs to be combined in such a way as to fully and appropriately characterise the uncertainty inherent in the evidence (i.e. parameter uncertainty), and hence uncertainty in the adoption decision (i.e. decision uncertainty). It is therefore highly unlikely that a single RCT, even with a piggybacked economic evaluation, will be sufficient for decision making and that as a consequence, decision modelling will always be required, for example when considering long-term outcomes or adverse events (see also, *inter alia*, Chapters 2, 3 and 9).[11,14]

Approaches to setting research priorities

It has been argued that a research prioritisation mechanism should be consistent with the objective of the system within which it operates.[15] In the health care field, this is assumed to be the maximisation of health gain, subject to budget and equity considerations

(see also Chapter 6). A number of approaches to research priority setting within the health care field are proposed and/or practised by various funding bodies, which we group into 'non-economic' and 'economic' approaches (see Box 12.1).

Non-economic approaches

Subjective judgement is perhaps the means most commonly used to prioritise research projects. However, due to its lack of replicability and explicit quantification of the value of research, it is unlikely to be consistent with the health system objective stated above.

Burden of disease approaches assume a direct link between the size of a problem and the value of research into it.[16,17] However, this need not necessarily be the case, as there may be very little uncertainty regarding the effectiveness of a treatment for a highly burdensome disease. Research into such treatments would have very little chance of changing policy and hence very little impact on health gain.

Priority setting according to the estimated welfare loss from clinical variations in practice argues that the reason for variation in practice (after adjustment for case-mix, demographics, etc.) is disagreement as to the effectiveness of interventions. However, this approach does not distinguish between variation that is due to uncertainty in the effectiveness of a treatment and variation due to lack of dissemination of existing knowledge. Under this approach, a further trial could be recommended even in circumstances where there is little uncertainty regarding the effectiveness of a treatment. Fleurence & Torgerson argue that, in these circumstances, there are probably more efficient means of changing practice than undertaking a new RCT.[15]

Box 12.1 Approaches to setting research priorities

Non-economic
   Subjective judgement/'gut feeling'
   Burden of disease
   Welfare loss from variation in practice
   Trial sequential analysis
Economic
   Payback
   Value of information

Finally, trial sequential analysis has been proposed as a method for establishing when sufficient evidence has been gathered.[18] This approach is an extension of group sequential analysis – a means of adjusting hypothesis tests to account for repeated testing (thus avoiding spurious rejection of hypotheses).[19,20] As this does not take into account the opportunity cost of conducting research, it cannot assess the relative value of investments in alternative research projects.

In summary, the limitations of 'non-economic' approaches are that they are unlikely to be consistent with the objectives of the health system to which they contribute, and that they do not consider the issue of the opportunity cost of research: namely, that resources invested in research may have generated more health for the population had they been spent either in alternative research projects or in direct care provision.

Economic approaches

The 'payback' approach involves the use of scenario analysis to estimate the likely cost-effectiveness of a proposed trial. As with the 'clinical variations' approach described above, this is a function of not only the results of a trial but also any change in policy resulting from that trial. That is, following publication and dissemination of a trial result, clinical practice may change, resulting in changes in costs and health gain (QALYs) within the population. The expected change in costs (including the cost of conducting the trial itself) divided by the expected change in QALYs gives the expected cost-effectiveness of the trial, expressed in terms of the incremental cost per QALY gained. This approach has been used to determine the likely cost-effectiveness of an RCT of the long-term effects of hormone replacement therapy (HRT).[21]

Expression of the results in terms of the incremental cost per QALY gained allows direct comparison with the cost-effectiveness of other health care interventions, and/or the expected cost-effectiveness of further trials of other health care interventions (and application of the same willingness-to-pay thresholds). However, the payback approach assumes policy changes will be determined by the result of one new 'definitive' trial, rather than a synthesis of all available evidence. This is a potential limitation, since it may be preferable to base decisions on the formal combination of all previous evidence as well as evidence from the new trial.

In the following section, we present (VoI) analysis as an economics-based approach to research prioritisation that is fully compatible with the iterative approach to evidence gathering and decision making and the objective of health gain maximisation.

Value of information analysis

Information theory has its origins in the early 1960s in the work of Raiffa & Schlaifer.[4] Recent applications have been in the areas of, for example, agriculture, environmental economics and finance.[22–26] However, recent interest has also grown in its application to health care research prioritisation.

Value of information analysis provides justification for whether future research should be conducted, and if so, on which uncertain parameters, and provides an estimate of the appropriate sample size for such a study.[5–7] Essentially, VoI values the returns from investment in further research to reduce decision uncertainty, and provides an alternative to conventional power calculations used to estimate the appropriate sample size for future trials, based on a comparison of the return from the marginal trial participant and the associated marginal cost of including her/him in the research. Pilot studies have been undertaken to inform future research priorities in the UK NHS Health Technology Assessment programme and for the UK National Institute for Health and Clinical Excellence, and VoI analyses are beginning to appear alongside published economic evaluations.[27–39]

The key statistics in VoI analysis are the:
- expected value of perfect information (EVPI)
- expected value of perfect parameter information (EVPPI)
- expected value of sample information (EVSI), and the
- expected net benefit of sampling (ENBS).

Expected value of perfect information (EVPI)

The EVPI provides an upper boundary for all expenditure on research into a decision question. As stated in the introduction to this chapter, the decision rule is to choose the option which maximises expected NB for a given population (see Appendix, equation A4). This equation is based on current information.

As a result of uncertainty (i.e. imperfect information), there is a probability that the decision will be wrong, in which case there will be a loss to society (i.e. foregone health gain). If we had perfect information we would always choose the correct option, so there would be no loss. The expected loss from uncertainty is equivalent to the expected gain from eliminating uncertainty (i.e. the EVPI). Mathematically, it is the difference between the expected maximum NB and the maximum expected NB (see Appendix, equation A5). The second term on the right hand side of equation A5 is simply equation A4 (i.e. the maximum expected net benefit with current information). The first term is the expected maximum net benefit with perfect information. Thus the EVPI is the difference between the two.

Example

Suppose the current treatment for disease X is called 'Old' and patients currently treated have an annual risk of death of P_o. A new treatment 'New' is developed which reduces the relative risk of death by RR_N compared to 'Old', but 'New' is also more expensive. The attendant decision question is whether to adopt 'New' in place of 'Old'. A systematic review and meta-analysis have yielded point estimates and distributions around P_o and RR_N: assume current data comprises a study of 200 patients in total, randomised to 'Old' and 'New', and that it estimated a 20% annual probability of death with 'Old' and a relative risk of death with 'New' of 0.75. Based on this information, the baseline probability of death (on 'Old') is

characterised as a beta distribution and relative risk as lognormal with parameters as per equations 1 and 2, below.

$$P_O \sim Beta(20, 80) \qquad (1)$$

$$LN(RR_N) \sim Normal(-0.29, 0.097) \qquad (2)$$

A simple decision model based on a two-state Markov chain is developed incorporating these as well as other data (such as the 'up-front' cost of 'Old' and 'New', changes in subsequent resource use and costs associated with 'Old' and 'New' and health state utility values), over an appropriate time horizon (see Figure 12.2). The model combines these input parameters into estimates of the net benefit from each treatment (NB_o and NB_N) and a PSA is used to derive an expected net benefit with 'Old', $E(NB_o)$ and expected net benefit with 'New', $E(NB_N)$.

Table 12.1 shows the results of the PSA (note that only five iterations are shown in this illustrative example; several thousands would typically be necessary, depending on the complexity of the model). The expected net benefit of 'Old' is £84,178 and of 'New', £92,153 ('E(.)' is the expectation in Table 12.1). The maximum expected net benefit (see Appendix, equation A4) is thus £92,153 and 'New' should be adopted. However, for iterations 2, 3 and 5, 'Old' has the highest net benefit, and therefore as 'New' is the chosen option, there is an opportunity loss equal to the difference in net benefit (£16,677, £15,026 and £315 respectively). The expected loss over all iterations is

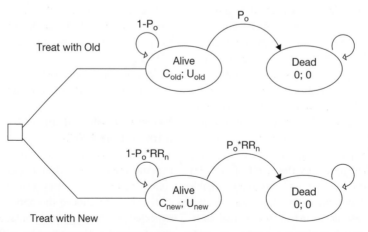

Figure 12.2 Decision model (Markov chain): 'Old' and 'New', where C_j and U_j are cost per year and utility of patient with treatment j (j = 'Old', 'New').

Table 12.1 EVPI illustration.

Iteration	NB$_O$	NB$_N$	D	Max	Loss
1	£67,913	£119,013	N	£119,013	£0
2	£110,199	£93,522	O	£110,199	£16,677
3	£77,624	£62,598	O	£77,624	£15,026
4	£68,291	£89,083	N	£89,083	£0
5	£96,863	£96,548	O	£96,863	£315
E(.)	£84,178	£92,153	N	£98,556	£6403

therefore £6403, which is the gain from eliminating all uncertainty (i.e. the EVPI).

The per-patient EVPI is £6403. This should be scaled up to the current and future population to provide an upper limit for the budget for future research into the technology in question (see Appendix, equation A6).

Thus if the incidence of disease X is 10,000 per annum, for a 10-year time horizon and with a discount rate of 3.5%, the population EVPI is:

$$£6403^* \sum_{t=0}^{9} \frac{10,000}{1.035^t} = £551m$$

The maximum budget for research into the cost-effectiveness of 'Old' versus 'New' should therefore be set at (the rather high figure of) £551m. This does not mean that such a budget *should* be allocated! What this does state is that if a particular research project will cost more than the EVPI, then it will definitely not be cost-effective: the funds should be spent elsewhere (e.g. direct patient care or in an alternative research area). The cost of a research project being less than the EVPI is therefore a necessary but not sufficient condition.

Expected value of perfect parameter information (EVPPI)

The EVPPI provides an upper boundary to research expenditure with respect to a particular parameter or group of parameters (see Appendix, equation A7). As such, the EVPI is a special case of the EVPPI where the parameters of interest are all parameters in the model. Again, this should be multiplied by the incident population over an 'appropriate' time horizon to calculate the population EVPPI (see Appendix, equation A8).

Note the sum of EVPPIs will not be equal to the EVPI due to the potential for interactions between variables; for example, collecting information on one parameter may affect the value of collecting further information on another with which it is closely correlated.

Example

In our example, we now consider the EVPPI associated with the single parameter, P$_o$ (although we could consider other variables or groups of related parameters). We first sample a value from the distribution

Table 12.2 EVPPI illustration.

Iteration	P$_o$	NB$_O$	NB$_N$	D	Max	Loss
1	0.23	£101,323	£105,554	N	£105,554	£0
2	0.19	£67,466	£70,849	N	£70,849	£0
3	0.19	£105,311	£92,888	O	£105,311	£12,423
4	0.20	£58,946	£77,969	N	£77,969	£0
5	0.21	£106,624	£99,337	O	£106,624	£7287
E(.)		£87,934	£89,319	N	£93,261	£3942

of P_o as a possible realisation of the 'true' parameter value. We then run the PSA for a 'large' number of iterations, holding P_o constant, and record the expected net benefits of 'Old' and 'New' respectively (see Table 12.2). The next step is to sample another value from the distribution of P_o, repeat the PSA and record the expected net benefits. This is repeated a large number of times. As before, we take the expectations of the columns 'NB$_o$', 'NB$_N$' and 'Max'. The expected value of perfect information on P_o is then the expected maximum net benefit (£93,261) less the maximum expected net benefit (= max (£87,934, £89,319)), yielding an EVPPI for P_o of £3942 and a population EVPPI for P_o of:

$$£3942 * \sum_{t=0}^{9} \frac{10,000}{1.035^t} = £339.3m$$

Repeating the EVPPI calculation for a number of parameters provides an indication of what further research may be most useful (or, rather, efficient) to reduce decision uncertainty. However, as per EVPI, the EVPPI provides the necessary but not sufficient condition for deciding whether or not to carry out a research project.

Expected value of sample information (EVSI) and expected net benefit of sampling (ENBS)

The EVSI provides the sufficient condition as to whether to undertake a particular data collection exercise (whether RCT, prospective case series, retrospective database analysis, etc.) by estimating the value of the return from a study of sample size n. For a particular parameter or group of parameters, this is the expected maximum expected net benefit with the new information less the maximum expected net benefit with current information (see Appendix, equations A9 and A10).

The ENBS is the difference between the EVSI with sample size n and the cost of conducting the research with sample size n. The point at which this is maximised is the efficient sample size for the proposed study. If there is no positive sample size for which the ENBS is greater than zero, then additional research is not warranted, and decisions should be based on current information only (i.e. the cost of future research outweighs the benefit).

Example

Figures 12.3 and 12.4 show the steps in calculating the EVSI and ENBS for the parameter P_o. Figures 12.3 and 12.4 each show three tables labelled A to C. Table B will contain the output of the standard decision model PSA. Table A will contain the summaries of each of these and Table C will contain the EVSI estimated for each sample size.

With current information, our meta-analysis determined the prior distribution of P_o as $P_o \sim Beta(20,80)$. We have already established that the EVPPI associated with this parameter is greater than zero (£339m) and so now want to calculate the EVSI and ultimately the ENBS.

We first decide on a possible sample size for our proposed study, say n = 10. We then sample a value from the prior distribution of P_o. This represents one possible realisation of the world. Let us say that value is 0.24. So this is a world where the true population baseline mortality rate is 24%. We fill this value in cell (row 3, column 2) of Figure 12.3, Table A. The results of the study (call this P_{os}) therefore must be a binomial random variable with mean 0.24 and sample size 10 (i.e. $P_{os} \sim Bin(0.24,10)$).

We now sample from this distribution as a possible realisation of the study results. Suppose we sample the value 3. That is, one possible result is that three patients died and seven survived to 1 year. The next step is to use Bayes' theorem to combine our prior distribution and the 'new' data to a (pre)posterior distribution.[40] Call this P_o'. For the beta distribution this is simply:

$$P_o' \sim Beta(A + P_{os}, B + n - P_{os})$$

$$=> P_o' \sim Beta(20 + 3, 80 + 10 - 3)$$

$$=> P_o' \sim Beta(23, 87)$$

This equation is entered in cell (r1, c2) of Figure 12.3, Table B. We then run the PSA for a 'large' number of iterations (only 5 shown for demonstration purposes), each time sampling from the distributions of P_o' as well as the other model inputs, and record the net benefit obtained from each treatment in Figure 12.3, Table B, cells (r3, c3) to (r7, c4).

After all the iterations, we estimate the expected net benefit from 'Old' at £98,453, and from 'New', £85,395 (Table B, cells (r2, c3) and (r2, c4)). We then transfer these estimates to cells (r3, c3) and (r3, c4) of Table A.

A. Iteration summaries

Run					
Average	Po ~ Beta(20,80)	NBo	NBn	Max	
1	0.24	**£98,453**	**£85,395**		
2					
3					
4					
5					

C. EVSI

n	EVSI
10	
20	
30	
40	
50	
...	

$$P_{OS} \sim Bin(0.24,10)$$

$$P_{OS} = 3$$

B. Model iterations

MODEL	Po' ~ Beta(23,87)	NBo	NBn
Mean		**£98,453**	**£85,395**
1	0.23	£118,651	£95,671
2	0.22	£118,873	£78,423
3	0.24	£73,682	£92,143
4	0.23	£104,719	£73,621
5	0.23	£76,339	£87,116

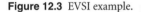

Figure 12.3 EVSI example.

The next step is to sample from the prior distribution of P_o again. Let us say the result this time is 0.18. We record this in Table A (Figure 12.4, Table A, cell (r4, c2)). The results of the hypothesised study are now a binomial random variable with a Bin(0.18,10) distribution. Sampling from this distribution, we get a possible study result of, say, one death and nine survivors. Adding these new data to the prior gives us Po' ~Beta(21,89), providing us with the new (pre)posterior distribution. The model is then run a large number of times, sampling each time from this new distribution along with the remaining model inputs, and the expected net benefit from each treatment is recorded. In this case we get £72,814 and £84,599 respectively (Figure 12.4, Table A, cells (r4, c3) and (r4, c4)). This process is repeated a large number of times.

After running the iterations, we record the maximum expected net benefit from each run in the final column of Figure 12.4, Table A, and take the mean of each column (recorded in the top row of Table A:

£81,324, £88,396 and £91,008). The EVSI is the expected maximum net benefit with perfect information about P_o less the maximum expected net benefit with current information. The former is simply the expectation of the final column of Table A (£91,008). The latter is approximated by the maximum of the expectations of columns 3 and 4 (= max (£81,324, £88,396)). Thus the EVSI on parameter P_o from a study of size n = 10 is:

£91,008 − max (£81,324, £88,396) = £2612.

This is the EVSI of a study of sample size 10. We now need to repeat the entire process for studies with a range of sample sizes. Table 12.3 shows the results for calculating EVSI for sample sizes of 0–500 patients. As with EVPI and EVPPI, this is the per-patient EVSI, so we need to multiply by the present and (discounted) future population of patients (column 3 of Table 12.3; see Appendix, equation A11). We then need to net off the costs of conducting the study, which we have split into a

A. Iteration summaries

Run		£81,324	£88,396	£91,008
Average	Po ~ Beta(20,80)	NBo	NBn	Max
1	0.24	**£98,453**	**£85,395**	**£98,453**
2	0.18	£72,184	£84,599	**£84,599**
3	0.19	£76,439	£94,157	**£94,157**
4	0.19	£75,368	£85,677	**£85,677**
5	0.21	£84,178	£92,153	**£92,153**

C. EVSI

n	EVSI
10	**£2612**
20	
30	
40	
50	
...	

$$P_{OS} \sim Bin(0.21,10)$$

$$P_{OS} = 2$$

B. Model iterations

MODEL	Po' ~ Beta(22,88)	NBo	NBn
Mean		**£84,178**	**£92,153**
1	0.23	£100,584	£120,634
2	0.23	£67,527	£73,963
3	0.23	£108,340	£99,127
4	0.22	£57,498	£61,501
5	0.23	£86,941	£105,540

Figure 12.4 EVSI example (continued).

Table 12.3 EVSI and ENBS illustration.

n	Per-patient EVSI	Population EVSI (£ms)	Cost of sampling (fixed costs, £ms)	Cost of sampling (variable costs, £ms)	£ sampling (£ms)	ENBS (£ms)
0	0	£0.00	£0.00	£0.00	£0.00	£0.00
10	£2612	£224.83	£0.15	£0.15	£0.30	£224.53
20	£3400	£292.66	£0.15	£0.30	£0.45	£292.21
30	£3654	£314.52	£0.15	£0.45	£0.60	£313.92
40	£3765	£324.08	£0.15	£0.60	£0.75	£323.33
50	£3820	£328.81	£0.15	£0.75	£0.90	£327.91
100	£3880	£333.98	£0.15	£1.50	£1.65	£332.33
150	£3930	£338.28	£0.15	£2.25	£2.40	£335.88
200	£3945	£339.57	£0.15	£3.00	£3.15	£336.42
250	£3947	£339.75	£0.15	£3.75	£3.90	£335.85
500	£3949	£339.92	£0.15	£7.50	£7.65	£332.27

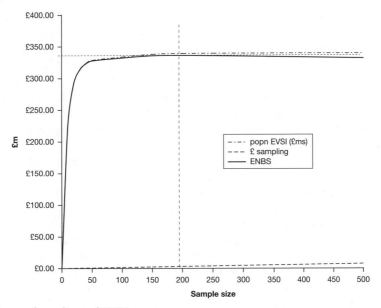

Figure 12.5 EVSI, cost of sampling and ENBS.

fixed and variable component (Table 12.3, columns 4–6; see Appendix, equation A12). The difference is the ENBS (Table 12.3, final column). The sample size at which this is maximised is the optimum sample size for the study. In this example, the optimum sample size is approximately 195 patients (see Figure 12.5).

Discussion

The preceding section showed a worked example of how VoI can be applied to determine the optimum sample size for a study on the single model parameter, P_0, a probability with a beta distribution. Applying the techniques to other parameters with alternative distributions such as relative risk (lognormal) and resource use or costs (usually gamma) is possible with appropriate modifications to the algorithm (see Ades *et al.* for these algorithms[7]).

An appropriate study design to estimate P_0 would be a prospective case series; however, the methods can just as easily be applied to determine appropriate study endpoints and follow-up length for an RCT, and even the optimum allocation of patients between arms and any patient subgroup for investigation.[41] Nevertheless, there are a number of limitations and underlying assumptions to VoI analysis and these are discussed below.

Structural uncertainty and characterisation of parameter uncertainty

The validity of the VoI approach to research prioritisation rests on two critical assumptions. First, that the assumed structure of the decision model is correct, and second, that the uncertainty around each of the parameter inputs is appropriately characterised.

The first point is a question of 'structural uncertainty', a type of uncertainty which conventional sensitivity analyses do not commonly address, other than through a range of scenario analyses from which the decision maker is invited to choose the most plausible.[42] An alternative is to employ a model-averaging approach based either on model fit to the data or by adding parameters to the model to represent the choice between the alternative scenario analyses. Each iteration of the PSA then selects one of the scenarios based on some distribution of the likelihood of each.[42]

The second point relates to the use and combining of evidence (i.e. systematic review and meta-analysis). Economic evaluations, including decision models, should ideally make use of 'all appropriate evidence'.[43] This is to ensure consistency with the principles of evidence-based medicine, defined as 'the conscientious, explicit and judicious use of current best evidence in making decisions about the care of individual patients'.[44] Although in the current context we are concerned with the population level (i.e. policy decision making) rather than an individual patient, the latter statement is equally valid for informing economic evaluations upon which to base policy decisions.

The thorny question is what constitutes appropriate evidence. The *Cochrane Handbook for Systematic Reviews of Interventions* states that the primary difference between a *systematic* as opposed to a *narrative* review is the 'pre-specification of eligibility criteria for including and excluding studies in the review', defined as a statement of the clinical question and specification of the types of study that will be included.[45] The Handbook suggests that a review should seek 'all rigorous studies of a particular comparison of interventions'. For estimating measures of the effects of health care interventions, a focus on RCTs, as the study design least prone to bias, is suggested.

The result is that systematic reviews, such as those produced by the Cochrane Collaboration, focus on establishing the best estimate of one particular parameter or group of related parameters (i.e. beneficial and adverse effects). They provide a valuable input into decision models, but are highly unlikely to provide data for every parameter included in a model (see also, *inter alia*, Chapters 7 and 8).

For example, a systematic review of early versus delayed laparoscopic cholecystectomy for acute cholecystitis reported statistics relating to risk of peri- and postsurgical complications, conversion to open procedure and mortality.[46] A subsequent decision model drew heavily on this review, but in addition required data on the probability of a patient becoming symptomatic, prognosis of pancreatitis, as well as resource use, unit costs and utilities.[47]

To be classed as using all appropriate evidence, these model inputs should also be based on careful reviews of evidence (see also, *inter alia*, Chapters 7 and 8). However, these are often not available for every parameter (especially resource use estimates), so as a last resort, model inputs are sometimes based simply on researcher or expert estimates. It is therefore unclear whether the probability distribution assigned around such point estimates adequately reflects parameter uncertainty.

Incorrect specification of parameter uncertainty will lead to incorrect estimation of the value of further research. The only practical solution is to ensure that care is taken to fully characterise parameter uncertainty, for example, by replacement of author, researcher or expert estimates with a formal elicitation technique.[48] Ultimately, a 'comprehensive decision-modelling' approach is desirable in which systematic review, parameter estimation, sensitivity analysis and economic evaluation are carried out within a single modelling framework.[49]

Defining the relevant patient population

The value of additional research into a decision question is a function of not only the current but also future patient population estimated over an 'appropriate' time horizon. Whilst it may be possible to estimate the future incidence and prevalence of a disease with a reasonable degree of certainty, it is far from clear exactly what an 'appropriate' time horizon is, and the value of information is extremely sensitive to the time horizon selected.[50]

One approach would be to adopt an infinite time horizon. This will yield a finite value of information for any positive discount rate, and so may provide an upper limit of the value of information (although this ceases to be true once uncertainties associated with technological change and future prices are incorporated).[50] However, an infinite time horizon is not intuitively plausible. Current methods guidelines recommend that the selected time horizon should reflect the 'effective lifetime of the technology'. One could treat this as an unknown parameter for which further information could be sought.[7] An alternative time horizon would be one that equates to the 'time over which the decision question remains relevant'. In other words, the expected time to the next major development in the disease area that would render the current decision question obsolete. 'Horizon scanning' of new technologies in early stage development may be a means to estimate this.

A review of applied studies employing VoI techniques found that such studies have tended to select a time horizon of either 10 or 20 years, with no clear justification in either case.[50] The review authors argue that adopting a single cut-off is essentially an approximation of a more complex process of changes to the decision problem through time, where changes in relative prices, information and development of new technologies each affect the VoI attributable to different model parameters to differing degrees.[50] They do not, however, recommend simultaneous modelling of all these aspects for pragmatic reasons. Instead, they recommend consideration of the information needs of decision makers; in essence, the analysis has to be sophisticated enough to incorporate all relevant influences but simple enough to be delivered within a reasonable timeframe and comprehensible to those making the decision. The decision to pursue additional research will be made with or without formal analysis and the purpose of decision analysis is to improve the quality of the decision (i.e. to increase the probability of a decision being the 'correct' one), and not to capture in minute detail every nuance of the decision problem.

Those patients who participate in a primary research study will not normally be able to benefit from the information obtained from that study, although this is not always the case. For example, study participants may benefit from the study where the disease is characterised by well-defined periods of relapse and remittance, and the treatment provides symptomatic relief of relapses. Therefore, when multiplying the per-patient EVSI to the population level, the population should be adjusted for this consideration, if applicable.[3] Furthermore, there is inevitably a delay between any decision to carry out new research and the results being acted upon, which carries an opportunity cost borne by the entire patient population, requiring further adjustment to the population EVSI.[51]

Computational burden

It will be evident from the worked example presented in this chapter that VoI calculations can be 'computationally expensive'. In our commentary on the example, we suggested sampling only once from the distribution of P_{os} for each iteration, but intuitively it would be preferable to sample from this distribution repeatedly. This adds yet another loop to the process and thus increases the number of iterations performed by an order of magnitude. Whilst improvements in the power of computers may partially solve the problem, there is a tendency for programmers to develop more sophisticated models as a result, thus counteracting the increase in modern computer processor speed. Alternative shortcuts have been proposed, including linear approximations of non-linear models, meta-models and search algorithms, which

may provide an appropriate compromise between computational speed and loss of accuracy.[52–56]

Independence of the adoption and research decisions

The iterative approach to evidence gathering and decision making involves an important conceptual distinction between the decision to adopt a new technology and the decision to pursue further research (to inform a future revision of the adoption decision).

Whilst separate, the adoption and research decisions are not truly independent of one another, for two reasons. First, if the adoption decision is delayed whilst new research is undertaken, there is likely to be an opportunity cost to those who could have benefited (assuming the technology in question has a positive INB) and vice versa.[57] Second, there may be considerable costs associated with reversing a decision.[58]

For example, suppose a new technology has a positive mean INB compared with current practice, but with sufficient uncertainty to warrant further research. The recommendation from this would be to adopt the technology for the present and gather new evidence. If the new evidence suggests that the original adoption decision was wrong (i.e. expected INB is now negative), the decision should be reversed at that point. But if the cost of reversing that decision is greater than the benefit from reversal (e.g. retraining of staff, construction of new facilities, etc.), the expected value of the 'adopt and research' recommendation becomes zero (it cannot affect the adoption decision): the optimal recommendation would in fact have been to 'delay and research', even when current evidence suggests a mean positive INB.[58] The cost of reversal should therefore be incorporated in the VoI analysis.[57]

Multiple jurisdictions

Information is a public good: once in the public domain, it is 'non-rival' and 'non-excludable', meaning consumption by one individual or group neither diminishes consumption by another, nor can that individual or group prevent another from consuming it. This leads to free riding, since there is no reason for one jurisdiction (e.g. a state research funder) to pay for research when another can do so. Therefore, whilst the EVSI may suggest that a particular study should be carried out, it may be strategically optimal to wait for another jurisdiction to undertake the research instead, depending on the likelihood that the results will be generalisable or transferable to the local jurisdiction (see also, *inter alia*, Chapters 3 and 5).[59]

Study design

The VoI approach described in this chapter estimates the return from gathering information on a (group of) variable(s). It does not explicitly specify the 'best' study design to elicit that variable. Different study designs are subject to differing degrees of bias: a retrospective case series may be less expensive than a prospective RCT, but has been shown to be more prone to bias, although the direction and magnitude of the bias are uncertain.[60,61] At issue is whether the bias is sufficient to affect the decision, and whether it is worth investing in a less biased (and potentially more expensive) study design.[62]

Value of information has the potential to influence study design through analyses of a study's interim results. For example, an interim analysis of effects data collected in a trial of long-term HRT (oestrogen plus progestin) found a significantly increased risk of breast cancer in the intervention group, at which point the study was terminated.[63] Similarly, VoI analyses have the potential to be used at the interim analysis stage to trigger 'stopping rules' based on consideration of both costs and effects (i.e. cost-effectiveness). This could also be extended to the incorporation of new external information emerging during the conduct of a study. For example, the results of a newly published, separate study may be incorporated and used to determine whether it is efficient to continue the current study.

Conclusion

Value of information analysis is an approach used to assist research priority setting by valuing the return on investment in research in terms of a reduction in the probability of making the 'wrong' decision, and hence increasing the expected value of that decision. If the cost of gathering the new information exceeds this value, the research is not worthwhile; the research

resources would be better spent elsewhere (e.g. direct service provision or other research projects).

Intrinsic to this approach is the iterative approach to evidence gathering and decision making, beginning with systematic review and economic evaluation, followed by adoption and research decisions, and ending with new information being gathered using a new primary research study and reappraised within an updated review and evaluation. VoI analysis can therefore inform the efficient allocation of scarce research resources.

Appendix

Incremental cost-effectiveness ratio (ICER)

$$\frac{C_2 - C_1}{E_2 - E_1} < \lambda \qquad (A1)$$

where C_j and E_j are the expected cost and outcome respectively of option j. The decision rule is to adopt option 2 if the ICER is below some threshold, λ.

Incremental net benefit (INB)

Rearranging the ICER to the incremental net (monetary) benefit (INB):

$$\lambda(E_2 - E_1) - (C_2 - C_1) > 0 \qquad (A2)$$

Maximum expected net benefit (NB)

This generalises to choosing the option j, with the highest (expected) net benefit:

$$Max_j[E(\lambda E_j - C_j)] \qquad (A3)$$

If E_j and C_j are a function of a set of parameters θ (e.g. effectiveness of the technologies, utility weights, unit costs and resource counts), then we can rewrite the decision rule as:

$$Max_j\{E_\theta[NB(j, \theta)]\} \qquad (A4)$$

where:

j = intervention (e.g. 1 = current treatment, 2 = new treatment)

θ = input parameters to model

$NB(j, \theta)$ = net benefit of intervention j with parameter set θ.

Expected value of perfect information (EVPI)

$$EVPI = E_\theta\{\max_j[NB(j,\theta)]\} - \max_j\{E_\theta[NB(j,\theta)]\} \tag{A5}$$

where j, θ and $NB(j, \theta)$ are as above.

Population expected value of perfect information

$$PopnEVPI = EVPI. \sum_{t=0}^{T} \frac{I_t}{(1+r)^t} \tag{A6}$$

where:

I_t = incident population in time t

r = discount rate.

Expected value of perfect parameter information (EVPPI)

$$EVPPI_\varphi = E_\varphi\{\max_j[E_{\Psi|\varphi}NB(j,\varphi,\psi)]\} \\ -\max_j\{E_\theta[NB(j,\theta)]\} \tag{A7}$$

where:

$$\varphi \cup \psi = \theta$$

(φ is a parameter or subset of parameters of interest, ψ is all the others in set θ).

Population expected value of perfect parameter information

$$PopnEVPPI = EVPPI. \sum_{t=0}^{T} \frac{I_t}{(1+r)^t} \tag{A8}$$

Expected value of sample information

$$EVSI_{\theta,n} = E_D\{\max_j[E_{\theta|D}NB(j,\theta)]\} \\ -\max_j\{E_\theta[NB(j,\theta)]\} \tag{A9}$$

where

θ = single uncertain parameter

D = sampled value of θ from trial of size n.

And similarly for groups of parameters:

$$EVSI_{\psi,n} = E_D\{\max_j[E_{\psi,\varphi|D}NB(j,\varphi,\psi)]\} \\ -\max_j\{E_\theta[NB(j,\theta)]\} \tag{A10}$$

Population expected value of sample information

$$PopnEVSI_{\theta,n} = EVSI_{\theta,n}. \sum_{t=1}^{T} \frac{I_t}{(1+r)^t} \tag{A11}$$

where:

Expected net benefit of sampling

$$ENBS_{\theta,n} = EVSI_{\theta,n} - TC_{\theta,n} \tag{A12}$$

where:

$TC_{\theta,n}$ = total cost of a study estimating parameter θ with sample size of n.

How this chapter should be cited

Wilson E, Abrams K. Chapter 12: From evidence-based economics to economics-based medicine: using systematic review to inform the design of future research. In: Shemilt I, Mugford M, Vale L, Marsh K, Donaldson C (editors). *Evidence-based decisions and economics: health care, social welfare, education and criminal justice.* Oxford: Wiley-Blackwell, 2010.

References

1 National Institute for Health and Clinical Excellence (NICE). *Guide to the Methods of Technology Appraisal.* London: National Institute for Health and Clinical Excellence, 2008.

2 Fenwick E, Claxton K, Sculpher M. Representing uncertainty: the role of cost-effectiveness acceptability curves. *Health Economics* 2001; 10(8): 779–787.

3 Claxton K. The irrelevance of inference: a decision-making approach to the stochastic evaluation of health care technologies. *Journal of Health Economics* 1999; 18(3): 341–364.

4 Raiffa H, Schlaifer R. *Applied Statistical Decision Theory.* Boston: Harvard Business School, 1961.

5 Claxton K, Posnett J. An economic approach to clinical trial design and research priority-setting. *Health Economics* 1996; 5(6): 513–524.

6 Willan AR, Pinto EM. The value of information and optimal clinical trial design. *Statistics in Medicine* 2005; 24(12): 1791–1806.

7 Ades AE, Lu G, Claxton K. Expected value of sample information calculations in medical decision modeling. *Medical Decision Making* 2004; 24(2): 207–227.

8 Banta HD, Thacker SB. The case for reassessment of health care technology: once is not enough. *Journal of the American Medical Association* 1990; 264(2): 235–240.

9 Fenwick E, Claxton K, Sculpher M, Briggs A. *Improving the Efficiency and Relevance of Health Technology Assess ment: the role of decision analytic modelling (CHE Discussion Paper No. 179).* York: Centre for Health Economics, 2000.

10 Sculpher M, Drummond M, Buxton M. The iterative use of economic evaluation as part of the process of health technology assessment. *Journal of Health Services Research and Policy* 1997; 2(1): 26–30.

11 Sculpher MJ, Claxton K, Drummond M, McCabe C. Whither trial-based economic evaluation for health care decision making? *Health Economics* 2006; 15(7): 677–687.

12 Griffin S, Claxton K, Sculpher M. Decision analysis for resource allocation in health care. *Journal of Health Services Research and Policy* 2008; 13(S3): 23–30.

13 Briggs AH. Handling uncertainty in cost-effectiveness models. *Pharmacoeconomics* 2000; 17(5): 479–500.

14 Buxton MJ, Drummond MF, van Hout BA, *et al.* Modelling in economic evaluation: an unavoidable fact of life. *Health Economics* 1997; 6(3): 221–227.

15 Fleurence RL, Torgerson DJ. Setting priorities for research. *Health Policy* 2004; 69(1): 1–10.

16 Gross CP, Anderson GF, Powe NR. The relation between funding by the National Institutes of Health and the burden of disease. *New England Journal of Medicine* 1999; 340(24): 1881–1887.

17 Michaud CM, Murray CJ, Bloom BR. Burden of disease – implications for future research. *Journal of the American Medical Association* 2001; 285(5): 535–539.

18 Wetterslev J, Thorlund K, Brok J, Gluud C. Trial sequential analysis may establish when firm evidence is reached in cumulative meta-analysis. *Journal of Clinical Epidemiology* 2008; 61(1): 64–75.

19 Armitage P. Sequential analysis in therapeutic trials. *Annual Review of Medicine* 1969; 20: 425–430.

20 Pocock S. Group sequential methods in the design and analysis of clinical trials. *Biometrika* 1977; 64(2): 191–199.

21 Townsend J, Buxton M. Cost effectiveness scenario analysis for a proposed trial of hormone replacement therapy. *Health Policy* 1997; 39(3): 181–194.

22 Eppel T, von Winterfeldt D. Value-of-information analysis for nuclear waste storage tanks. *Decision Analysis* 2008; 5(3): 157–167.

23 Yokota F, Thompson KM. Value of information analysis in environmental health risk management decisions: past, present, and future. *Risk Analysis* 2004; 24(3): 635–650.

24 Yokota F, Gray G, Hammitt JK, Thompson KM. Tiered chemical testing: a value of information approach. *Risk Analysis* 2004; 24(6): 1625–1639.

25 Forsberg O, Guttormsen A. The value of information in salmon farming. Harvesting fish at the right time. *Aquaculture Economics and Management* 2006; 10(3): 183–200.

26 Oksendal B. The value of information in stochastic control and finance. *Australian Economic Papers* 2005; 44(4): 352–364.

27 Claxton K, Ginnelly L, Sculpher M, Philips Z, Palmer S. A pilot study on the use of decision theory and value of information analysis as part of the NHS Health Technology Assessment programme. *Health Technology Assessment* 2004; 8(31): 1–103.

28 Claxton K, Eggington S, Ginnelly L, *et al. A Pilot Study of Value of Information Analysis to Support Research Recommendations for NICE (CHE Research Paper No. 4)*. York: Centre for Health Economics, 2005.

29 Colbourn TE, Asseburg C, Bojke L, *et al.* Preventive strategies for group B streptococcal and other bacterial infections in early infancy: cost effectiveness and value of information analyses. *British Medical Journal* 2007; 335(7621): 655.

30 Bojke L, Hornby E, Sculpher M. A comparison of the cost effectiveness of pharmacotherapy or surgery (laparoscopic fundoplication) in the treatment of GORD. *Pharmacoeconomics* 2007; 25(10): 829–841.

31 Wailoo AJ, Sutton AJ, Cooper NJ, *et al.* Cost-effectiveness and value of information analyses of neuraminidase inhibitors for the treatment of influenza. *Value in Health* 2008; 11(2): 160–171.

32 Grant A, Wileman S, Ramsay C, *et al.*, on behalf of the REFLUX Trial Group. The effectiveness and cost-effectiveness of minimal access surgery amongst people with gastro-oesophageal reflux disease – a UK collaborative study. The REFLUX Trial. *Health Technology Assessment* 2008; 12(31): 1–181.

33 Castelnuovo E, Thompson-Coon J, Pitt M, *et al.* The cost-effectiveness of testing for hepatitis C in former injecting drug users. *Health Technology Assessment* 2006; 10(32): 1–93.

34 Garside R, Pitt M, Somerville M, Stein K, Price A, Gilbert N. Surveillance of Barrett's oesophagus: exploring the uncertainty through systematic review, expert workshop and economic modelling. *Health Technology Assessment* 2006; 10(8): 1–158.

35 Ginnelly L, Claxton K, Sculpher MJ, Golder S. Using value of information analysis to inform publicly funded research priorities. *Applied Health Economics and Health Policy* 2005; 4(1): 37–46.

36 Henriksson M, Lundgren F, Carlsson P. Informing the efficient use of health care and health care research resources – the case of screening for abdominal aortic aneurysm in Sweden. *Health Economics* 2006; 15(12): 1311–1322.

37 Iglesias CP, Claxton K. Comprehensive decision-analytic model and Bayesian value-of-information analysis: pentoxifylline in the treatment of chronic venous leg ulcers. *Pharmacoeconomics* 2006; 24(5): 465–478.

38 Philips Z, Claxton KP, Palmer S, Bojke L, Sculpher MJ. Priority setting for research in health care: an application of value of information analysis to glycoprotein IIb/IIIa antagonists in non-ST elevation acute coronary syndrome. *International Journal of Technology Assessment in Health care* 2006; 22(3): 379–387.

39 Robinson M, Palmer S, Sculpher M, *et al.* Cost-effectiveness of alternative strategies for the initial medical management of non-ST elevation acute coronary syndrome: systematic review and decision-analytical modelling. *Health Technology Assessment* 2005; 9(27): 1–158.

40 Spiegelhalter DJ, Abrams KR, Myles JP. Bayesian approaches to clinical trials and health care evaluation. In: Senn S, Barnett V (eds) *Statistics in Practice*. Chichester: John Wiley, 2004.

41 Claxton KP, Sculpher MJ. Using value of information analysis to prioritise health research: some lessons from recent UK experience. *Pharmacoeconomics* 2006; 24(11): 1055–1068.

42 Bojke L, Claxton K, Palmer S, Sculpher M. *Defining and Characterising Structural Uncertainty in Decision Analytic Models (CHE Research Paper No. 9)*. York: Centre for Health Economics, 2006.

43 Drummond M, Sculpher M, Torrance G, O'Brien B, Stoddart G. Chapter 9.2.2: Economic evaluation using decision analytic modelling: the need to reflect all appropriate evidence. In: *Methods for the Economic Evaluation of Health care Programmes*, 3rd edn. Oxford: Oxford University Press, 2005.

44 Sackett DL, Rosenberg WM, Gray JA, Haynes RB, Richardson WS. Evidence based medicine: what it is and what it isn't. *British Medical Journal* 1996; 312(7023): 71–72.

45 O'Connor D, Green S, Higgins JPT (eds). Defining the review question and developing criteria for including studies. In: Higgins JPT, Green S (eds) *Cochrane Handbook of Systematic Reviews of Interventions*. Version 5.0.1 (updated September 2008). Oxford: Cochrane Collaboration, 2008.

46 Gurusamy K, Samraj K, Gluud C, Wilson E, Davidson BR. Meta-analysis of randomised controlled trials on the safety and effectiveness of early versus delayed laparoscopic cholecystectomy for acute cholecystitis. *British Journal of Surgery* 2010; 97(2):141–50.

47 Wilson EC, Gurusamy K, Samraj K, Davidson BR. Cost-utility and value of information analysis of early versus delayed laparoscopic cholecystectomy for acute cholecystitis. *British Journal of Surgery* 2010; 97(2):210–9

48 O'Hagan A, Oakley J. *SHELF: the Sheffield Elicitation Framework*. Sheffield: SHELF, 2008. Available from: http://tonyohagan.co.uk/shelf.

49 Cooper NJ, Sutton AJ, Abrams KR, Turner D, Wailoo A. Comprehensive decision analytical modelling in economic evaluation: a Bayesian approach. *Health Economics* 2004; 13(3): 203–226.

50 Philips Z, Claxton K, Palmer S. The half-life of truth: what are appropriate time horizons for research decisions? *Medical Decision Making* 2008; 28(3): 287–299.

51 Eckermann S, Willan AR. Time and expected value of sample information wait for no patient. *Value in Health* 2008; 11(3): 522–526.

52 Brennan A, Kharroubi S, O'Hagan A, Chilcott J. Calculating partial expected value of perfect information via Monte Carlo sampling algorithms. *Medical Decision Making* 2007; 27(4): 448–470.

53 Tappenden P, Chilcott JB, Eggington S, Oakley J, McCabe C. Methods for expected value of information analysis in complex health economic models: developments on the health economics of interferon-beta and glatiramer acetate for multiple sclerosis. *Health Technology Assessment* 2004; 8(27): 1–78.

54 Karnon J. Planning the efficient allocation of research funds: an adapted application of a non-parametric Bayesian value of information analysis. *Health Policy* 2002; 61(3): 329–347.

55 Stevenson MD, Oakley J, Chilcott JB. Gaussian process modeling in conjunction with individual patient simulation modeling: a case study describing the calculation of cost-effectiveness ratios for the treatment of established osteoporosis. *Medical Decision Making* 2004; 24(1): 89–100.

56 Griffin S, Claxton K, Hawkins N, Sculpher M. Probabilistic analysis and computationally expensive models: necessary and required? *Value in Health* 2006; 9(4): 244–252.

57 Eckermann S, Willan AR. The option value of delay in health technology assessment. *Medical Decision Making* 2008; 28(3): 300–305.

58 Eckermann S, Willan AR. Expected value of information and decision making in HTA. *Health Economics* 2007; 16(2): 195–209.

59 Eckermann S, Willan AR. Globally optimal trial design for local decision making. *Health Economics* 2009; 18(2): 203–216.

60 Deeks JJ, Dinnes J, d'Amico R, *et al.*, for the International Stroke Trial Collaborative Group, European Carotid Surgery Trial Collaborative Group. Evaluating non-randomised intervention studies. *Health Technology Assessment* 2003; 7(27): 1–173.

61 MacLehose RR, Reeves BC, Harvey IM, Sheldon TA, Russell IT, Black AM. A systematic review of comparisons of effect sizes derived from randomised and non-randomised studies. *Health Technology Assessment* 2000; 4(34): 1–154.

62 Shavit O, Leshno M, Goldberger A, Shmueli A, Hoffman A. It's time to choose the study design! Net benefit analysis of alternative study designs to acquire information for evaluation of health technologies. *Pharmacoeconomics* 2007; 25(11): 903–911.

63 Rossouw JE, Anderson GL, Prentice RL, *et al.*, for the Writing Group for the Women's Health Initiative Investigators. Risks and benefits of estrogen plus progestin in healthy postmenopausal women: principal results from the Women's Health Initiative randomized controlled trial. *Journal of the American Medical Association* 2002; 288(3): 321–333.

CHAPTER 13

Complex problems or simple solutions? Enhancing evidence-based economics to reflect reality

Chantale Lessard[1], Stephen Birch[2]

[1]Department of Health Administration, University of Montreal, Montreal, Canada
[2]Centre for Health Economics and Policy Analysis, McMaster University, Hamilton, Ontario, Canada

Introduction

As demand for new health care technologies increases in environments of cost containment, choices must be made about which interventions to fund. Similar problems arise in other sectors as decision makers struggle to determine the most productive ways of deploying the resources available to them. The evidence-based approach has drawn on economics with the aim of providing analytical frameworks to inform decision makers about effectiveness and efficiency of resource use. Such frameworks increasingly form the basis for resource allocation decisions. For example, several countries have adopted formal requirements and guidelines for economic evaluation in health care.[1–4]

In 2002, Donaldson and colleagues recognised the need for the application of evidence-based principles in the practice of economic evaluation.[5] However, the importance of adopting evidence-based approaches in health economics is not confined to the economic evaluation of new technologies. Health economics encompasses a much broader range of influences and constraints on the production of health, illness and recovery in populations.[6] Moreover, under an evidence-based approach, the methods and processes

used, as well as the principles and assumptions on which they are based, must themselves be compatible with the concepts of economics.[5]

The evidence-based approach to decision making draws its foundations from clinical epidemiology. The focus of attention is establishing 'evidence' of effectiveness (i.e. providing information on whether a technology works or not).[7] This has led to the development and use of research methods which devalue the complexity of social reality and exclude the consideration of context.[8] As a result, the research undertaken answers questions about whether the intervention 'works' on average in the sample of the population selected for study. The addition of economics into the evidence-based approach has generally been constrained by the traditional confines of clinical epidemiology. Economic evaluations use health outcomes to compare the average incremental costs and incremental effects resulting from use of a new intervention in place of the current standard treatment for a given patient population. In this way, the economic question remains 'acontextual' and evaluations often overlook important aspects of patient-relevant consequences, as well as important modifying factors.[6,9] The 'science' of controlling for 'other factors' undermines the 'social' nature of the problem. For research to be decision informing, it must reflect decision makers' needs for information and knowledge about the problems they face and the contexts in which they are faced.

Evidence-Based Decisions and Economics, 2nd edition. Edited by I. Shemilt, M. Mugford, L. Vale, K. Marsh and C. Donaldson.
© 2010 Blackwell Publishing.

Current methods emerge from a scientific paradigm which is generally not compatible with either the economics discipline or the needs of decision makers. The prevailing paradigm involves breaking down complex problems (e.g. what is the best way for this individual's health problem to be addressed?) into smaller ones (e.g. what works best, on average, in a patient population with this health problem?) in order to analyse, understand and solve the problem by rational deduction. It assumes that associations between technologies and health outcomes demonstrated in 'highly controlled environments' (e.g. randomised controlled trials (RCTs), systematic reviews) are linear and causal in the real world, regardless of place, culture or other contextual circumstances.[10] However, economic frameworks underpin the notion of the production of health, illness and recovery in populations.[11,12] These frameworks identify the large range of health determinants and the complex pathways in which health is produced.

This chapter focuses attention on the importance of incorporating complexity into economic evaluations, which employ evidence synthesis methods. Complexity is increasingly identified as a priority for research in public health, health services research and health policy.[9,13–20] The concept of complexity refers to the difficulty associated with analysing and understanding a problem. So a complex problem may lie beyond the capacity of traditional analytic techniques.[21] However, complexity is not a dichotomous concept; that is, it is not simply a question of describing quantitatively the level of difficulty in a relative sense (where something is more or less complicated than something else). As an example, the Medical Research Council defines complex interventions as 'interventions that contain several interacting components'.[22,23] Complexity science seeks to understand complex adaptive systems, which are systems characterised by a large number of agents interacting in open and dynamic environments, whose actions are interconnected among all agents in the system. The focus is on relations and interactions (i.e. interactive causality) and not on components and structures. Complexity emphasises the importance of context, uncertainty, multiple objectives, multiple perspectives and broader stakeholder involvement.[9,24] This way of thinking focuses attention on explanation and understanding (why and how a technology works

and under what conditions it works best) as opposed to simply whether an intervention works 'on average' (see also Chapter 3).

This chapter first describes complexity in health and health care, and identifies current approaches to dealing with complexity in economic evaluations that utilise evidence synthesis (e.g. decision modelling) methods (see also Chapters 2 and 5). It then introduces the perspective of complexity as an alternative approach to conceptualising both the production of health, illness and recovery, and the system of planning, managing and delivering health care. This leads to a discussion of the implications of adopting a complexity perspective for the field of economic evaluation. Finally, the chapter concludes with the original contributions that the complexity approach could make to this field. Although this chapter focuses on health, we believe that the same principles would apply to social welfare, education and crime and justice.

Reality and complexity in health care decision making

Complexity in health and health care

Complexity in health embodies two elements: the production of health, illness and recovery and the system of planning, managing and delivering of health care (a third element of complexity, the decision-making process, lies beyond the scope of this chapter – see Chapters 3, 4 and 5 for coverage of this issue). The production of health, illness and recovery in populations occurs through multiple dynamic, interacting systems. The human body is inherently complex while individuals are part of wider social systems made up of complex social relationships and institutions.[20] Although the uncertainty associated with the effects and costs of health care interventions is already recognised in economic evaluation methodology, investigations of influences on the expected distribution of effects and costs are limited to a small number of largely biomedical markers (e.g. age and sex). This fails to acknowledge the wider range of social factors and their interactions that influence the distribution of outcomes. Without such careful consideration, the outcomes of health care at the individual level are much less predictable.[20]

The system of planning, managing and delivering health care is embedded in the wider society and shaped by society's principles and values. The health care system involves a large variety of actors and activities interacting in diverse and complex settings that change over time.[16] Social and professional networks have a key impact on health care professionals' behaviours, attitudes and practices.[25] All of these factors influence the way in which problems are defined and analysed and solutions developed and delivered. As a result, there is a system influence on the association between interventions and outcomes that lies beyond statistical variations. For example, social scientific and epidemiological researchers have observed that providers' diagnostic and management strategies are influenced by providers' personal and professional characteristics, patients' physical and psychosocial characteristics, practice settings, and organisational and structural features of health care systems.[26-31] All these factors are influential in determining costs and effects of interventions.[31-33] The implication for economic analysis is that the efficiency of an intervention for identical patients might differ between different providers (see also Chapter 3). So, what provider characteristics, either taken alone or when interacting with patient characteristics, are associated with greater levels of efficiency? Some might argue that these issues may be addressed by using decision-modelling techniques; however, the next section will highlight the main limitations of such approaches.

In addition to information generation, there is the problem of implementation that needs to recognise that health care decision making spans different levels of the health care system: macro (policy), meso (administrative) and micro (clinical). Health care decisions are often interdependent both within and across these levels. The evidence-based approach often assumes a linear, rational decision-making process.[34-36] However decision makers use a variety of processes, depending upon, *inter alia*, the nature of the problem.[14,37] Health care decisions emerge from complex, dynamic and often non-linear processes involving many stakeholders and the dynamic interactions among stakeholders have a significant impact on the outcome of a decision.[14]

Complexity in economic evaluation

Systematic reviews have shown the limited influence of economic evaluations on health care decisions.[38-43] Although there is a trend towards greater use of

economic evaluation, as jurisdictions introduce requirements for economic evaluations and guidelines for the methods and conduct of those evaluations at the macro level, the use of this 'economic evidence base' at the meso and micro levels remains low.[39] For example, in the National Health Service (NHS) in England and Wales, the National Institute for Health and Clinical Excellence (NICE) makes explicit use of economic evaluation for technology appraisal, but local decision makers often follow different decision-making approaches.[43-45]

Several barriers to the use of economic evaluation in decision making have been identified. As with any type of information, decision makers may not have the time and other resources to understand the concepts on which the evaluations are based or the implications of the findings for the decisions they face. But even if the evaluations are understood by the decision makers, the design of the economic evaluation may fail to reflect the nature of the decision makers' problem.[39,43,46-49] Alternatively, the methodology may not reflect the decision makers' context of constrained maximisation.[50-53] In other words, the simple questions being addressed by the economic evaluation are not the complex questions faced by decision makers. Patient groups are not homogeneous and neither are the providers responsible for their care. Moreover, decision makers operate in a budget-constrained environment. They do not have an infinite stream of resources that can be used to implement cost-effective interventions irrespective of their total additional cost. Decision problems therefore cannot be reduced to consideration of the incremental cost-effectiveness ratio (ICER) of different interventions and comparison of the ICER with some arbitrary cost-effectiveness threshold.

Decision modelling is used in many economic evaluations to evaluate complex health care decisions under conditions of uncertainty.[54-57] Proponents of this approach claim that it allows explicit representation of the 'real world' in a more simple and comprehensible structure.[54] Mathematical and statistical models are often developed to synthesise information from different sources to determine the relative cost-effectiveness of alternative interventions.[55,57-59] Decision-modelling techniques are used to:

- extrapolate primary data beyond a trial follow-up period
- link intermediate endpoints to final outcomes

- synthesise and compare interventions when no 'head-to-head' trials exist
- generalise from trial populations to specific target groups
- generalise data gathered in one setting to other settings and countries
- investigate uncertainty in the knowledge base
- identify priorities and designs for future studies
- provide more precise and reliable estimates of cost-effectiveness.[54,55,58,60]

However, current decision-modelling techniques in economic evaluation are inadequate to address the many problems and decisions that decision makers face. They suffer from a number of limitations, including the structural assumptions made and the sources of data inputs.[56,58,59] They depend on effectiveness estimates produced by systematic reviews and RCTs. Hence, although the model structure may initially reflect the decision makers' needs, final models may be refined in accordance with the limitations of the data. In this way, the models risk being driven by the data rather than by the problem facing the decision makers. Many of these analyses are focused on narrowly defined populations, and driven by expertise and opinion.[56] Many health care problems are complex, involving substantial uncertainty and ambiguity, and numerous inter-related systems, stakeholders and possible alternative solutions. Decisions are dynamic in the sense that their contexts change constantly, decisions are not independent, decisions have to be made in real time, and preferences do not remain constant over time. Most economic evaluation methods are presented as a series of neutral and decontextualised procedures, and thus as taking place in a social vacuum.[9] Implicit assumptions about actors' interests and interactions ignore social reality. Understanding the preferences and behaviours of stakeholders requires serious attention to social reality.[61,62] Because the nature of reality is relative and socially constructed, identical findings can lead to different interpretations.

Decision modelling cannot be used as a substitute for explanation and understanding of a problem. The method does not reduce the uncertainty faced by decision makers.[59] It attempts to represent reality through the use of mathematical and statistical relationships.[60] In economic evaluations, including those using decision-modelling methods, the emphasis is on cause and effect (causal relationships). Applying mathematics to solve health care decision problems may grant a pseudo-scientific aura of objectivity and truth to economic evaluation results.[46] But decision modelling may oversimplify complex decisions. Decision-modelling techniques are based on the assumptions of the mechanistic paradigm. The response to the challenge of complex health problems has therefore been to emphasise more sophisticated analytical and technical tools, simply adding up the data of isolated parts without considering interactions between them.[18,21] These 'reduce and resolve' approaches emphasise problem solving, prediction and control. The goal of decision analysis is to find the optimum solution to a problem, assuming that predictions can be made. These research methods provide information on whether an intervention works or not, not on the conditions under which an intervention works best. This fails to reflect the complex pathways for the production of health, illness and recovery in populations, and the social contexts in which problems faced by decision makers occur. Decisions based on the findings of the research generated under this narrow paradigm may be associated with reductions in efficiency of use of health care resources and increasing inequalities in health.[63] This hints at the requirement for a broader scientific paradigm, together with research methods, to consider the complexity in the health field and the contextual 'embeddedness' of decision-making processes.

Changing research paradigms: reversing reductionist thinking to enhance problem solving

The term 'evidence-based decision making' has been defined as 'the systematic application of the best available evidence to the evaluation of options and to decision making in clinical, management and policy settings'.[64] The methods of the evidence-based approach are primarily epidemiological and statistical. The approach grades research findings according to the level of internal validity, with results from systematic reviews and RCTs generally being given precedence over information gathered from studies using other methods, such as observational studies and qualitative research.[65,66] Although Coyle and colleagues propose a hierarchy relating to the quality of data sources in decision models (see Chapter 9), while others are increasingly using Bayesian methods to combine information from heterogeneous sources, these developments remain within the same philosophical framework as the evidence-based approach, which has been criticised for promoting a positivist-empiricist conception of the term 'evidence'.[66] This reflects the underlying research paradigm on which the evidence-based approach is based.

Newtonian paradigm and the positivist perspective

The prevailing paradigm in evidence-based approaches to health economics has problems in both its descriptive and prescriptive powers.[62,67] Under the evidence-based approach, there is a predominant reliance on the Newtonian paradigm, which incorporates doctrines of *reductionism* and *universality*. The machine is the dominant metaphor of how the world works. Machines, although complicated, are characterised by high levels of control in the environment in which they operate and low levels of uncertainty in their performance. The Newtonian paradigm is based on *reducing* phenomena into smaller divisions, and considering parts in isolation in order to analyse and understand each part separately by rational deduction. The understanding of each part is aggregated to achieve an understanding of the whole phenomenon. These *universal* models of science are deterministic and objective, and consider researchers as independent observers. Relationships between causes (e.g. interventions) and effects are linear and causal in the real world, regardless of time, place or other contextual factors. A BMW car will perform the same whether it is in Canada or Mongolia and it will perform better than a Lada car in both settings.

This logical positivism has extended to medical and biomedical sciences with empirical observations (i.e. scientifically verifiable propositions) being the basis for evidentiary claims.[66,68–70] The application of economic evaluation to this field has been based on this form of positivism, founded on empirical observations provided by experiments designed to maximise internal validity.[67,71] Such empirical knowledge is considered more important, reliable and useful to decision making than other kinds of knowledge and information.[65] However, under contemporary theory of knowledge, all scientific knowledge is constructed

and reflects the researchers' ontological and epistemological stances (i.e. their attitudes towards the nature of reality, truth and knowledge), thus undermining the notion of a neutral observation.[70,72] Decisions about research designs, implementation and interpretation are all value influenced. For example, the choice of 5-year survival as an outcome measure may be made to ease the task of outcome measurement for researchers, but it implies that all survival durations less than 5 years are of equal value, and that all survival durations exceeding 5 years are of equal value. But is anyone indifferent to the choice between surviving 5 years and surviving 10 years?

Complexity perspective

The perspective of complexity offers an alternative model for conceptualising the relationships between health care and health outcomes as complex processes composed of and operating within multiple dynamic and interacting systems. Complex adaptive systems are characterised by large numbers of agents interacting and exchanging information in open and dynamic environments, whose actions are interconnected among all agents in the system.[13–16,73] The immune system and primary health care organisations are two examples of complex adaptive systems. The human body is composed of multiple inherently complex systems, including physiological, biochemical, molecular and psychological systems. Individuals are themselves nested in social systems.[20,68] Complexity conceptualises a situation as a function of interacting and interdependent agents. Interactions occurring at a local level can have consequences for the whole system. At one level of analysis, an individual's emotional well-being will affect and be affected by changes at other levels.[74] No single agent knows or controls the whole system so one cannot understand the system by examining individual components.[13–16,73] The behaviour of an individual cannot be described simply by summing up the behavioural outcome of each constituent process (e.g. physiological, biochemical, etc.).

Interactions may be *non-linear*, meaning that small changes within, or external to, the system can lead to large changes to the system. Conversely, major changes can have little effect on overall system behaviour.[13–16,73] For example, among type 2 diabetic patients with drug treatment failure, add-on drug therapy may either have little effect on blood glucose levels or cause a potentially dangerous reaction.[75] There are often positive and negative feedback loops in the interactions.[13–16,73] Complex systems are highly adaptive and resilient, attempting to balance seemingly opposing forces in ways that maintain system stability in response to perturbations.[14,15] Feedback may help to maintain stability in the system or may lead to the amplification of perturbations, moving the system away from its current state.

Decision modelling may accommodate aspects of non-linear relationships. However, it fails to recognise the synergism of interactions (the whole is greater than the sum of its constituent parts) as an *emergent property* of the complex system. For example, in palliative care, the patient's overall feeling of pain may be an emergent phenomenon, arising from the interactions of physical pain, emotional distress, anger, social isolation and other factors.[76] Consequently, the effectiveness of an intervention, for example, will be influenced by these interactions.

Over time, the overall behaviour of the system emerges through *self-organisation* which arises under conditions of disequilibrium.[13–16,73] Complex adaptive systems create or change their structures and behaviours, via the interactions of system elements, in order to meet the changing demands of internal and external environments.[13–16,73] For example, variation in primary care practices is inevitable as each practice is a unique self-organised system that emerges through dynamic relationships and interactions among particular agents (e.g. family practitioners, office staff, patients and their families) with their unique preferences, interests, goals and priorities within the context of a particular community setting, given specific regional and global influences (e.g. culture, regulations, health care systems).[77] In complex adaptive systems, individuals act and respond to the environment according to their own internal rules or mental models.[14,15] For example, in their daily practice, many primary care practitioners rarely directly access, appraise and make use of knowledge from research or other formal sources, relying instead on *mindlines* – 'collectively reinforced, internalised, tacit guidelines'.[78] Although there may be a lack of detailed predictability, complex adaptive systems can form specific types of behavioural patterns around 'attractors' and follow overall predictable paths.[13–16,73] For example, professional traditions, values and behavioural norms are

attractors that determine and regulate medical practice.[79] This suggests that a small number of rules may underpin the system behaviour.[14]

Complex adaptive systems have fuzzy boundaries. System membership can change, and agents can be members of multiple systems at the same time.[15] Complex adaptive systems are open systems characterised by agents interacting and exchanging information with others beyond the system boundaries. For example, individuals interact with other individuals in their social networks within social, cultural, economic and political systems which can influence behaviours and health outcomes.[20] The systems, the agents within them, and their environments change and *co-evolve* through these interactions. Because complex adaptive systems are dependent on initial conditions, the system's history is important in understanding its current and future behaviour.[13–16,73] For example, health care systems are embedded within and bounded by the broader (often country-specific) societal contexts with which they co-evolve. Developments in contemporary health care systems cannot be understood without considering their historical context.

Implications for the field of economic analysis

Economics provides a set of principles for the exploration of efficiency in the use of scarce resources. However, the addition of economics into the evidence-based approach has been constrained by the traditional confines of clinical epidemiology – what has been described as 'dolly economics'.[5] Thus, questions about the efficient use of resources confronting decision makers have remained acontextual.[6] Nevertheless, the application of economics principles would suggest that the effectiveness and efficiency of a technology will depend on the preferences and circumstances of health care patients and providers, as well as on the various contexts in which these actors operate.[7]

Grossman's model of the demand for health[11] and Evans & Stoddart's framework for the determinants of health[12] are two economic approaches that accommodate the complexities and contexts discussed above. Both of these models particularly underpin the complex pathways to health, illness and recovery involving interactions among a large range of health determinants. The relation between intervention and health status is captured in the health production function. Grossman has shown that social, economic and environmental factors constitute inputs to the health production function.[11] Evans & Stoddart have proposed a dynamic framework for considering the factors that influence health in a community. The framework adopts a systems approach in which health outcomes are the products of complex dynamic interactions between health determinants. The framework's feedback loops link the different components of health determinants (e.g. social environments, genetic endowments, etc.). These interactions are potentially as important as the actions of any single factor. What is not yet available is an understanding of how and why the interactions occur. This framework helps to:

- refocus health improvement efforts towards the broad social determinants of health
- emphasise the importance of considering both biological and behavioural responses to physical and social environments
- underscore the interdisciplinarity of health production
- recognise and make explicit the possible trade-offs involved between different determinants of health (e.g. health care versus social support).[12]

This multidimensional perspective reinforces the value of systems thinking and holistic approach to health, illness and recovery.

Under complexity thinking, the emphasis is on relations and networks between different determinants (interactive causality). This recognises that systems, and the individuals within them, do not exist in isolation but interact and co-evolve with other systems. This does not imply that problems are too complex to be tackled but instead argues that problems should be approached differently.

For example, smoking represents a complex health problem, one which could be addressed by the application of complexity thinking. Individual behaviour is influenced by individual characteristics (e.g. age, gender, occupation, socio-economic status). But individuals are embedded in networks of relationships that have a significant impact on their beliefs, behaviours and choices (e.g. smoking in the family or among friends

or colleagues). Environments in which individuals live may also influence behaviour (e.g. smoking behaviour may be facilitated or impeded by the tobacco tax policies and advertising laws). But these levels of influence need not be independent or separate. The relationship between gender and smoking might depend on family context and political environment. We might therefore expect the effectiveness of smoking cessation interventions to be highly dependent on local and wider contexts. So, for example, the poor economic circumstances of unemployed single mothers might be an important part of exploring the effectiveness of particular interventions among women (e.g. smoking cessation programmes or medications), not simply statistical 'noise' to be controlled for in intervention studies.[7]

Similarly, the interaction between health professionals and individuals may also affect smoking behaviour. Providers' choices of smoking cessation interventions are influenced by their personal and professional characteristics and the contexts in which they work (e.g. practice organisation, remuneration policies, etc.) as well as by patients' physical and psychosocial characteristics. Hence, what works best for a particular patient may depend on these supply-side factors, and the efficient treatment for a given patient (or group of patients) may vary across different provider types and settings.

The proposed perspective would suggest consideration of a wide array of 'policy' targets. A better understanding of the 'smoking issue' would require a multidimensional approach focusing on various stakeholders' involvement. This would contribute to developing awareness of the issue of 'transdisciplinarity' in the field of economic evaluation. The transdisciplinary perspective is collaborative and inclusive, being open to incorporation of multiple perspectives, values, approaches and experiences in defining and solving complex problems.[80] It allows creativity and innovative thinking in dealing with the challenges of producing and delivering contextually relevant knowledge. Because of the uncertainty and ambiguity of complex health problems, one 'best' solution simply does not exist. For economic evaluation, this means creatively expanding the range of possible solutions, with a view to understanding why and how a technology works and under what conditions it works best as opposed to simply whether it works 'on average' (see also Chapter 3).

The complexity perspective suggests that, through observation over time, it may be possible to identify what factors are important in bringing about a change in a system. It points to the existence of recurring patterns and suggests that a small number of rules may underpin system behaviour.[14] Explanation and understanding are achieved through a contextual approach (observation or narrative analysis) to study the dynamics of interactions and search for order in patterns over time, focusing on non-linear effects, unintended consequences, emergent and holistic properties, self-organisation and historical development of the system. Various analytical approaches to complexity science are being used or developed in many fields of research.[13,16,81,82] Division of the determinants of behaviour into multiple levels would be of fundamental importance in this new model. For economic evaluation, viewing systems through multilevel models could accommodate the neoclassical economic framework while recognising that all action is socially situated and cannot be explained by individual motives alone.[17]

Lastly, complexity thinking does not reject the Newtonian framework of modern science or its claim to reliable knowledge altogether. Rather, it sees reductionist thinking in the context of a much broader framework. For simple problems where there is a high degree of certainty and agreement among stakeholders, reductionism and rational analysis are appropriate. In such situations, systems are close to equilibrium, displaying fewer emergent properties.[14,15,17] However, few situations in health and health care have high levels of certainty and agreement. Systems change and evolve constantly and remain far from equilibrium.[17] As problems become more complex with insufficient certainty and agreement, complexity thinking is more appropriate. For economic evaluation, this would alert researchers to the importance of considering the system as a whole and selecting the approach best suited to the complexities of the problem.

Conclusion

Current approaches to economic evaluation depart from the intellectual tradition of economics, and hence

they provide simple solutions (e.g. ICERs) to inherently complex problems.[52,53] A complex set of priorities, responsibilities, objectives, values and preferences drives national and local debates about health care resource allocation. In order to be useful for health care decision making, the theory and practice of economic evaluation must expand to include different types of knowledge and methodologies, and must adapt to the practical realities and needs of patients, decision makers, health care systems, and ultimately society.

New paradigms that incorporate a dynamic and emergent view of the world must replace reductionist approaches to health care. Complexity thinking offers an alternative model for conceptualising both the production of health, illness and recovery in populations, and the system of planning, managing and delivering health care, as expressions of parts of complex, dynamics and interacting systems. It suggests that many types of knowledge are valid and useful for evaluation, not just knowledge produced by traditional methodological approaches. For economic evaluation, this involves the acknowledgement of complex, interdependent relationships and broader contextual factors.[24] An approach based on complexity, uncertainty and a plurality of legitimate perspectives, values and interests would more firmly ground economic evaluations in the economics discipline as well as with the experiences of people engaging with health care systems.[67] This would provide a means of informing policy aimed at a more equitable and efficient use of health care resources because allocation decisions would be based on improved knowledge and understanding of health problems.

Complexity thinking would thus expand the scope of economic evaluation and increase its real-world applicability.[9] What is at issue is whether economists and systematic reviewers are ready to rise to the challenge.

How this chapter should be cited

Lessard C, Birch S. Chapter 13: Complex problems or simple solutions? Enhancing evidence-based economics to reflect reality. In: Shemilt I, Mugford M, Vale L, Marsh K, Donaldson C (editors). *Evidence-based decisions and economics: health care, social welfare, education and criminal justice*. Oxford: Wiley-Blackwell, 2010.

References

1 American Managed Care Pharmacy (AMCP). *The AMCP Format for Formulary Submissions. A format for submission of clinical and economic data in support of formulary consideration by health care systems in the United States (Version 2.1).* Alexandria, VA: Foundation for Managed Care Pharmacy, 2005.

2 Canadian Agency for Drugs and Technologies in Health (CADTH). *Guidelines for the Economic Evaluation of Health Technologies: Canada,* 3rd edn. Ottawa: Canadian Agency for Drugs and Technologies in Health, 2006.

3 Commonwealth Department of Health and Aging (CDHA). *Guidelines for the Pharmaceutical Industry on Preparation of Submissions to the Pharmaceutical Benefits Advisory Committee, Including Major Submissions Involving Economic Analyses.* Canberra: Commonwealth of Australia, 2002.

4 National Institute for Health and Clinical Excellence (NICE). *Guide to the Methods of Technology Appraisal.* London: National Institute for Health and Clinical Excellence, 2008.

5 Donaldson C, Mugford M, Vale L (eds). *Evidence-Based Health Economics: from effectiveness to efficiency in systematic review.* London, BMJ Books, 2002.

6 Birch S, Gafni A. Evidence-based health economics. Answers in search of questions? In: Kristiansen IS, Mooney G (eds) *Evidence-Based Medicine in Its Place.* Adington: Routledge, 2004.

7 Birch S. As a matter of fact: evidence-based decision-making unplugged. *Health Economics* 1997; 6(6): 547–559.

8 Carr-Hill R. Welcome? To the brave new world of evidence based medicine. *Social Science and Medicine* 1995; 41(11): 1467–1468.

9 Lessard C. Complexity and reflexivity: two important issues for economic evaluation in health care. *Social Science and Medicine* 2007; 64(8): 1754–1765.

10 Biswas R, Umakanth S, Strumberg J, Martin CM, Hande M, Nagra JS. The process of evidence-based medicine and the search for meaning. *Journal of Evaluation in Clinical Practice* 2007; 13(4): 529–532.

11 Grossman M. On the concept of health capital and the demand for health. *Journal of Political Economy* 1972; 80(2): 223–255.

12 Evans RG, Stoddart GL. Producing health, consuming health care. *Social Science and Medicine* 1990; 31(12): 1347–1363.

13 Holt TA (ed). *Complexity for Clinicians.* Abingdon: Radcliffe Medical Press, 2004.

14 Kernick D (ed). *Complexity and Health care Organisation: a view from the street.* Abingdon: Radcliffe Medical Press, 2004.

15 Plsek PE, Greenhalgh T. Complexity science: the challenge of complexity in health care. *British Medical Journal* 2001; 323(7313): 625–628.

16 Sweeney K, Griffiths F (eds). *Complexity and Health care: an introduction.* Abingdon: Radcliffe Medical Press, 2002.

17 Kernick D. Health economics and insights from complexity theory. In: Kernick D (ed) *Getting Health Economics into Practice.* Adington: Routledge, 2002.

18 Sanderson I. Complexity, 'practical rationality' and evidence-based policy making. *Policy and Politics* 2006; 34(1): 115–132.

19 Shiell A, Hawe P, Gold L. Complex interventions or complex systems? Implications for health economic evaluations. *British Medical Journal* 2008; 336(7656): 1281–1283.

20 Wilson T, Holt T, Greenhalgh T. Complexity science: complexity and clinical care. *British Medical Journal* 2001; 323(7314): 685–688.

21 Standish RK. Concept and definition of complexity. In: Yang A, Shan Y (eds) *Intelligent Complex Adaptive Systems.* Hershey, PA: IGI Publishing, 2008.

22 Medical Research Council (MRC). *Developing and Evaluating Complex Interventions: a new guidance.* London: Medical Research Council, 2008.

23 Craig P, Dieppe P, Macintyre S, Mitchie S, Nazareth I, Petticrew M. Developing and evaluating complex interventions: the new Medical Research Council guidance. *British Medical Journal* 2008; 337: 979–983.

24 Healy SA. Changing science and ensuring our future. *Futures* 1997; 29(6): 505–517.

25 Ferlie E, Fitzgerald L, Wood M. Getting evidence into clinical practice: an organisational behaviour perspective. *Journal of Health Services Research and Policy* 2000; 5(2): 96–102.

26 Arber S, McKinlay J, Adams A, Marceau L, Link C, O'Donnell A. Patient characteristics and inequalities in doctors' diagnostic and management strategies relating to CHD; a video-simulation experiment. *Social Science and Medicine* 2006; 62(1): 103–115.

27 Landon BE, Reschovsky J, Reed M, Blumental D. Personal, organizational, and market level influences on physicians' practice patterns: results of a national survey of primary care physicians. *Medical Care* 2001; 39(8): 889–905.

28 Lutfey KE, Campbell SM, Renfrew MR, Marceau LD, Roland M, McKinlay JB. How are patient characteristics relevant for physicians' clinical decision making in diabetes? An analysis of qualitative results from a cross-national factorial experiment. *Social Science and Medicine* 2008; 67(9): 1391–1399.

29 McKinlay J, Link C, Arber S, Marceau L, O'Donnell A, Adams A. How do doctors in different countries manage the same patient? Results of a factorial experiment. *Health Services Research* 2006; 41(6): 2182–2200.

30 Von dem Knesebeck O, Bönte M, Siegrist J, *et al.* Country differences in the diagnosis and management of coronary heart disease – a comparison between the US, the UK and Germany. *BMC Health Services Research* 2008; 8: 198.

31 Harris MI. Health care and health status and outcomes for patients with type 2 diabetes. *Diabetes Care* 2000; 23(6): 754–758.

32 Watkins C, Harvey I, Carthy P, Moore L, Robinson E, Brawn R. Attitudes and behaviour of general practitioners and their prescribing costs: a national cross sectional survey. *Quality and Safety in Health care* 2003; 12(1): 29–34.

33 Rubin RR, Peyrot M, Siminerio LM. Health care and patient-reported outcomes: results of the cross-national Diabetes Attitudes, Wishes and Needs (DAWN) study. *Diabetes Care* 2006; 29(6): 1249–1255.

34 Coyle D. *Increasing the Impact of Economic Evaluations on Health Care Decision-Making. Discussion Paper 108.* York: Centre for Health Economics, 1993.

35 Haines A, Donald A (eds). *Getting Research Findings into Practice*, 2nd edn. London: BMJ Publishing Group, 2004.

36 Straus SE, Richardson WS, Glasziou P, Haynes RB. *Evidence-Based Medicine: how to practice and teach EBM*, 3rd edn. Edinburgh: Churchill Livingstone, 2005.

37 Greenhalgh T. Intuition and evidence – uneasy bedfellows? *British Journal of General Practice* 2002; 52(478): 395–400.

38 Drummond M, Brown R, Fendrick AM, *et al.*, for the ISPOR Task Force. Use of pharmacoeconomics information – report of the ISPOR Task Force on use of pharmacoeconomic/health economic information in health care decision making. *Value in Health* 2003; 6(4): 407–416.

39 Eddama O, Coast J. A systematic review of the use of economic evaluation in local decision-making. *Health Policy* 2008; 86(2–3): 129–141.

40 Späth HM, Allenet B, Carrère MO. L'utilisation de l'information économique dans le secteur de la santé: le choix des médicaments à inclure dans les livrets thérapeutiques hospitaliers. *Journal d'Economie Médicale* 2000; 18(3–4): 147–161.

41 Van Velden ME, Severens JL, Novak A. Economic evaluations of health care programmes and decision making: the influence of economic evaluations on different health care decision-making levels. *Pharmacoeconomics* 2005; 23(11): 1075–1082.

42 Walkom E, Robertson J, Newby D, Pillay T. The role of pharmacoeconomics in formulary decision-making. *Formulary* 2006; 41(8): 374–386.

43 Williams I, McIver S, Moore D, Bryan S. The use of economic evaluations in NHS decision-making: a review and empirical investigation. *Health Technology Assessment* 2008; 12(7).

44 Buxton MJ. Economic evaluation and decision making in the UK. *Pharmacoeconomics* 2006; 24(11): 1133–1142.

45 Eddama O, Coast J. Use of economic evaluation in local health care decision-making in England: a qualitative investigation. *Health Policy* 2009; 89(3): 261–270.

46 Coast J. Is economic evaluation in touch with society's health values? *British Medical Journal* 2004; 329(7476): 1233–1236.

47 Menzel P, Gold MR, Nord E, Pinto-Prades JL, Richardson J, Ubel P. Toward a broader view of values in cost-effectiveness analysis of health. *Hastings Center Report* 1999; 29(3): 7–15.

48 Nord E, Pinto JL, Richardson J, Menzel P, Ubel P. Incorporating societal concerns for fairness in numerical valuations of health programmes. *Health Economics* 1999; 8(1): 25–39.

49 Stolk EA, van Donselaar G, Brouwer WBF, Busschbach JJV. Reconciliation of economic concerns and health policy. Illustration of an equity adjustment procedure using proportional shortfall. *Pharmacoeconomics* 2004; 22(17): 1097–1107.

50 Birch S, Gafni A. Information created to evade reality (ICER): things we should not look to for answers. *Pharmacoeconomics* 2006; 24(11): 1121–1131.

51 Birch S, Gafni A. The biggest bang for the buck or bigger bucks for the bang: the fallacy of the cost-effectiveness

threshold. *Journal of Health Services Research and Policy* 2006; 11(1): 46–51.

52 Gafni A, Birch S. Inclusion of drugs in provincial drug benefit programs: should 'reasonable decision' lead to uncontrolled growth in expenditures? *Canadian Medical Association Journal* 2003; 168(7): 849–851.

53 Gafni A, Birch S. Incremental cost-effectiveness ratios (ICERs): the silence of the lambda. *Social Science and Medicine* 2006; 62(9): 2091–2100.

54 Buxton MJ, Drummond MF, van Hout BA, *et al.* Modelling in economic evaluation: an unavoidable fact of life. *Health Economics* 1997; 6(3): 221–227.

55 Soto J. Health economic evaluations using decision analytic modeling. Principles and practices – utilization of a checklist to their development and appraisal. *International Journal of Technology Assessment in Health care* 2002; 18(1): 94–111.

56 Lee RC, Donaldson C, Cook LS. The need for evolution in health care decision modeling. *Medical Care* 2003; 41(9): 1024–1033.

57 Philips Z, Ginnelly L, Sculpher M, *et al.* Review of guidelines for good practice in decision-analytic modelling in health technology assessment. *Health Technology Assessment* 2004; 8(36).

58 Cooper NJ, Coyle D, Abrams K, Mugford M, Sutton A. Use of evidence in decision models: an appraisal of health technology assessments in the UK since 1997. *Journal of Health Services Research and Policy* 2005; 10(4): 245–250.

59 Sheldon TA. Problems of using modelling in the economic evaluation of health care. *Health Economics* 1996; 5(1): 1–11.

60 Brennan A, Akehurst, R. Modelling in health economic evaluation. What is its place? What is its value? *Pharmacoeconomics* 2006; 24(11): 1043–1053.

61 Bourdieu P. *The Social Structures of the Economy.* Oxford: Polity Press, 2005.

62 Small N, Mannion R. A hermeneutic science: health economics and Habermas. *Journal of Health Organisation and Management* 2005; 19(3): 219–235.

63 Hall J, Birch S, Haas M. Creating health gains or widening gaps: the role of health outcomes. *Health Promotion Journal of Australia* 1996; 6(1): 4–6.

64 National Forum on Health. *Canada Health Action: building on the legacy. Final Report Volume II: Creating a culture of evidence-based decision making.* Ottawa: Health Canada, 1997. Available from: www.hc-sc.gc.ca/hcs-sss/pubs/renewal-renouv/1997-nfoh-fnss-v2/ legacy_heritage5-eng.php.

65 Cohen AM, Stavri PZ, Hersh WR. A categorization and analysis of the criticisms of evidence-based medicine. *International Journal of Medical Informatics* 2004; 73(1): 35–43.

66 Goldenberg MJ. On evidence and evidence-based medicine: lessons from the philosophy of science. *Social Science and Medicine* 2006; 62(11): 2621–2632.

67 Mannion R, Small N. Postmodern health economics. *Health care Analysis* 1999; 7(3): 255–272.

68 Herman J. Beyond positivism: a metaphysical basis for clinical practice? *Medical Hypotheses* 1992; 39(1): 63–66.

69 Kneebone R. Total internal reflection: an essay on paradigms. *Medical Education* 2002; 36(6): 514–518.

70 Malterud K. Reflexivity and metapositions: strategies for appraisal of clinical evidence. *Journal of Evaluation in Clinical Practice* 2002; 8(2): 121–126.

71 Richardson J, McKie J. Empiricism, ethics and orthodox economic theory: what is the appropriate basis for decision-making in the health sector? *Social Science and Medicine* 2005; 60(2): 265–275.

72 Latour B, Woolgar S. *Laboratory Life: the construction of scientific facts.* Princeton: Princeton University Press, 1986.

73 Cilliers P. *Complexity and Postmodernism: understanding complex systems.* London: Routledge, 1998.

74 Frijda NH. The laws of emotions. *American Psychologist* 1988; 43(5): 349–358.

75 Vinik A. Advancing therapy in type 2 diabetes mellitus with early, comprehensive progression from oral agents to insulin therapy. *Clinical Therapeutics* 2007; 29(6, part 1): 1236–1257.

76 Munday DF, Johnson SA, Griffiths FE. Complexity theory and palliative care. *Palliative Medicine* 2003; 17(4): 308–309.

77 Miller WL, McDaniel RR Jr, Crabtree BF, Stange KC. Practice jazz: understanding variation in family practices using complexity science. *Journal of Family Practice* 2001; 50(10): 872–878.

78 Gabbay J, Le May A. Evidence based guidelines or collectively constructed 'mindlines?'. Ethnographic study of knowledge management in primary care. *British Medical Journal* 2004; 329(7473): 1013–1017.

79 Freidson E. *Profession of Medicine: a study of sociology of applied knowledge.* Chicago: University of Chicago Press, 1988.

80 Albrecht G, Freeman S, Higginbotham N. Complexity and human health: the case for a transdisciplinary paradigm. *Culture, Medicine and Psychiatry* 1998; 22(1): 55–92.

81 Moss S. Policy analysis from first principles. *Proceedings of the National Academy of Sciences of the United States of America* 2002; 99(suppl 3): 7267–7274.

82 Seely AJ, Macklem PT. Complex systems and the technology of variability analysis. *Critical Care* 2004; 8(6): R367–R384.

CHAPTER 14

Evidence-based decisions and economics: lessons for practice

Luke Vale

Health Economics Research Unit, University of Aberdeen, Aberdeen, UK

Introduction

This chapter aims to summarise key implications for the application of approaches to combine economics and systematic review methods. These form lessons for future research practice for the evidence synthesis community, based on what we already know in this area.

The first edition of this book focused almost exclusively on health and health care.[1] Indeed, the focus was primarily on the evaluation of health care treatments. Within this volume, the focus has widened to consider social welfare, education and criminal justice as well as health. It has also drawn lessons from other policy domains. For example, Stanley[2] uses a case study of an issue in labour economics, while Lessard & Birch[3] present arguments about why consideration of complexity is relevant to any economic analysis. These two examples illustrate the first lessons for practice from this book.

Economics is a rich and active research area and problems in one policy area may have been faced within another area. The first lesson is not to forget to reflect back to the parent discipline of economics. It may provide a practical solution or provide fresh insight and help us to continually reassess whether the approaches we adopt can truly inform decisions about how best to allocate resources. This is not easy to achieve in practice, but regular interaction and consultation with colleagues, facilitated by use of email discussion lists and the burgeoning array of other communication technologies, may help. The second lesson for practice is to be open to looking beyond economics to other disciplines for ways that can be used to improve the relevance and applicability of approaches to combine economics and systematic review methods.

In part, it was the desire to learn these lessons that prompted the production of this book. There is much that we can learn from each other and also that we can learn together. Some specific lessons are highlighted in this volume but there are many more to be learned and the challenge for a researcher is to be open to them.

The remainder of this chapter presents a reading of the main lessons for practice to be drawn from all the preceding chapters in this volume. These are grouped around the following themes.

- Using existing evidence on efficiency to derive new evidence on efficiency
- Using decision models to derive evidence on relative efficiency
- Making efficient decisions about the need for further research
- Assessing the distribution of costs and benefits

These are not the only lessons for practice; there are several other gems sprinkled throughout the book and the reader is invited to draw further lessons from each individual chapter.

Evidence-Based Decisions and Economics, 2nd edition. Edited by I. Shemilt, M. Mugford, L. Vale, K. Marsh and C. Donaldson. © 2010 Blackwell Publishing.

Using existing evidence on efficiency to derive new evidence on efficiency

In the first edition of this book, various options for obtaining evidence about the relative efficiency of interventions were suggested. Briefly, these options ranged over various permutations of systematic review of the existing economic evidence to the development of a new evaluation typically based on a decision model. Within this edition, the authors of various chapters have argued that the review of existing economic analyses may have limited scope and limited value if a principal objective is to estimate relative efficiency based solely on evidence collected from included studies. However, as outlined below, this does nothing to mitigate the important role such reviews can play in informing new evaluations and decision making. It simply highlights that reviews of existing economic analyses conducted to provide evidence on relative efficiency are likely to represent a mis-specification of research design in most cases.

Various reasons for the limited scope for systematic reviews of economic analyses have been advanced, including the following.

- *The lack of existing analyses.* Byford and colleagues observe that this may be particularly acute in social welfare, education and criminal justice, but also that even in health there typically exist less than a handful of economic analyses comparing specific interventions.[4]
- *Fundamental methodological limitations of the existing economic analyses.* Individual analyses vary widely in terms of methodological quality and although they may have been fit for their original purpose, they might be of limited use to inform researchers adopting a different perspective or in other jurisdictions.
- *Transferability, complexity and relevance.* This issue is highlighted in several chapters. Walker and colleagues[5] and Anderson & Shemilt[6] consider which factors might vary between settings and outline the need to understand which parameters vary between settings. Lessard & Birch identify a more conceptual approach to understanding the complexity inherent in any policy decision.[3]

The latter considerations remind us that while a review not considering issues related to the transferability, complexity and relevance of identified studies may be limited, by the same token a review that is explicitly designed to think about these factors may be extremely valuable. They also point to the need for careful consideration and clear specification of the objectives for a review of existing economic analyses and the alignment of objectives with methodological choices at each stage of the review process. Anderson & Shemilt address both of these issues.[6] They suggest a set of main roles or objectives for such reviews, as follows: justifying and informing model development; identifying the most relevant study (for the decision problem); or understanding the key economic trade-offs and causal relationships in a decision problem or treatment area. They also align the first and (especially) the third objectives to their proposal for a more explanatory approach that involves application of 'realist synthesis' methods to explore how and why observed levels and configurations of resources appear to be related to observed levels and types of outcomes, and what contextual factors affect these relationships.[6]

Thus, there is relatively little support in this book for the use of reviews of existing evidence to draw firm policy conclusions about relative efficiency, costs or other objectives (e.g. equity) that economic methods can usefully inform. Anderson & Shemilt suggest that this might conceivably be possible if relatively consistent cost or cost-effectiveness results were observed across studies, but that this will not be the norm; as such, the most that can be expected is that review findings indicate interventions that are promising in terms of their relative efficiency. There are few examples even in health where quantitative synthesis of relative efficiency has been performed, and although there have been rather more examples synthesising elements of cost or benefits, such analyses often do not explore the importance of contextual factors.

Stanley, however, reminds us that quantitative synthesis might be possible; specifically, that meta-regression (or moderator analysis, as it is known in some areas of research) can be used.[2] Conceptually, key aspects of a decision problem that are hypothesised to be of importance, such as contextual factors, may be included as explanatory variables within this type of economic analysis. A further lesson for practice is to at least consider whether such analysis is possible. A related lesson is that extreme caution is required before using simple methods of meta-analysis, such as use of a routine fixed or random effects model. Practical arguments have been advanced against this in several chapters, which all relate to the issue of complexity.

Using decision models to derive evidence on relative efficiency

Given the limitations of existing evidence, Marsh argues that decision models will typically be required to evaluate the relative efficiency of interventions.[7] Researchers therefore need, or should have access to, the skills necessary to design, populate and analyse a decision model. Access to relevant research skills is all the more important as models are simplifications of a complex issue. The design of the model therefore needs to reflect the key issues that make a decision problem complex. As noted above, there is a need to understand the causal relationships that exist and the context in which a decision is being made.[3,5,6] This information might come from the review of existing economic evidence or through discussion with key experts in the relevant area.

Given that a modelling approach is likely to be necessary, several chapters have considered how to assemble data for use in decision models. Glanville & Paisley stress the need to use different search strategies for each of the different types of parameter needed to populate a model.[8] The focus of Glanville & Paisley's chapter is on health and several implications for practice are identified.

• Search for economic evaluations in available collections of economic evaluations before progressing to searches of larger general databases.
• Search filters are available for identifying economic evaluations in a range of databases in health care, but should be used with caution outside health care.
• Documenting the search process makes an important contribution to the transparency of reviews and models.
• Searching to inform the development and population of decision models is organic, varied and likely to be pragmatic and non-exhaustive.
• Searching to inform decision models requires access to a wider range of resources and types of evidence than for searches to identify economic analyses.

The first two bullet points are specific lessons for researchers working in the area of health, but the others provide general principles to guide searching within a range of policy areas.

Coyle and colleagues reinforce some of these points. For example, they recommend that it is: 'imperative that the reporting of the methods of determining the data sources adopted within any model should be explicitly stated'.[9] Similarly, related to the fourth bullet point, they provide an example showing the types of data to which the results of an economic analysis were most sensitive. Whilst, as the authors acknowledge, the results of their example are not necessarily transferable to other interventions or policy areas, the key lesson for practice is that, as part of developing the model, the researcher should seek to identify, in discussion with experts and using sensitivity analysis, the most important model parameters and devote more effort to obtaining reliable and precise estimates for those parameters than others.

Coyle and colleagues also consider possible hierarchies for the different types of evidence used in decision models (e.g. relative effect sizes, baseline risks of clinical events, resource use, costs and outcome valuations – which in their case are health state utility values).[9] The hierarchies were advanced for health to prompt debate and would need to be developed to make them applicable to other policy domains. Nevertheless, the underlying rationale behind these hierarchies is that, for any given decision-making context, data derived from certain sources for each of the different types of information would be most applicable. The lesson for practice, relevant to all the policy domains, is to consider at the outset (and provide justification for) what hierarchies of evidence are relevant for each type of information for the specific policy question being addressed.

Brazier and colleagues focus on how to identify one type of information required for a decision model – the valuations of outcomes.[10] Their chapter focuses solely on health state valuations, used to derive quality-adjusted life-years (QALYs). As such, its specific lessons are most relevant to the health field. In other policy domains (and arguably in health as well), relevant beneficial (and adverse) outcomes of alternative policy interventions are often much wider than the effects on health. Brazier and colleagues argue that analysts should use 'the most appropriate values for the mean [*outcome valuation*] and the uncertainty surrounding them based on all relevant evidence, rather than just the best known study'. They emphasise the importance of context, which means outcome values need to be relevant to the population considered within the model and the decision-making process.[10]

In the absence of data with which to value the outcomes of an intervention (a common problem in analyses across all policy domains), the development of balance sheets to present the pros and cons of alternative courses of action may be helpful. Brunetti and colleagues present the use of one particular sort of balance sheet, advocated by the GRADE Working Group.[11] They argue that the summaries of outcomes and resource use included in a balance sheet can be used to weigh up whether the benefits, harms and costs of an intervention are worthwhile compared with an alternative course of action.

The primary focus of Brunetti and colleagues' chapter is on how to present information to decision makers to inform judgements about the best use of resources.. Features of this approach are that only important outcomes should be included in the balance sheet, to avoid information overload, and that outcomes should be quality assessed. Quality criteria may need to be developed to reflect specific features of other policy domains. For example, within the GRADE system data derived from randomised controlled trials (RCTs) start as being considered high quality, although this can be downgraded if there is a risk of bias, the results between trials are inconsistent, there are concerns about generalisability of the trials to the specific policy context, results are imprecise and finally, if there is publication bias. Observational studies start as low quality but can be upgraded if they are felt to be more applicable to the decision-making context.

As noted in some chapters, there is no consensus across policy domains that RCTs are at the top of an evidence hierarchy, primarily because of the difficulties of conducting a trial to evaluate alternatives in some circumstances. Because of the difficulty (and perhaps impossibility) of overcoming these problems, trial results might be treated with scepticism. In the absence of clear guidance for researchers in policy domains other than health, the practical lesson is that if quality is to be judged, the methods used should be transparent and justification given.

This will allow more constructive critique of the approach adopted which in turn may lead to an improvement in methodology.

A further issue with respect to preparing balance sheets is how a researcher can know what outcomes are most important to present within a balance sheet. Some practical guidance on this issue is provided by Anderson & Shemilt,[6] who suggest that analysts should identify key economic trade-offs (i.e. in what factors would plausible changes most likely change a conclusion?), and also by Coyle and colleagues,[9] who suggest that analysts should identify the most important model parameters (in terms of driving conclusions and those most sensitive to plausible changes). In addition to these approaches, it can be useful to elicit from policy makers, practitioners and/or consumers, at the outset of a project, which outcomes are considered likely to be important for decision making.

Making efficient decisions about the need for further research

Evidence-based approaches that incorporate economic analysis can be used to inform judgements about which interventions should be used in practice. Rarely, however, is a researcher or a decision maker certain that the judgement made is the correct one. An essential component of research is to explore what further research is required. Even during a research project, there is an ongoing process to develop and refine the methods of analysis and the data used. Wilson & Abrams recommend that there should be an iterative process between evidence synthesis and primary research, allowing for continual revision of an economic analysis and an attendant policy decision.[12]

Wilson & Abrams outline an approach that can be used to aid this iterative process by eliciting the value of future research. Their example relies on placing a value on society's willingness to pay for a QALY. QALYs may not be suitable for all health interventions and will have limited relevance in other policy domains. However, other outcomes such as a single natural measure (e.g. proportion of reoffenders or willingness-to-pay estimates) could in practice be used in place of a QALY. There are a number of software packages that might be used for decision modelling and some of these have built-in features that allow the calculation of the value of information (VoI). However, extensions of this process are analytically demanding and in practice, a researcher may need to seek training or expert advice.

One important point to remember about VoI analysis is that it does not actually place a value on removing the uncertainty surrounding a given policy decision. Rather, it identifies the value of removing uncertainty in a decision model which, as noted above, is a simplification of reality, used to inform a policy decision. This returns us to the issue of complexity. As noted above, the decision model is used to estimate relative efficiency and therefore value of information must be structured in such a way as to account for the complexity of the decision problem, the context of the system and the circumstances in which a policy decision is being made.[3]

Assessing the distribution of costs and benefits

The efficient use of resources is only one potential policy objective amongst several. Another objective is equity or, more specifically, the reduction of inequalities in the access, use or benefits from services. McDaid & Sassi argue that this is an under-researched area, particularly in the context of evidence synthesis.[13] As McDaid & Sassi show, reducing inequalities may involve a trade-off between equity and efficiency. However, it is also argued that provision of evidence on this trade-off requires an adaption and development of methods. McDaid & Sassi identify three areas in which there are lessons on how equity considerations can be included in evidence synthesis.

- *Identify what information is important.* First, are equity issues likely to be important? This can be informed by discussions with subject experts and decision makers. If equity is important then contextual factors need to be investigated, including the effects of demographic and socio-economic differences.
- *Identify the evidence.* McDaid argues that a broad search may be required to identify relevant information to inform considerations of equity and that these data may come from qualitative, quantitative, geographical and epidemiological studies. Box 6.2 in McDaid & Sassi's chapter illustrates equity considerations that might be used to assess the effect of distributional issues.

- *Use the evidence to refine analysis.* Analyses can be refined to reflect the impacts on different subgroups of interest. However, consideration should be given to whether the data relevant to a specific subgroup for each of the categories of data highlighted by Coyle and colleagues differ from those that might be used to reflect an average effect within a population.

Conclusion

Within this book, methodological approaches and lessons learned from work conducted in health care, social welfare, education and criminal justice have been presented. Not all the lessons for practice that can be drawn from individual chapters are applicable to all these policy arenas. However, there are many lessons about how to conduct research in practice that *are* common across policy domains. These lessons cover the scope and role of synthesis of existing economic evidence, the value of decision models and how data to populate models might be obtained. They also cover how economic evidence might be used to provide information about equity and how evidence might be presented to decision makers so that evidence-based decisions can be made about future policy, practice and research.

How this chapter should be cited

Vale L. Chapter 14: Evidence-based decisions and economics: lessons for practice. In: Shemilt I, Mugford M, Vale L, Marsh K, Donaldson C (editors). *Evidence-based decisions and economics: health care, social welfare, education and criminal justice.* Oxford: Wiley-Blackwell, 2010.

References

1 Donaldson C, Mugford M, Vale L (eds). *Evidence-Based Health Economics: from effectiveness to efficiency in systematic review.* London: BMJ Books, 2002

2 Stanley TD. Meta-regression models of economics and medical research. In: Shemilt I, Mugford M, Vale L, Marsh K, Donaldson C (eds) *Evidence-Based Decisions and Economics: health care, social welfare, education and criminal justice.* Oxford: Wiley-Blackwell, 2010.

3 Lessard C, Birch S. Complex problems or simple solutions? Enhancing evidence-based economics to reflect reality. In: Shemilt I, Mugford M, Vale L, Marsh K, Donaldson C (eds) *Evidence-Based Decisions and Economics: health*

care, social welfare, education and criminal justice. Oxford: Wiley-Blackwell, 2010.

4 Byford S, Barrett B, Dubourg R, Francis J, Sisk J. The role of economic evidence in formulation of public policy and practice. In: Shemilt I, Mugford M, Vale L, Marsh K, Donaldson C (eds) *Evidence-Based Decisions and Economics: health care, social welfare, education and criminal justice.* Oxford: Wiley-Blackwell, 2010.

5 Walker DG, Teerawattananon Y, Anderson R, Richardson G. Generalisability, transferability, complexity and relevance. In: Shemilt I, Mugford M, Vale L, Marsh K, Donaldson C (eds) *Evidence-Based Decisions and Economics: health care, social welfare, education and criminal justice.* Oxford: Wiley-Blackwell, 2010.

6 Anderson R, Shemilt I. The role of economic perspectives and evidence in systematic review. In: Shemilt I, Mugford M, Vale L, Marsh K, Donaldson C (eds) *Evidence-Based Decisions and Economics: health care, social welfare, education and criminal justice.* Oxford: Wiley-Blackwell, 2010.

7 Marsh K. The role of review and synthesis methods in decision models. In: Shemilt I, Mugford M, Vale L, Marsh K, Donaldson C (eds) *Evidence-Based Decisions and Economics: health care, social welfare, education and criminal justice.* Oxford: Wiley-Blackwell, 2010.

8 Glanville J, Paisley S. Searching for evidence for cost-effectiveness decisions. In: Shemilt I, Mugford M, Vale L, Marsh K, Donaldson C (eds) *Evidence-Based Decisions and Economics: health care, social welfare, education and criminal justice.* Oxford: Wiley-Blackwell, 2010.

9 Coyle D, Lee KM, Cooper NJ. Use of evidence in decision models. In: Shemilt I, Mugford M, Vale L, Marsh K, Donaldson C (eds) *Evidence-Based Decisions and Economics: health care, social welfare, education and criminal justice.* Oxford: Wiley-Blackwell, 2010.

10 Brazier JE, Papaioannou D, Cantrell A, Paisley S, Herrmann KH. Identifying and reviewing health state utility values for populating decision models. In: Shemilt I, Mugford M, Vale L, Marsh K, Donaldson C (eds) *Evidence-Based Decisions and Economics: health care, social welfare, education and criminal justice.* Oxford: Wiley-Blackwell, 2010.

11 Brunetti M, Ruiz F, Lord J, Pregno S, Oxman AD. Grading economic evidence. In: Shemilt I, Mugford M, Vale L, Marsh K, Donaldson C (eds) *Evidence-Based Decisions and Economics: health care, social welfare, education and criminal justice.* Oxford: Wiley-Blackwell, 2010.

12 Wilson E, Abrams K. From evidence-based economics to economics-based evidence: using systematic review to inform the design of future research. In: Shemilt I, Mugford M, Vale L, Marsh K, Donaldson C (eds) *Evidence-Based Decisions and Economics: health care, social welfare, education and criminal justice.* Oxford: Wiley-Blackwell, 2010.

13 McDaid D, Sassi F. Equity, efficiency and research synthesis. In: Shemilt I, Mugford M, Vale L, Marsh K, Donaldson C (eds) *Evidence-Based Decisions and Economics: health care, social welfare, education and criminal justice.* Oxford: Wiley-Blackwell, 2010.

CHAPTER 15

Evidence-based decisions and economics: an agenda for research

Michael Drummond

Centre for Health Economics, University of York, York, UK

Introduction

This book has been about the interactions between evidence synthesis, systematic review, economic analysis and decision making in the arena of health and social policy and practice. At the time of the first edition of this book, which focused solely on health care, there was considerable uncertainty about whether such interactions would produce positive results.[1] Many imperfections in the existing research were noted and an agenda for future research was specified.[2] Eight years on, it is time to assess whether the interactions have been positive and whether many of the research challenges have been met. It is also time to assess whether the experience in health care is relevant to other areas of public policy, such as social welfare, education and criminal justice.

The earlier research agenda, which (like the first edition of this book) focused exclusively on health care, was organised under three general headings. The main research needs identified under each heading were as follows.

Using systematic reviews in economic evaluation
- In what ways should the inclusion criteria for studies in systematic reviews be modified to accommodate the needs of economic evaluation?
- Can quality criteria be developed for non-randomised, or observational, studies?

Evidence-Based Decisions and Economics, 2nd edition. Edited by I. Shemilt, M. Mugford, L. Vale, K. Marsh and C. Donaldson. © 2010 Blackwell Publishing.

- How can non-randomised controlled trial (RCT) data best be incorporated in systematic reviews?
- Is it possible, or desirable, for systematic reviews to give an estimate of the clinical effect size for subgroups of the patient population, as well as the average effect size?
- How can issues of external validity (generalisability) be better addressed in systematic reviews of clinical studies?

Undertaking systematic reviews of economic evaluations
- What are the possible objectives in undertaking systematic reviews of economic evaluations and are these attainable?
- Can the really critical methodological features of economic evaluations be identified, so as to guide decisions on the inclusion of studies in systematic reviews?
- Can a quality score (or grading) system be developed for economic evaluations, and how would such a system be validated?

Obtaining evidence about the effects of broader health policies and interventions
- What are the real (and imagined!) problems of conducting RCTs of policy measures?
- Would more pragmatic designs for clinical trials address some of the concerns about unnecessary simplification of problems and increase the practical relevance of study results?
- In which situations would RCTs not be the preferred approach and can these situations be easily identified?

- Can we define more clearly the limits of the evidence-based medicine (EBM) paradigm and specify more fully the alternatives?

In this chapter, the contribution of the current set of papers is assessed in the context of the earlier research agenda and a new research agenda is specified. The new research agenda (and reformulated general headings) reflect both the methods proposals and controversies covered in this volume and also the extension of the scope of this volume to encompass other spheres of social policy and practice alongside health care.

A new agenda for research

Using systematic reviews in economic analysis

Many economic evaluations are undertaken by building a decision model, whereby data from a range of sources are synthesised. As Coyle and colleagues illustrate in their case study, in most situations the most important model parameter is the estimate of relative treatment (or intervention) effect and it is most appropriate that this estimate is obtained from a systematic review of the relevant literature.[3]

In general, this is the area where economic evaluation is best served by systematic review. However, in his chapter in this volume, Marsh points out that the use of systematic review to measure treatment effect in decision models is far from universal across several policy domains including health care, so there is still considerable room for improvement in this respect.[4] This point is emphasised in the chapter by Coyle and colleagues, who demonstrate that the quality of data inputs varies and that this can have a major impact on the cost-effectiveness estimates.[3]

In addition, decision models also require estimates of other parameters, such as long-term outcomes, that are not often available from standard systematic reviews, which may only consider evidence drawn from certain study designs (e.g. RCTs) to the exclusion of other evidence (e.g. from observational studies). Finally, decision models require estimates of resource use, unit costs and valuations of outcomes of programmes, which may not typically be included in systematic reviews of effectiveness.

Several of the chapters in this volume tackle these issues. Glanville & Paisley stress the need for different search strategies to identify evidence needed to populate decision models.[5] As well as providing considerable practical advice on what those strategies might consist of in the health care field, this chapter suggests several important research needs that are common to all policy domains. These include:

- the need for evidence on the performance of search filters to identify economic analyses and other evidence required for decision models
- the need to investigate whether publication bias (and other forms of reporting bias) is an issue for reviews of economic evaluations; and
- the need to develop standardised search methods for the identification of evidence for decision models, so that search processes are transparent.

The chapter by Brazier and colleagues focuses specifically on the challenges of identifying health state utility values for populating decision models for health economic evaluation.[6] They discuss how search strategies can be developed, identify key sources of health utility data, and discuss how these data can be synthesised and adapted for use in decision models.

In their discussion, they identify several deficiencies in existing approaches and specify several research needs. These include:

- the need to improve the sensitivity and specificity of search filters for quality of life, health utility and other data required to populate decision models; and
- the development of formal synthesis methods for health state utility values.

Furthermore, if the interest is in outcomes of policies in areas such as social welfare, education and criminal justice, search strategies may have to be even more sophisticated, as there may not be sources equivalent to Medline, which contains a high percentage of the literature on medical outcomes.

In their chapter, Coyle and colleagues respond to one of the research needs identified in the first edition of this book.[2,3] Recognising that decision models synthesise data from a wide range of sources, they develop and test a hierarchy of data quality for five common categories of data in health economic evaluations: clinical effect sizes, baseline clinical data, resource use, costs and utilities. The test of the hierarchy, on an existing decision model for osteoporosis, shows that choosing evidence of different quality levels can have a substantial effect on the results of economic studies.

This suggests several research needs common to all policy domains, including:

- the development of guidelines for economic evaluation that embody a prescriptive approach to the quality of sources for data elements within decision models
- further analyses, in different clinical and policy areas, to confirm the impacts of using different data sources; and
- the development of Bayesian methods for updating results as more data become available and for the pooling of data from disparate sources of differing quality.

Undertaking systematic reviews of economic analyses

Several chapters in the volume discuss various aspects of the systematic review of economic evaluations and other forms of economic analysis. Responding to one of the research needs specified in the first edition of this book, Brunetti and colleagues discuss approaches for grading economic evidence.[7] Specifically, they describe the application of a new system – Grading of Recommendations Assessment Development and Evaluation (GRADE) – to economic study results. The GRADE approach is becoming widely used in health care applications for assessing the quality and applicability of clinical studies and generates an evidence profile that includes assessments of study limitations, inconsistency of results, directness of evidence, imprecision and publication bias.

The authors argue that the GRADE evidence profile is not suitable for summarising estimates of costs or cost-effectiveness derived from decision models. However, since modelling is ubiquitous in economic evaluation, some users of the GRADE system have developed an approach for presenting modelled economic evidence alongside GRADE evidence profiles, including the approach developed for use in the National Institute for Health and Clinical Excellence (NICE) clinical guidelines programme that is profiled in the chapter.

It will therefore be important to evaluate the application of the new economic evidence profiles in future NICE clinical guidelines. Also, the GRADE approach, which, unlike some approaches for grading evidence, is not based exclusively on study type (e.g. RCT, observational study, etc.), would potentially be useful in the other policy domains discussed in this volume, where controlled experiments are less common. Therefore,

a major research need would be to explore its use in grading the quality of evidence in social welfare, education and criminal justice.

In their chapter, Anderson & Shemilt discuss the possibility of producing pooled estimates of costs and cost-effectiveness when conducting systematic reviews of economic evaluations.[8] This issue was raised in the first edition of this book, where it was suggested that 'the real contribution of a systematic review of economic evaluations may not be to produce a single authoritative result, but to help decision makers understand the structure of the resource allocation problem they are addressing and the impact, on the overall result, of the main parameters'.[2]

The analysis conducted by Anderson & Shemilt largely supports this assertion. Specifically, they argue that in some circumstances, a review of all full economic evaluations relating to a particular policy comparison may provide a fairly consistent cost-effectiveness answer, but that such examples will not be the norm. Rather, reviews of economic studies are likely to be more useful in: (i) justifying and informing decision model development, (ii) identifying the most relevant study (for the decision problem being faced) or (iii) understanding the key economic trade-offs and causal relationships in a decision problem or policy area.

Bearing this in mind, there may be a role for reviews that seek to explain how and why particular levels and configurations of resources appear to be related to the levels and types of outcomes observed in different settings. This may help us understand better how relationships between interventions and contextual factors affect costs and outcomes. Lessard & Birch elaborate on this theme in their chapter in this volume.[9] Within the health care field, contextual factors are likely to be more important the further one moves from narrowly defined clinical outcomes to broader public health measures. Such contextual factors are also likely to be very important in some of the other policy areas discussed in this volume. For example, in their review of interventions for adolescent substance abuse, Homer and colleagues found that contextual factors were very important in interpreting the results of particular economic evaluations.[10]

Therefore, two central research needs implied by these chapters are to:
- look beyond the established methodological conventions of systematic reviewing, which are particularly

dominant in evidence-based medicine, focusing less on producing a pooled estimate of outcomes and more on explaining why certain programmes work (and conversely, why, sometimes, they don't), or are more or less costly, or cost-effective; and to

- develop review methods that recognise that health and other outcomes are jointly produced by both the interventions themselves and the multilevel contexts in which they are placed (e.g. the underlying characteristics and social dynamics of the populations and communities which create or sustain the health or social problems being targeted).

Some of these issues are explored in the chapter by Walker and colleagues, on generalisability, transferability, complexity and relevance, in which the authors discuss factors affecting the results of economic analyses that are likely to vary from setting to setting.[11] These factors can limit the generalisability of economic analyses and call into question the production of pooled estimates of cost or cost-effectiveness. Indeed, a pooled estimate, whilst possibly being more precise, might not apply in any setting!

The implication is that more research is needed on:
- which parameters vary between settings;
- how much variation in the levels of these parameters influences resultant variations in costs; and
- the conditions under which the cost structure can be assumed to be the same, so that costs can be applied from one setting to another.

Finally, two chapters discuss methods, primarily developed within economics research, which could be used to improve systematic reviews and economic analyses in the future. First, Stanley discusses the use of meta-regression models in economics and medical research.[12] He argues that the development of such models is necessary because economics deals largely with observational data. He goes on to suggest that these approaches have been especially helpful in identifying and correcting for publication bias, a problem that also plagues medical research. The need for these methods in policy areas such as education and criminal justice is also self-evident, as in these areas it is often difficult to conduct RCTs or other controlled experiments.

Research needs arising from this chapter include:
- the need to explore and refine variants of funnel asymmetry and precision effect tests to correct for publication bias; and

- the need to investigate alternative multivariate meta-regression analysis models to better explain the systematic variation routinely found in economic and medical research.

Second, Wilson & Abrams explore the use of value of information (VoI) analysis to set research priorities.[13] VoI analysis has so far been applied mainly within the context of decision models for health economic evaluation, in order to identify those parameters for which the value, in reducing the probability of making the 'wrong' decision, is greatest. The VoI can then be compared with the cost of undertaking further research to obtain better estimates of the parameters concerned. Wilson & Abrams argue that this type of analysis is intrinsic to an iterative approach to decision making, beginning with systematic review and economic evaluation, followed by adoption of the intervention and research decisions, and ending with new information being gathered and reappraised within an updated review and evaluation.

This chapter suggests several research needs, including:
- research into the appropriate time horizon for VoI analysis or the incorporation of time horizon as an additional source of uncertainty in the analysis;
- research into the costs of reversing treatment adoption decisions and how these affect the value of information and subsequent research decisions; and
- research into the utility of VoI in guiding decisions on data collection and study design.

Also, since VoI analysis has been applied primarily in the context of health care, research is needed to assess how easy it would be to apply the same methods to decision analysis in the social welfare, education and criminal justice fields. This is unlikely to be straightforward, since the approach is predicated on the notion of a threshold of social willingness to pay for the outcome of interest. Such a threshold has been specified for the quality-adjusted life-year (QALY) but there is no comparable figure for the social willingness to pay for the social benefits of programmes in the other policy domains covered in this volume.

Obtaining evidence about broader health and other social and behavioural interventions and policies

At the time of the first edition of this book, which focused on evidence-based medicine and health economics, a major criticism was that most published literature on the use of systematic reviews in health economic evaluation related to narrowly defined clinical interventions.[1,2] In contrast, there was little evidence that this approach would be successful in conducting evaluations in social welfare or evaluations of more complex public health interventions. This is because, in the latter situations, treatment effects may be more dependent on the context in which the intervention is delivered, and hence less generalisable. In turn, this would limit the usefulness of a pooled estimate of treatment effect obtained using a systematic review and meta-analysis.

Several papers in this volume discuss these issues in more detail. Marsh discusses the role of review and synthesis methods in producing decision models in both health and non-health fields.[4] He points out that use of systematic reviews for this specific purpose is currently limited outside the health field and also that there are relatively few RCTs of non-health interventions. Therefore, economic analyses are more likely to be based on quasi-experimental or observational data. He therefore argues that research is required to:

- inform the development of guidance on the size of bias produced by different study designs. For example, when is a good-quality quasi-experimental study better than a poor quality RCT?
- determine how outcomes from non-health care interventions should be measured and valued.

Byford and colleagues review the role of economic evidence in formulating public policy and practice within and across the health care, social welfare, education and criminal justice fields.[14] They also comment briefly on the role of economic evidence in low- and middle-income countries. The latter issue is also explored in the chapters by Anderson & Shemilt[8] and Walker and colleagues.[11]

Byford and colleagues conclude that whilst the health sector is leading the field in the conduct and use of economic evaluations, other parts of the public sector are making considerable efforts to bridge the gap between the demand for good-quality evidence and its availability. They argue that, to a large extent, limitations in the availability of primary studies incorporating economic analysis in some sectors outside health currently limit the scope for systematic review and synthesis of such studies. However, they also suggest that the potential for such secondary analyses is likely to be realised more rapidly if greater attention is focused on addressing methodological complexities inherent in the social welfare, education and criminal justice sectors, which are sometimes distinct from those present in the health care sector.

Several research needs can be identified, including:

- further research into methods for valuing the economic impact of policy decisions on service users and their families;
- further research to develop sector-appropriate measures of outcome capable of capturing the full impact of policy decisions on societal well-being; and
- further research to explore appropriate study designs for economic evaluation in situations where experimental designs are infeasible.

The most fundamental concerns about the role of approaches to evidence synthesis that combine systematic review and economics methods are raised in the chapter by Lessard & Birch,[9] which echoes several of the themes introduced by Anderson & Shemilt.[8] Lessard & Birch argue that health, health care and social systems are highly complex and that the systems of planning, managing and delivering health care, social welfare, education and criminal justice are embedded in the wider society and shaped by society's principles and values.[9] For example, whilst systematic review and economic evaluation focus on clinical and cost-effectiveness, many of society's concerns relate to the distributional issues surrounding health and health care.

Therefore, they argue that systematic review and economic evaluation, with their focus on a small range of measureable outcomes, are inadequate for increasing our understanding of a broader range of complex interactions. Essentially, these methods simplify a complex problem, in order to be able to offer a solution.

Lessard & Birch identify several research needs, including:

- the expansion of economic evaluation to include different types of knowledge and methodologies, so that it can better adapt to practical realities and the needs of patients, decision makers, health care and social systems and ultimately society; and
- the use of new paradigms, such as complexity thinking, that incorporate a dynamic and emergent view of the world, rather than the reductionist approaches embodied in systematic review and economic evaluation.

Some of the concerns raised by Lessard & Birch are discussed in the chapter by McDaid & Sassi.[15] They acknowledge that there have been few attempts to consider equity within or alongside economic evaluations. There is therefore a need for primary research on the extent to which a range of policy interventions, such as improvements in the environment, housing and the alleviation of poverty, help tackle underlying causes of inequality and hence inequalities in health, educational and crime outcomes. McDaid & Sassi also recognise, like others in this volume, that insufficient attention has been paid to the fact that the success or otherwise of these policies may be context specific, since they rely on an adequate behavioural response from the recipients of the interventions.

They argue that systematic review and economic evaluation, as currently practised, have some way to go to tackle these issues. For example, in the health field, existing critical appraisal checklists do not contain items related to equity issues, and existing databases, such as the NHS Economic Evaluation Database, do not have a domain relating to equity. This means that the reviews of economic evaluations are unlikely to focus much on equity issues. Outside the health care field, there are not even databases of studies comparable to NHS EED and information retrieval is generally more difficult.[5,15]

Several research needs are apparent from McDaid & Sassi's chapter, including:

- the development of an equity and context checklist for use within the context of systematic reviews of the effectiveness and cost-effectiveness literature, building on existing efforts; and
- more modelling to assess the cost-effectiveness of interventions in different population subgroups, as a precursor to understanding better the role of contextual factors in determining the success of various health and social policies.

Conclusion

The papers contained in this volume contribute to the development of methodological approaches to evidence synthesis that combine systematic review and economics methods by addressing some of the research needs identified in the earlier book by Donaldson and colleagues.[1,2] In particular, methods have been developed to search for the data required to populate decision models and to assess the quality of data sources. Also, there is now more experience in the use of systematic review and economic analysis beyond narrowly defined clinical interventions and also in the other social policy areas covered in this volume.

There has been considerable progress in understanding better the role of systematic reviews of previously published and unpublished economic analyses and in the grading of economic evidence identified using such reviews. There is also growing agreement that the primary purpose of such reviews is *not* to produce summary estimates of cost or cost-effectiveness, but arguably less agreement on what the ultimate purpose should be. However, several methods have been proposed for the identification and synthesis of appropriate economics literature.

Nevertheless, there remain doubts as to whether methods that have been most prevalent to date in the health economics and evidence-based paradigm are sufficient for the analysis of more complex health, social welfare, education and criminal justice policies, or those interventions where the outcomes are context specific. This volume suggests that, in order to tackle these issues, evidence synthesis will need to embrace a broader range of methods than economic evaluation and systematic review alone. Therefore, it is important that the new research needs identified here are tackled in the years to come.

How this chapter should be cited

Drummond, M. Chapter 15: Evidence-based decisions and economics: an agenda for research. In: Shemilt I, Mugford M, Vale L, Marsh K, Donaldson C (editors). *Evidence-based decisions and economics: health care, social welfare, education and criminal justice.* Oxford: Wiley-Blackwell, 2010.

References

1 Donaldson C, Mugford M, Vale L (eds). *Evidence-Based Health Economics: from effectiveness to efficiency in systematic review.* London: BMJ Books, 2002.
2 Drummond M. Evidence-based medicine meets economic evaluation: an agenda for research. In: Donaldson C, Mugford M, Vale L (eds) *Evidence-Based Health Economics: from effectiveness to efficiency in systematic review.* London: BMJ Books, 2002.
3 Coyle D, Lee KM, Cooper NJ. Use of evidence in decision models. In: Shemilt I, Mugford M, Vale L, Marsh K,

Donaldson C (eds) *Evidence-Based Decisions and Economics: health care, social welfare, education and criminal justice.* Oxford: Wiley-Blackwell, 2010.

4 Marsh K. The role of review and synthesis methods in decision models. In: Shemilt I, Mugford M, Vale L, Marsh K, Donaldson C (eds) *Evidence-Based Decisions and Economics: health care, social welfare, education and criminal justice.* Oxford: Wiley-Blackwell, 2010.

5 Glanville J, Paisley S. Searching for evidence for cost-effectiveness decisions. In: Shemilt I, Mugford M, Vale L, Marsh K, Donaldson C (eds) *Evidence-Based Decisions and Economics: health care, social welfare, education and criminal justice.* Oxford: Wiley-Blackwell, 2010.

6 Brazier JE, Papaioannou D, Cantrell A, Paisley S, Herrmann K. Identifying and reviewing health state utility values for populating decision models. In: Shemilt I, Mugford M, Vale L, Marsh K, Donaldson C (eds) *Evidence-Based Decisions and Economics: health care, social welfare, education and criminal justice.* Oxford: Wiley-Blackwell, 2010.

7 Brunetti M, Ruiz F, Lord J, Pregno S, Oxman AD. Grading economic evidence. In: Shemilt I, Mugford M, Vale L, Marsh K, Donaldson C (eds) *Evidence-Based Decisions and Economics: health care, social welfare, education and criminal justice.* Oxford: Wiley-Blackwell, 2010.

8 Anderson R, Shemilt I. The role of economic perspectives and evidence in systematic review. In: Shemilt I, Mugford M, Vale L, Marsh K, Donaldson C (eds) *Evidence-Based Decisions and Economics: health care, social welfare, education and criminal justice.* Oxford: Wiley-Blackwell, 2010.

9 Lessard C, Birch S. Complex problems or simple solutions? Enhancing evidence-based economics to reflect reality. In: Shemilt I, Mugford M, Vale L, Marsh K, Donaldson C (eds) *Evidence-Based Decisions and Economics: health care, social welfare, education and criminal justice.* Oxford: Wiley-Blackwell, 2010.

10 Homer JF, Drummond MF, French MT. Economic evaluation of adolescent addiction programs: methodological challenges and recommendations. *Journal of Adolescent Health* 2008; 43(6): 529–539.

11 Walker DG, Teerawattananon Y, Anderson R, Richardson G. Generalisability, transferability, complexity and relevance. In: Shemilt I, Mugford M, Vale L, Marsh K, Donaldson C (eds) *Evidence-Based Decisions and Economics: health care, social welfare, education and criminal justice.* Oxford: Wiley-Blackwell, 2010.

12 Stanley TD. Meta-regression models of economics and medical research. In: Shemilt I, Mugford M, Vale L, Marsh K, Donaldson C (eds) *Evidence-Based Decisions and Economics: health care, social welfare, education and criminal justice.* Oxford: Wiley-Blackwell, 2010.

13 Wilson E, Abrams K. From evidence-based economics to economics-based evidence: using systematic review to inform the design of future research. In: Shemilt I, Mugford M, Vale L, Marsh K, Donaldson C (eds) *Evidence-Based Decisions and Economics: health care, social welfare, education and criminal justice.* Oxford: Wiley-Blackwell, 2010.

14 Byford S, Barrett B, Dubourg R, Francis J, Sisk J. The role of economic evidence in formulation of public policy and practice. In: Shemilt I, Mugford M, Vale L, Marsh K, Donaldson C (eds) *Evidence-Based Decisions and Economics: health care, social welfare, education and criminal justice.* Oxford: Wiley-Blackwell, 2010.

15 McDaid D, Sassi F. Equity, efficiency and research synthesis. In: Shemilt I, Mugford M, Vale L, Marsh K, Donaldson C (eds) *Evidence-Based Decisions and Economics: health care, social welfare, education and criminal justice.* Oxford: Wiley-Blackwell, 2010.

CHAPTER 16

Glossary of terms

Asmaa Abdelhamid[1], Ian Shemilt[2]
[1]Research Associate, University of East Anglia, Norwich, UK
[2]Senior Research Associate, University of East Anglia, Norwich, UK

Administrative data are data collected for any administrative purpose that can be used to assess the 'real-world' prevalence and incidence of a condition, events and/or use of resources (e.g. drug use data contained in prescription databases, hospitalisation data contained in hospital databases, attendance or attainment data contained in school databases, or crime statistics contained in police databases, etc.).

Allocation concealment refers to processes used to prevent prior knowledge of which comparison group an individual will be randomly assigned to in a randomised controlled trial. Inadequate concealment of allocation may lead to selection bias.

Allocative efficiency refers to decisions about the distribution of resources across a range of interventions within a given system (e.g. a health care system, a criminal justice system, etc.); that is, decisions about whether to invest resources in a particular intervention versus another and/or how much to invest. In contrast to technical efficiency, when an allocative efficiency decision is made, one group of stakeholders (e.g. patient, service users) gains at the expense of another. Allocative efficiency is achieved within a given system when the outcomes achieved with the total available resources match the priorities of society.

Balance sheets are tools used to present research findings in a simple, tabular format that are designed to help decision makers develop an accurate understanding of the important consequences of two or more options (e.g. interventions) being compared, for example, their beneficial and adverse effects and/or resource consequences. Balance sheets present 'raw information' to which decision makers need to apply their own judgements about the trade-offs between benefits, harms and use of resources. The GRADE evidence profile described in Chapter 10 is as example of a specific form of balance sheet.

Bayes' rule is a mathematical formula that shows how existing beliefs, formally expressed as probability distributions, are modified by new information.[1] The formula expresses the theory that the posterior probability distribution of an event is proportional to the product of a prior probability distribution and a likelihood measure evaluated with respect to observed evidence. This allows new information to be used to update the conditional probability of occurrence of an event.

Bayesian methods are a class of modelling approaches to statistical analysis that draw on Bayesian probability theory – see *Bayes' rule*. This involves the interpretation of data collected from one or more studies in the light of external evidence and judgement, resulting in estimates of the probability of predicting an observation conditional on the model and its assumptions. In the context of health technology assessment, Bayesian methods have been defined as 'the explicit

Evidence-Based Decisions and Economics, 2nd edition. Edited by I. Shemilt, M. Mugford, L. Vale, K. Marsh and C. Donaldson. © 2010 Blackwell Publishing.

quantitative use of external evidence in the design, monitoring, analysis, interpretation, and reporting of a health technology assessment'.[1] Advantages of using Bayesian methods in decision models for economic evaluation include that they allow the synthesis of external data collected from multiple sources and study designs to produce conclusions in a form that is argued to contribute naturally to support policy decisions.[2]

Bias refers to systematic error or deviation in the results or inferences of a research study, leading to a distortion of the results and/or inferences based on results. Biases can operate in either direction: different biases may lead to underestimation or overestimation of a 'true' effect. Biases can vary in magnitude: some are small (and trivial compared with the observed effect) and some are substantial (so that an apparent finding may be entirely due to bias). Because the results of a study may be unbiased despite a methodological flaw, it is more appropriate to consider risk of bias.[3]

Blinding is the concealment of the assignment of participants, in an experiment, to intervention or control groups. The concealment can be from participants only or from participants, personnel and outcome assessors (referred to as 'double blinding').

Budgetary constraint describes the limit of expenditure and consumption options available to a specific agent (e.g. individual, service provider, government, etc.), given the types and amounts of resources available to be allocated to the production of a set of goods or services.

Case-mix is a system that classifies people (e.g. patients, service users) into groups that are homogeneous in their use of resources within a specific jurisdiction and over a specific time period (e.g. in health care, the mix of clinically homogeneous patient groups, based on the collection of clinical and administrative data on treatment and associated costs).

Clinical data are data related to or derived from observations and treatment of patients.

Comparator refers to the alternative course of action that the intervention under investigation is compared

to. For example, in a randomised controlled trial, the intervention under investigation (i.e. the experimental intervention) is compared to one or more comparators (also known as control or counterfactual conditions), where the alternative course of action (s) may be another intervention (that ideally reflects current standard practice in the study setting), a placebo or no intervention (i.e. a 'do nothing' alternative).

Complex intervention refers to an intervention consisting of several components that seem essential to its proper functioning, although the 'active ingredient' of the intervention is difficult to specify, as the components may act either independently or interdependently.[4] The components usually include behaviours and resources, parameters of behaviours and resources (e.g. frequency and timing), and methods of organising those behaviours and resources (e.g. type(s) of practitioner, service setting and geographical location).[5] Since almost all interventions contain several interacting components, the level of complexity of an intervention is conceptualised on a continuum, influenced by the nature of the problems and interventions under evaluation and dependent upon: the number of interacting components; the number and difficulty of behaviours required by those delivering or receiving the intervention; the number of groups or organisational levels targeted by the intervention; the number and variability of outcomes; and the degree of flexibility or tailoring of the intervention.[4,6]

Context (contextual factors) refers to the current broad set of organisational and cultural environments, conditions, structures, processes and settings in which actions and decisions take place, and which thus influence, specify or explain their meaning, inputs and outcomes.

Cost(s) refer to the value of resources that have an opportunity cost as a result of being used in the provision of an intervention – see *Opportunity cost*.

Cost analysis is a type of partial economic evaluation – see *Partial economic evaluation*.

Cost-benefit analysis (CBA) is a type of full economic evaluation in which measures of both resource use and beneficial (and adverse) effects are valued in commensurate (often monetary) units, so that the costs and benefits of alternative interventions can be directly compared to assess the extent to which interventions may be judged favourably from an economic point of view. Results may be expressed in terms of an incremental cost-benefit ratio or incremental net benefit.

Cost-consequences analysis is a form of cost-effectiveness analysis which sets out both the costs (resource use) and consequences (beneficial and adverse effects) associated with intervention(s) and comparator(s), but which does not include formal analysis of the relationship between costs and consequences (i.e. the joint distribution of costs and effects). In this respect, it is analogous to a 'balance sheet approach' to economic evaluation, in which decision makers need to apply their own judgements about the trade-offs between benefits, harms and use of resources – see *Balance sheets*.

Cost-effective refers to the point at which an intervention may be judged favourably from an economic point of view, based on estimates of the joint distribution of costs (resource use) and outcomes (beneficial and adverse effects).

Cost-effectiveness refers to the relationship between the costs (resource use) and outcomes (beneficial and adverse effects) associated with interventions.

Cost-effectiveness acceptability curve (CEAC) is a graphical representation of estimates of the joint distribution of costs (resource use) and outcomes (beneficial and adverse effects) associated with interventions and their associated uncertainty, which allows assessment of the probability of the assessed interventions being cost-effective at various threshold levels of willingness to pay for an additional unit of health outcome.

Cost-effectiveness analysis (CEA) is a type of full economic evaluation in which the results are expressed in terms of the incremental cost per measured unit of each outcome (i.e. measures of resource use are valued, usually in monetary terms, but outcomes are not). Comparisons are thus limited to services or treatment

options that produce the same outcome, which is measured strictly in one-dimensional, naturally occurring units. Interventions producing the same outcome are compared to assess the extent to which they may be judged favourably from an economic point of view. Cost-effectiveness analyses primarily address decisions relating to technical efficiency – see *Technical efficiency*.

Cost-effectiveness threshold refers to the maximum cost a specified stakeholder (or group of stakeholders) is willing to pay for a specified unit of outcome. The choice of cost-effectiveness threshold is a value judgement that depends on several factors.[7,8] For example, in the context of a cost-utility analysis, the cost-effectiveness threshold is a politically and strategically defined value of the maximal willingness to pay to gain one quality-adjusted life-year (QALY). If the cost per QALY associated with an intervention falls below the threshold value, it is judged cost-effective and the intervention is likely to be adopted, contingent upon trade-offs with other considerations that may influence a decision. Based on analysis of the preferences revealed in its resource allocation decisions, the National Institute of Health and Clinical Excellence in England and Wales appears to use a cost-effectiveness threshold of approximately £20–30,000 per QALY as a benchmark threshold to inform health technology adoption decisions.[9]

Cost-of-illness study is a form of economic analysis that aims to describe, measure and value the total resource use (economic impact) associated with the management of a specific medical condition or within a specific patient group, from the perspective of a specified stakeholder group, or society as a whole.

Cost per quality-adjusted life-year (cost per QALY) is a metric used to express the results of a cost-utility analysis in terms of the monetised value per unit of health gain, where the health gain is valued in terms of QALYs – see *Cost-utility analysis* and *Quality-adjusted life-year*.

Cost-utility analysis (CUA) is a type of full economic evaluation in which the results are expressed in terms of the incremental cost per quality-adjusted life-year (QALY) (i.e. measures of resource use are valued in monetary terms and outcomes are valued in terms of QALYs – see *Quality-adjusted life-years*) to allow comparisons of interventions within a given health system, in order to assess the extent to which they may be judged favourably from an economic point of view.

Covariate (co-variate) is an independent variable that may affect or be predictive of the outcome(s) under investigation.

Criminal justice economics is a subdiscipline of economics applied to the study of crime, justice and related interventions, policies and systems.

Decision model is an analytic tool comprising a model structure and set of parameters used to support systematic approaches to evaluating the impact of alternative interventions on costs and other outcomes under conditions of uncertainty.[10,11] All types of full economic evaluation can be conducted using a decision model – see *Full economic evaluation*. Decision models are typically used to synthesise a number of different types of evidence, collected from several different sources, in order to inform a specific resource allocation decision.

Deterministic sensitivity analysis is a form of sensitivity analysis in which the input parameters are assigned point estimate values.[12]

Disability-adjusted life-year (DALY) is a measure of the value of health outcomes in relation to a specific disease or health condition, calculated as the sum of the years of life lost due to premature mortality in a specified population and the years lost due to disability for incident cases of the health condition in the specified population.

Discount rate is the percentage rate used in discounting – see *Discounting*.

Discounting is the process of adjusting costs or outcomes incurred or received at different points in the future to their present value, so that they can be compared in commensurate units as if they all occurred at the same point in time. Discounting is used in economic evaluations to adjust for social or individual preferences for the timing of costs and outcomes.

Dominant is a term used in full economic evaluation to describe an intervention that is both more effective and costs less than one or more specified comparators.

Dominated is a term used in full economic evaluation to describe an intervention that is both less effective and costs more than one or more specified comparators.

Dummy variable is a term used in regression analysis or meta-regression analysis to indicate a variable that takes the value 0 or 1 to indicate the absence or presence of some categorical effect that may be expected to influence the outcome(s) or phenomena of interest.

Econometrics is a set of quantitative techniques for economic analysis that combines economic theory with statistics to build mathematical models which describe economic relationships, test the validity of hypotheses about economic relationships and estimate specified parameters in order to obtain measures of the strengths of the influences of different explanatory variables upon dependent variables.[13]

Economic analysis is a broad term used to describe the full range of analytical approaches to the investigation of economic phenomena or issues relating to the supply, demand or allocation of resources. Examples include, *inter alia*, full economic evaluations (including decision models), partial economic evaluations, econometric analyses, cost-of-illness studies, utility studies, and so on.

Economic evaluation – see *Full economic evaluation* and *Partial economic evaluation*.

Economic evidence is a broad term used to describe the full range of types of evidence that may be used to inform an economic analysis, including, *inter alia*, evidence on beneficial and adverse effects, baseline risks of events, resource use, unit costs, utilities or other measures of the value of outcomes, and so on.

Economics is the study of the optimal allocation of limited resources for the production of benefit to society.[14]

Economies of scale are the long run cost advantages that an organisation obtains due to expansion, causing the 'per unit' costs of production to decrease as the volume of production increases.

Education economics is a subdiscipline of economics applied to the study of education and related interventions, policies and systems.

Effectiveness refers to the extent to which a given intervention produces beneficial outcomes in individuals who receive the intervention in 'real-world' settings. Intervention effectiveness is a function of intervention efficacy, complexity, acceptability and compliance, and may be influenced by a wide range of contextual factors.

Effect size is a relative or absolute measure of the difference in outcome observed between intervention and control groups in a controlled experimental study.

Efficacy refers to the capacity or power of a given intervention to produce intended, beneficial outcomes in individuals who receive (and fully comply with) the intervention in ideal, carefully controlled conditions and settings.

Efficiency refers to the optimal allocation and use of scarce resources. There are two (related) types of efficiency: technical and allocative efficiency – see *Allocative efficiency* and *Technical efficiency*.

Elasticity is a measure of responsiveness of a dependent variable to an associated explanatory variable. Specifically, it is the percentage change in the dependent variable that is observed in response to a 1% change in the associated explanatory variable.

Empirical economic evaluation refers to a full or partial economic evaluation conducted alongside a single, primary study (e.g. a randomised controlled trial) and utilising individual-level primary data on outcomes (beneficial and adverse effects) and/or resource use (costs), collected prospectively or retrospectively, on participants in that study.

Epidemiology is a field of study that examines the frequency, distribution, determinants and control of diseases and medical conditions in populations.

Equity refers to the equal distribution of variations in final outcomes (e.g. health, social welfare, education or crime-related outcomes) between defined population subgroups.

Evidence-based medicine (EBM) is the conscientious, explicit and judicious use of current 'best evidence' in making decisions about the care of individual patients.[15]

Exchange rate is the rate at which a currency unit of one country can be exchanged for a unit of the currency of another country – see also *Purchasing Power Parities*.

Expenditure is the payment of cash or cash-equivalent for goods or services, or a charge against available funds in settlement of an obligation, as evidenced by an invoice, receipt or other similar document.

External validity refers to the degree to which the findings of a study are generalisable or transferable to populations or settings other than those in which the study was conducted.

Extrapolation refers to a set of mathematical procedures in which the values of a variable are estimated over a time horizon that has not been observed, using predictions based on observed data points.

Full economic evaluation is the comparative analysis of alternative courses of action (e.g. interventions) in terms of both their costs (resource use) and consequences (outcomes).[16] Principal types of full economic evaluation are cost-effectiveness analysis (CEA), cost-utility analysis (CUA) and cost-benefit analysis (CBA). These can be conducted alongside empirical, primary studies or using a decision model.

Grey literature refers to documents and other research-based material issued in limited amounts outside formal channels of publication and distribution. Examples include scientific and technical reports, government documents, doctoral theses and unpublished material.

Health economics is a subdiscipline of economics applied to the study of health and related interventions, policies and systems.

Health technology assessment is the systematic evaluation of the properties, costs, effects and/or other impacts of health care interventions. It is designed to provide objective and unbiased evidence to support health care policy and practice decisions.

Incremental (e.g. incremental resource use, or costs, or effectiveness, or benefits, or cost-effectiveness) refers to the additional resource use, costs, effectiveness, benefit or cost-effectiveness associated with an intervention in comparison to a specified comparator.

Incremental cost-effectiveness ratio (ICER) is the ratio of the difference in costs between an intervention and a specified comparator to the difference in effectiveness between that intervention and specified comparator.

Indirect comparison refers to a set of analytical methods that may be used to compare the costs and/or effects of alternative interventions using data from separate primary studies when there is no, or insufficient, evidence from direct comparison 'head-to-head' trials. A common example of a situation in which no, or insufficient, evidence from direct comparison trials is available is where there is a class of several drugs, each of which has been studied in placebo-controlled randomised controlled trials, but there are no (or very few) trials in which the drugs have been directly compared with each other.[17]

Inflation refers to the increase in the general price level of goods and services and simultaneous decrease in the purchasing power of money over time.

Intention-to-treat (ITT) is a principle used in controlled experimental research when analysing the results of a study. An intention-to-treat analysis is based on participants' initial treatment assignment on entry to a study, regardless of whether or not they completed or received that treatment. It is conducted in order to avoid the effects of crossover, drop-outs and non-compliance, which may produce risk of bias if such effects are not randomly distributed between comparison groups.

Internal validity refers to the 'approximate truth' about inferences regarding cause-and-effect or causal relationships. Thus, internal validity is of relevance in studies that aim to establish a causal relationship. It is concerned with the rigor of (and the degree of control the investigator has over) the study design and the extent to which the study is conducted in a manner free from risk of bias, eliminating or controlling for potentially confounding variables, such that the potential for an alternative explanation for the observed effects of an intervention is minimised.

Intervention refers to the deliberate act of intervening or interceding with the intent of modifying health, social welfare, education or crime-related outcomes at the individual, group or population level. The term 'intervention' is used more or less interchangeably with the terms 'programme', 'policy', 'treatment', 'technology' and 'service' throughout this volume.

Log-log model is a regression model in which both the dependent variable and the explanatory variables are transformed into algorithms.

Log odds ratio is the natural log of the odds ratio – see *Odds ratio*.

Markov model is a specific form of decision model used in health economic evaluation, in which patients can exist in a finite set of health states, between which they can move over time. Movement between health states occurs over a discrete time interval (known as a Markov cycle), based on preset transition probabilities.

Meta-analysis is a statistical method for combining the numerical results of two or more independent studies to yield an overall statistic (together with its confidence interval) that summarises the effect size of an experimental intervention compared with a control intervention, in terms of measures of outcome. Meta-analysis is typically a two-stage process. In the first stage, a summary statistic is calculated for each study, to describe the observed intervention effect. In the second stage, a summary (pooled) intervention effect estimate is calculated as a weighted average of the intervention effects estimated in the individual studies. By combining information from all relevant studies, meta-analyses can provide more precise estimates of the effects than those derived from the individual studies included in a systematic review. They can also facilitate investigations of the consistency of evidence across studies, and the exploration of differences across studies.[18,19]

Meta-regression analysis (MRA) involves the use of a multivariate statistical model to analyse data collected from several studies, in order to investigate the impact of study characteristics on study results. In principle, this allows the effects of multiple characteristics to be investigated simultaneously. MRA is similar in essence to simple regression analysis, in which a dependent variable is predicted according to the values of one or more explanatory variables. However, in MRA the dependent variable is a study-level estimate of a specific effect and the explanatory variables are characteristics of studies that may influence estimates of the dependent variable (sometimes referred to as 'potential effect modifiers' or co-variates). The regression coefficient obtained from an MRA describes how the dependent variable changes given a unit increase in an explanatory variable.[18] See Chapter 11 for discussion and examples of MRA applications in economics and medical research.

Mis-specification bias is a term used in econometrics to refer to a variety of model mis-specification errors that may lead to biased estimates of effects and the relationships between dependent and explanatory variables. These include omission of potential effect modifiers, incorrect function form, and use of single equation models when a multiequation model is more appropriate.

Monte Carlo simulation is a probabilistic simulation technique used to evaluate the effects of uncertainty in the results of economic evaluations, including decision models, to random variation in the values of key parameters, using random numbers. The technique requires running a large number of simulations, for each of which values are drawn from distributions assigned to uncertain parameters, with the aim of constructing an empirical probability distribution for the overall results.[12]

Non-randomised studies is a broad collective term for quantitative studies estimating the effectiveness of an intervention that do not use randomisation to allocate units (e.g. individuals) to comparison groups. This includes studies where allocation occurs in the course of usual treatment decisions or people's choices (i.e. studies usually called observational). Types of non-randomised study include the case–control study, the cohort study, the controlled before-and-after study, the interrupted time-series study and some controlled trials that use inappropriate randomisation strategies (sometimes called quasi-randomised studies).[20]

Observational data are data derived from observational studies – see *Observational studies.*

Observational studies are a class of research study in which inferences are drawn or hypotheses tested about the possible effect of exposure to an intervention on specified outcomes, measured in a defined population, through use of observational methods. Intervention exposure occurs in the course of usual treatment decisions or people's choices; the investigator does not manipulate the use of, or deliver, an intervention but observes groups of individuals exposed to the intervention (and often groups of individuals who are not exposed, as a basis of comparison). Common types of observational study include the case–control study, the cohort study and the cross-sectional study.

Odds ratio is a measure of relative effect. In the context of econometric methods (e.g. a regression analysis or meta-regression analysis), the odds ratio (like the relative risk ratio) provides a measure of the estimated strength of association or non-independence between two binary variables and enables examination of the effects of other variables on that relationship.[21] In the context of a meta-analysis conducted as part of a systematic review, odds is defined as the ratio of the probability that a particular event will occur to the probability that it will not occur for binary outcomes, whilst the odds ratio describes the multiplication of the odds of the outcome that occurs with use of the experimental intervention (with confidence interval).[18] A value of 1 indicates that the estimated effect is the same for both the experimental intervention and the comparator. It is important to note that the interpretation of an odds ratio is different from the interpretation of a relative risk ratio – see *Relative risk ratio*.

Opportunity costs express the effects of an action in terms of the foregone benefits of the next best alternative use of the set of resources used to implement that action.[16]

Parameter is a measurable or quantifiable characteristic.

Parameter uncertainty refers to uncertainty regarding the 'true value' of a parameter, or group of parameters, used in an analysis (e.g. in a decision model).

Partial economic evaluation is a class of economic analysis comprising studies that: describe, measure and value resource use (costs) associated with alternative interventions (i.e. a cost analysis); describe, measure and value resource use (costs) associated with a single intervention, with no comparison between alternatives (i.e. a cost description); or describe, measure and value resource use (costs) and consequences (outcomes) associated with a single intervention, with no comparison between alternatives (i.e. a cost-outcome description). None of these types of economic analysis meets the strict definition of a full economic evaluation, as the latter involves the *comparative* analysis of *alternative* interventions in terms of *both* their costs (resource use) and consequences (outcomes).

Perspective (analytic perspective) refers to the viewpoint adopted in an economic analysis. The chosen analytic perspective will influence the relevant data that need to be collected for the analysis. For example, full economic evaluation is primarily a decision-informing class of economic analysis, so that the appropriate choices of type of full economic evaluation, and the detailed methods used, depend on characteristics of both the decision and the decision-making constituency that needs to be informed. The choice of analytical perspective will in turn influence the types of resource use (costs) and other outcome measures considered relevant for inclusion in the evaluation (i.e. depending on which stakeholder groups incur specific costs and/or receive specific benefits associated with the interventions being compared, and their relative importance in the

judgement of the decision maker and/or the analyst). Examples of analytical perspectives (or viewpoints) adopted in full (and partial) economic evaluations include: government (e.g. national government, local government); system (e.g. health system, social care system, etc.); multisector (e.g. the health and social care system); service provider (e.g. hospital, school, prison, etc.); third-party payers (e.g. insurance companies); service users (or other individuals) and their families (e.g. patients, victims of crime, caregivers, etc.) and societal (i.e. encompassing all stakeholder groups within a society).

Pharmacoeconomics is a subdiscipline of health economics concerned with assessments of the value and efficiency of pharmaceutical interventions.

Primary care refers to health services and professional groups that play a central role in local communities; for example, general practitioners/family doctors, pharmacists, dentists and midwives. Primary care providers are usually the first point of contact for a patient and may follow a patient through their care pathway.[22]

Primary research (primary study) is research that utilises original data collection to answer research questions.

Probabilistic sensitivity analysis is a form of sensitivity analysis in which probability distributions are applied to the ranges for a decision model's input parameters, and samples are drawn from these distributions to generate an empirical distribution of the relevant measure of cost-effectiveness.[12]

Probability is the statistical likelihood of an event, expressed as a value between 0 and 1.

Productivity is a measure of total output per unit of resource input.

Protocol is a prespecified template for a research study, often used for randomised controlled trials and systematic reviews, which fully describes the objectives and methods that will be used. In recent years, there has been increasing support for prospective registration of, and publication of protocols for, randomised controlled trials and systematic reviews. Prospective registration and publication of protocols aims to ensure that the research process is transparent, ethical and compliant with minimum standards, and that the evidence produced is reliable, complete and unbiased.

Publication bias is a form of reporting bias observed when studies suggesting a beneficial intervention effect or a larger effect size are selected for publication, while studies pointing in the other direction remain unpublished. In this situation a systematic review of published studies could identify a spurious beneficial intervention effect or miss an important adverse effect of an intervention.[23] Although risk of publication bias and other reporting biases are not specific to economic analyses, it is widely recognised that commercial and other pressures may affect the funding and publication of studies which focus on the economic value of interventions.[24,25] For example, a study by Gilbody and colleagues found that clinical effect sizes in randomised controlled trials of enhanced care for depression that published a full economic evaluation are systematically larger than those in randomised controlled trials that did not publish a full economic evaluation.[26] This finding is plausibly attributed to the presence of publication bias in favour of studies that cast enhanced care as comparatively attractive in terms of cost-effectiveness.

Purchasing Power Parities are exchange rates that adjust for differences in current price levels between countries, thus allowing comparisons based on a common set of average international prices. They have an advantage over pure exchange rate conversion and other (e.g. GDP per capita) approaches, since in effect they eliminate differences in price levels between countries in the process of conversion.[27]

Quality-adjusted life-year (QALY) is a measure of the value of health outcomes that combines quantity and quality of life. It assigns a weight corresponding to health-related quality of life (i.e. based on health state utility values) to each year of life.

Quasi-experimental study is a type of non-randomised study that has a design similar to an experimental study, but which lacks the necessary characteristic of random assignment to comparison groups.

Randomised controlled trial (RCT) is a form of experimental study in which units (i.e. individual participants, or defined groups of participants in a cluster RCT) are assigned at random (i.e. by chance alone) to receive either an experimental intervention (i.e. the intervention(s) that are the main focus of the investigation) or a control condition (i.e. a comparator or counterfactual condition(s)), in order to test the comparative efficacy or effectiveness of the experimental intervention in terms of a set of prespecified outcome measures.

Recall bias occurs when the accuracy of data collected from a respondent is influenced by the respondent's memory and ability to recall past events or experiences with accuracy.

Reference case refers to a core set of methods prescribed for use in the main analysis (or 'base case' analysis) of submissions to a specific organisation or decision-making constituency.

Relative risk ratio (or risk ratio, or relative risk) is a measure of relative effect. In the context of econometric methods (e.g. a regression analysis or meta-regression analysis), the relative risk ratio (like the odds ratio) provides a measure of the estimated strength of association or non-independence between two binary variables and enables examination of the effects of other variables on that relationship. In the context of a meta-analysis conducted as part of a systematic review, risk describes the probability that an outcome will occur, whilst the relative risk ratio describes the multiplication of the risk that occurs with use of the experimental intervention (with confidence interval).[18] A value of 1 indicates that the estimated effect is the same for both the experimental intervention and the comparator. It is important to note that the interpretation of a relative risk ratio is different from the interpretation of an odds ratio – see *Odds ratio*.

Resource(s) refer to components used in the production of an intervention, or impacted upon as a result of the effects of an intervention, such as human time and skills, drugs, equipment, buildings, energy and any other inputs. In Chapter 7, 'resources' refers to electronic literature databases, websites, libraries or any other sources or repositories containing records or copies of published or unpublished studies, or other research-based material, which may be searched as part of a systematic review or to inform development and population of a decision model.

Scenario analysis is a form of multiway analysis, which involves simultaneously substituting the parameter values and assumptions associated with an identifiable subgroup of interest.[28]

Search filter is a combined collection of search terms developed to capture specific themes, such as study design (e.g. randomised controlled trials, economic evaluations, etc.).

Secondary care often refers to acute health care (elective care or emergency care) provided by medical specialists in a hospital or other secondary care setting. Patients are often referred to secondary care services from a primary care professional, such as a general practitioner/family doctor.[22]

Secondary database refers to a searchable electronic database that indexes, organises and compiles bibliographic details, abstracts and/or citations to reports of original research studies first published in a primary source (e.g. journal articles, proceedings of meetings, conferences and symposia, technical reports, datasets). Secondary databases usually include literature and other research-based materials relevant to a specific field, discipline, subdiscipline or topic. Examples include Medline, Embase, PsychInfo, Social Sciences Citation Index, etc.

Secondary research is research that draws primarily on data collected from primary studies.

Selection bias is a form of bias that influences the results of a controlled experimental study (e.g. a randomised controlled trial) or quasi-experimental study, due to systematic differences between treatment groups in prognostic factors or responsiveness to treatment, which may be produced by the manner in which participants are selected into the study or assigned to treatment groups. In a randomised controlled trial, random allocation with adequate concealment of allocation is designed to protect against selection bias.

Sensitivity analysis refers to the range of methods used to determine whether and to what extent plausible changes in the values of uncertain parameters influence the main results of economic evaluations, including decision models.

Social welfare economics is a subdiscipline of economics applied to the study of social welfare and related interventions, policies and systems.

Statistical significance is the term used to indicate that a result of a comparative analysis is unlikely to have arisen due to chance alone. Statistical significance at the commonly cited 5% level ($p < 0.05$) means that the observed difference in outcome between compared groups would occur by chance (i.e. a type I error) in only 5% of cases (i.e. 1 of 20). However, if an observed difference is statistically significant, this does not necessarily mean it is important. Assessment of the importance of an observed difference requires further interpretation of the magnitude and meaning of the difference.

Structural uncertainty refers to uncertainty concerning structural assumptions employed in an analysis (e.g. the structure of a decision model).

Subgroup is a subset of a sample or population with one or more common characteristics.

Surrogate outcome is a measure that is used as a proxy for another outcome because it is believed to be an indicator or predictor of that outcome.

Systematic review is a form of secondary research that involves the use of explicit, reproducible and systematic methods to assemble, select, critically appraise and combine all empirical evidence that fits prespecified eligibility criteria in order to answer a specific research question.[19] The key characteristics of a systematic review are: a clearly stated set of objectives with predefined eligibility criteria for studies; an explicit, reproducible methodology; a systematic search that attempts to identify all studies that meet the eligibility criteria; an assessment of the validity of the findings of included studies, for example through the assessment of risk of bias and methodological quality; and a systematic presentation, and synthesis, of the characteristics and findings of the included studies.[19]

Technical efficiency refers to the aim of choosing the intervention which achieves a specified set and level of outcomes at the lowest overall cost.

Tertiary care refers to highly specialised health care services for patients with severe, complicated or unusual health conditions, usually provided in a specialist medical centre, teaching or research institution, and often requiring sophisticated technology and facilities and/or specialist medical and health professionals.

Tertiary database refers to a searchable electronic database containing records that draw primarily on the contents of secondary databases and original reports of studies to index, organise, abstract and compile bibliographic details, structured summaries, abstracts and/or citations to reports of original studies first published in a primary source (e.g. journal articles, proceedings of meetings, conferences and symposia, technical reports, datasets). Tertiary databases usually include literature and other research-based materials relevant to a specific field, discipline, subdiscipline or topic. Examples include the NHS Economic Evaluation Database (NHS EED), the Health Economic Evaluation Database (HEED) and the CEA Registry.

Time horizon usually refers to the time period specified in an economic analysis (e.g. economic evaluation) over which important differences in resource use (costs) and outcomes (beneficial and adverse effects) between compared interventions are expected to occur.

Unit cost is the cost per natural unit of a given resource.

Utility (health state utility value) is a measure of the strength of preference for a specific health outcome, which can be directly incorporated into calculations of quality-adjusted life-years in a cost-utility analysis – see *Cost-utility analysis* and *Quality-adjusted life-year*.

Utility study is a study in which measures of the strength of people's preferences for specific health states in relation to alternative health states are elicited.

Validity – see *External validity* and *Internal validity*.

Variance is a measure of the dispersion of a set of data points around their mean value. The variance of a distribution is the average of squares of the distances from the mean of the distribution.

Wald test is a statistical test used in econometric models to assess whether the coefficient of each independent variable in the model has a statistically significant relationship with the dependent variable. In the multivariate model, a test of the joint significance of a subset of variables at once may be carried out using a variance matrix.

Willingness to pay is an expression of the monetary value of the strengths of people's preferences for specified levels of benefits of interventions.

How this chapter should be cited

Abdelhamid A, Shemilt I. Chapter 16: Glossary of terms. In: Shemilt I, Mugford M, Vale L, Marsh K, Donaldson C (editors). *Evidence-based decisions and economics: health care, social welfare, education and criminal justice*. Oxford: Wiley-Blackwell, 2010.

References

1 Spiegelhalter DJ, Myles JP, Jones DR, Abrams KR. An introduction to Bayesian methods in health technology assessment. *British Medical Journal* 1999; 219(7208): 508–512.

2 Lilford RJ, Braunholtz D. The statistical basis of public policy: a paradigm shift is overdue. *British Medical Journal* 1996; 313 (7057): 603–607.

3 Higgins JPT, Altman DG. Assessing risk of bias in included studies. In: Higgins JPT, Green S (eds) *Cochrane Handbook for Systematic Reviews of Interventions*. Version 5.0.1 (updated September 2008). Oxford: Cochrane Collaboration, 2008.

4 Craig P, Dieppe P, Macintyre S, Mitchie S, Nazareth I, Petticrew M. Developing and evaluating complex interventions: the new Medical Research Council guidance. *British Medical Journal* 2008; 337(a1655): 979–983.

5 Medical Research Council. *A Framework for Development and Evaluation of Complex Interventions to Improve Health*. London: Medical Research Council, 2000.

6 Byford S, Sefton T. Economic evaluation of complex health and social care interventions. *National Institute Economic Review* 2003; 186(1): 98–108.

7 Owens DK. Interpretation of cost-effectiveness analyses. *Journal of General Internal Medicine* 1998; 13(10): 716–717.

8 Garber AM, Phelps CE. Economic foundations of cost-effectiveness analysis. *Journal of Health Economics* 1997; 16(1): 1–31.

9 Miners AH, Garau M, Fidan D, Fischer AJ. Comparing estimates of cost effectiveness submitted to the National Institute for Clinical Excellence (NICE) by different organisations: retrospective study. *British Medical Journal* 2005; 330(7482): 65–68.

10 Soto J. Health economic evaluations using decision analytic modelling. Principles and practices – utilization of a checklist to their development and appraisal. *International Journal of Technology Assessment in Health care* 2002; 18(1): 94–111.

11 Briggs A, Claxton K, Sculpher M. *Decision Modelling for Health Economic Evaluation*. Oxford: Oxford University Press, 2006.

12 Andronis L, Barton P, Bryan S. Sensitivity analysis in economic evaluation: an audit of NICE current practice and a review of its use and value in decision-making. *Health Technology Assessment* 2009; 13(29): 1–84.

13 Bannock G, Baxter R, Davis E. *Economist Dictionary of Economics*, 2nd edn. London: Economist Books, 1998.

14 Samuelson PA, Nordhaus WD. *Economics*. London: McGraw-Hill, 2005.

15 Sackett DL, Rosenberg WM, Gray JA, Haynes RB, Richardson WS. Evidence based medicine: what it is and what it isn't. *British Medical Journal* 1996; 312(7023): 71–72.

16 Drummond MF, Sculpher MJ, Torrance GW, O'Brien BJ, Stoddart GL. *Methods for the Economic Evaluation of Health care Programmes*, 3rd edn. Oxford: Oxford University Press, 2005.

17 Glenny AM, Altman DG, Song F, *et al.* Indirect comparison of competing interventions. *Health Technology Assessment* 2005; 9(26): 1–148.

18 Deeks JJ, Higgins JPT, Altman DG. Analysing data and undertaking meta-analyses. In: Higgins JPT, Green S (eds) *Cochrane Handbook for Systematic Reviews of Interventions*. Version 5.0.1 (updated September 2008). Oxford: Cochrane Collaboration, 2008.

19 Green S, Higgins JPT, Alderson P, Clarke M, Mulrow CD, Oxman AD. Introduction. In: Higgins JPT, Green S (eds) *Cochrane Handbook for Systematic Reviews of Interventions*. Version 5.0.1 (updated September 2008). Oxford: Cochrane Collaboration, 2008.

20 Reeves BC, Deeks JJ, Higgins JPT, Wells GA. Including non-randomized studies. In: Higgins JPT, Green S (eds) *Cochrane Handbook for Systematic Reviews of Interventions*. Version 5.0.1 (updated September 2008). Oxford: Cochrane Collaboration, 2008.

21 Bland JM, Altman DG. The odds ratio. *British Medical Journal* 2000; 320(7247): 1468.

22 Department of Health. *Health care: National policy, practical guidance and standards for the health care sector*. London: Department of Health, 2010. Available from: www.dh.gov.uk/en/ Health care/index.htm.

23 Sterne JAC, Egger M, Moher D. Addressing reporting biases. In: Higgins JPT, Green S (eds) *Cochrane Handbook for Systematic Reviews of Interventions*. Version 5.0.1 (updated September 2008). Oxford: Cochrane Collaboration, 2008.

24 Shemilt I, Mugford M, Byford S, *et al.* Incorporating economics evidence. In: Higgins JPT, Green S (eds) *Cochrane Handbook for Systematic Reviews of Interventions*. Version 5.0.1 (updated September 2008). Oxford: Cochrane Collaboration, 2008.

25 Drummond MF. Economic evaluation of pharmaceuticals: science or marketing? *Pharmacoeconomics* 1992; 1(1): 8–13.

26 Gilbody S, Bower P, Sutton AJ. Randomized trials with concurrent economic evaluations reported unrepresentatively large clinical effect sizes. *Journal of Clinical Epidemiology* 2007; 60(8): 781–786.

27 Shemilt I, Thomas J, Morciano M. A new web-based tool for adjusting costs to a common currency and price year. *Evidence and Policy*, submitted.

28 Berger ML, Bingefors K, Hedblom E, Pashos CL, Torrance G (eds). *Health care Cost, Quality and Outcomes: Ispor Book of Terms*. Lawrenceville, NJ: International Society for Pharmacoeconomics and Outcomes Research, 2003.

Index